Interprofessional Collaboration

Interprofessional collaboration in the health and social care services has become a commanding force, spear-headed by the Government's modernisation programme to improve partnership.

Interprofessional Collaboration highlights the benefits and factors arising from working together for patients, service users and carers through a review of theoretical models illustrated by relevant examples. Discussion of topical problems being faced by practitioners, managers and policy-makers in the health and social care sector covers:

- Policy issues from various interprofessional angles, including the place of management, ethical issues and technology
- The application of policy to practice in working together across professions, sectors and communities, giving an overview of teamwork, new primary care policies, interprofessional agendas for family support and mental health, as well as users' and carers' perspectives on collaboration in practice
- Policy and practice in learning together, including theoretical challenges and developments internationally.

Relevant for all those who have an interest in matters of health, social care, welfare and caring, *Interprofessional Collaboration* provides comprehensive coverage on interprofessional education and policy in the UK and abroad.

Interprofessional Collaboration

From Policy to Practice in Health and Social Care

Edited by Audrey Leathard

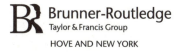

Brunner-Routledge
Taylor & Francis Group

HOVE AND NEW YORK

First published 2003 by Brunner-Routledge
27 Church Road, Hove, East Sussex BN3 2FA

Simultaneously published in the USA and Canada
by Brunner-Routledge
29 West 35th Street, New York, NY 10001

Brunner-Routledge is an imprint of the Taylor & Francis Group

Typeset in Times by RefineCatch Limited, Bungay, Suffolk
Printed and bound in Great Britain by MPG Books Ltd, Bodmin
Paperback cover design by Louise Page

British Library Cataloguing in Publication Data
A catalogue record for this book is available from the British Library

Library of Congress Cataloging-in-Publication Data
Interprofessional collaboration : from policy to practice in health
and social care / edited by Audrey Leathard.
        p. cm.
     Includes bibliographical references and index.
     ISBN 1–58391–175–8 – ISBN 1–58391–176–6 (pbk.)
      1. Medical cooperation. 2. Health care teams. 3. Interpersonal
relations. 4. Medical care. I. Leathard, Audrey.
   RA394.I585 2003
   362.1 – dc21
                                            2002034278

ISBN 1–58391–175–8 (hbk)
ISBN 1–58391–176–6 (pbk)

Contents

List of illustrations

List of tables

Contributors

Lesley Bainbridge, Head of the Division of Physical Therapy in the School of Rehabilitation Sciences, University of British Columbia, Canada.

Colin Barnes, Professor of Disability Studies at the Centre for Disability Studies, Department of Sociology and Social Policy, University of Leeds, Leeds, England.

Hugh Barr, Emeritus Professor of Interprofessional Education in the School of Integrated Health, University of Westminster; Chairman of the UK Centre for the Advancement of Interprofessional Education, London, England.

Alan Beattie, Professor of Health Promotion, St. Martin's College, Lancaster, England.

Paal Breivik, Assistant Professor in Sociology, Stavanger University College, Department of Health and Social Work Education, Stavanger, Norway.

Charles Engel, Professor, Centre for Higher Education Studies, Institute of Education, University of London, London, England.

Dr Marnie Freeman, Research Fellow, Centre for Nursing and Midwifery Research, University of Brighton, Brighton, Sussex, England.

Dr Della Freeth, Reader in Education for Health Care Practice, Institute of Health Sciences, City University, London, England.

Dr John Gilbert, Principal, College of Health Disciplines; Member of the Committee of Deans, University of British Columbia, Canada.

Caroline Glendinning, Professor of Social Policy, National Primary Care Research and Development Centre, University of Manchester, Manchester, England.

Sara Glennie, Member of the Professional Development Group, University of Nottingham; Independent Chair of the Cambridgeshire Area Child Protection Committee, Cambridgeshire, England.

Dr Rita Goble, Honorary Senior Lecturer, Institute of General Practice, School of Postgraduate Medicine and Health Sciences, University of Exeter, United Kingdom; Member of the Executive Committee of the Network: Community Partnerships for Health through Innovative Education, Service and Research, Maastricht, The Netherlands.

Dr Elin Gursky, Visiting Scholar, Department of Health Policy and Management, Bloomberg School of Public Health, The Johns Hopkins University, Baltimore, USA.

Richard Hugman, Professor of Social Work, University of New South Wales, Sydney, Australia.

Audrey Leathard (Editor), Visiting Professor of Interprofessional Studies, South Bank University, London, England.

Diana Lee, Professor, Nethersole School of Nursing, The Chinese University of Hong Kong, Hong Kong.

Dr Tony Leiba, Senior Research Fellow, South Bank University and North East London Mental Health Trust, London, England.

Jill Manthorpe, Reader in Community Care, Department of Social Work and Community Health, University of Hull, Hull, England.

Geoffrey Meads, Professor of Health Services Development, City University, London; Visiting Professor of Organisational Development, Centre for Primary Health Care Studies, University of Warwick, Warwick, England.

Professor Carolyn Miller, Head of Research, Centre for Nursing and Midwifery Research, University of Brighton, Brighton, Sussex, England.

Graham Park, Social Worker, from 1997–2001 managed *Under One Roof*, an experimental project designed to encourage greater cooperation between statutory and voluntary agencies providing services for homeless people in south London, England.

Scott Reeves, Research Fellow, Institute of Health Sciences, City University, London, England.

Kirstein Rummery, Lecturer in Health and Community Care, Department of Applied Social Science, University of Manchester, Manchester, England.

Lonica Vanclay (until recently) Service Manager, Family Welfare Association, London, England.

Andrew Wall, Senior Visiting Fellow, Health Services Management Centre, University of Birmingham, Birmingham, England.

Jenny Weinstein, Assistant Director Quality Assurance and Customer Care, Jewish Care, London, England.

Elisabeth Willumsen, Assistant Professor in Social Work, Stavanger University College, Department of Health and Social Work Education, Stavanger, Norway.

Foreword

This symposium reviews the difficult process of change towards partnership, coordination and maximum collaboration between professions and agencies in health and social services. The change is inevitable, if only because of the increasing capability, complexity and cost of the services, alongside the needs and developing expectations of patients, clients and carers. The alternative is confusion, duplication and inefficiency. But it is difficult for most of us to escape from tradition and adapt to change. It is difficult also to tolerate different beliefs and values, whether in other people or other institutions – especially difficult when professional traditions and boundaries are under attack, when professional people are under unusual pressure through short-ages and when policy-makers, in a hurry, harass those who have to carry out their next policy before the last one has been evaluated (a 'policy onslaught', as one contributor describes it, 'a systematic attempt, perhaps without parallel in a modern democratic state, to re-frame fundamentally the activities and attitudes of all the participants in a major public institution').

Faced by these challenges, how can this book help? It is concerned particularly with the ways, positive and negative, in which policies influence collaborative practice and teamwork. It offers theoretical models and illustrates them with existing examples, for instance in primary health care or in services for older people or in partnership with patients – successes to emulate and failures from which to learn. It is good that some chapters are from other countries; the problems are international.

Teamwork depends greatly on the wider context in which it is developed. Government and management polices are among the strongest determinants – they foster it or undermine it. As different writers analyse examples, the benefits of collaboration and the effectiveness of teamwork for patients/clients and carers are repeatedly confirmed, far outweighing any ill effects. Confirmed also are the benefits to trained professionals – shared knowledge and resources, widened perspectives, a more satisfying and supportive work environment, maximal opportunities for specialist skills. It is naive to think that these benefits will ensue without prior organisation and interprofessional education. Examples in this book confirm the depth of ignorance and the deep-rooted prejudices that one professional group can maintain about another. Yet they also reveal how the most important values are shared and how motivating is the experience of their convergence, given skilled facilitation. The purposes, methods and outcomes of interprofessional education are also critically examined in the final chapters.

The topic of this book is unavoidably complex at this time, but every author points in some way to one guiding ideal – 'think patients, clients, services users'. It is not only frontline workers, like my colleagues in general medical practice, who have to listen carefully within a trusted personal relationship, but those too who design or manage services for populations. Services also need to be trusted – by users and professional providers alike. It is between these two main groups that the most productive collaboration must develop.

John Horder
Past President of the Royal College of General Practitioners
Founding Chairman of the Centre for the Advancement of
Interprofessional Education

Part I

Policy and interprofessional issues

Chapter I

Introduction

Audrey Leathard

SUMMARY

The purpose of this book is outlined to acknowledge the professionals and people involved with interprofessional collaboration. An introduction to the authors and topic areas highlights the main theme from policy to practice in health and social care both in the UK and abroad. The background is set by considering the definition of terms alongside the negative then positive features of interprofessional working.

THE APPROACH TO THE PRESENT PUBLICATION

At the start of a new millennium, an updated review and new approaches to interprofessional collaboration are needed to perceive the twenty-first century with vision for the future. This book sets out to provide a balance between what can be gained from the past and present to enable future possibilities within the linked context of both policy and practice.

This book is therefore relevant for all who have an interest in matters of health (to include public health and health promotion), social care, welfare and caring, whether as policy-makers or politicians, educators, service users, commissioners or providers of care, as hospital doctors, nurses, members of the allied health professions (e.g., physiotherapists, speech therapists, radiographers, occupational therapists and osteopaths) as well as general practitioners, practice managers, practice nurses, community nurses (health visitors, district nurses and community psychiatric nurses), pharmacists, health educators, dental carers, informal carers, social workers, care managers, clergy, probation officers, police officers, housing officers and staff of voluntary organisations, private hospitals and nursing homes. Increasingly, the private sector has a significant part to play in partnership working with National Health Service (NHS) managers and chief executives in hospital trusts. Throughout, those involved with primary care trusts (PCTs), care trusts (from 2002) and local authority social services, all are variously involved in working together with others in health, social care and educational provision.

The first of three sections starts with a consideration of policy issues from various interprofessional angles. The sequence begins with a policy overview from the editor. Importantly, the place of management is next considered by Professor Charles Engel (from London) and Dr Elin Gursky (from the USA). In keeping with the international nature of the topic overall, Professor Richard Hugman then identifies the interprofessional dynamics in Australian health and welfare. Ethical issues have also become a key factor for interprofessional working that are addressed by Andrew Wall. At this point Scott Reeves and Dr Della Freeth introduce an innovative perspective, particularly relevant for the twenty-first century, in looking at new forms of technology for new forms of collaboration. This first section is then rounded up, by the editor, with the presentation of a range of models for interprofessional and interagency work in practice.

The second section seeks to apply policy to practice in working together across professions, sectors and communities. Professor Carolyn Miller and Dr Marnie Freeman provide an overview of teamwork, while Professor Geoffrey Meads looks at new primary care policies. Public health is next viewed through the relevance of metaphors for health alliances by Professor Alan Beattie. Moving then from the general to the particular, the sequence features specific groups across the policy and practice arenas, by addressing the interprofessional agenda for family support (from Lonica Vanclay); safeguarding children (by Sara Glennie); in developing services for older people (by Professor Caroline Glendinning and Kirstein Rummery); disability and user-led services (from Professor Colin Barnes); mental health within an interprofessional context (by Dr Tony Leiba); and an experimental interagency service for homeless single people (from Graham Park). Of central importance, Jill Manthorpe then highlights the users' and carers' perspectives on collaboration in practice. Jenny Weinstein completes this section with a questioning view on the place of the voluntary sector with respect to partnership.

The final section links policy to practice within the context of learning together. Professor Hugh Barr begins by 'unpacking' interprofessional education. The next three contributions all come from abroad with Dr John Gilbert and Lesley Bainbridge, from Canada, who consider theoretical challenges and practical solutions, while Professors Elisabeth Willumsen and Paal Breivik look at interprofessional education and practice for health and social care in Norway. In geographical contrast, Professor Diana Lee describes interprofessional work and education in Hong Kong. To complete the global perspective, Dr Rita Goble discusses various international developments with regard to multiprofessional education. The conclusion, from the editor, draws the perspectives together with a consideration of interprofessional issues overall for collaboration in policy and practice for the twenty-first century.

THE MEANING OF THE WORDS

Already various terms have been used to indicate the context of health and social care professionals working together. However, within an international arena, terminological variations become even more widespread. For example, lead writers from the USA have recently defined an interdisciplinary health care team as a group of colleagues from two or more disciplines who coordinate their expertise in providing care to patients (Farrell et al 2001). This perspective is shared by Marshall et al (1979) in the UK where both 'interdisciplinary' and 'multidisciplinary' are viewed as referring to a team of individuals, with different training backgrounds, who share common object-ives but make a different but complementary contribution. While for some, 'inter' means working between two groups only, so for them 'multidiscipli-nary' or 'multiprofessional' are preferable forms to denote a wider team of professionals. For others, the term 'interprofessional' is the key term that refers to interaction between the professionals involved, albeit from different backgrounds, but who have the same joint goals in working together. In contrast, the term 'intraprofessional' normally refers to different specialist groups, but from one profession as with different nursing specialisms. How-ever, as policy developments move apace, so an ever-expanding range of professionals, service users and carers have all become involved in interpro-fessional work as well as a variety of organisations and sectors. In academic parlance, multidisciplinary work usually refers to the coming together and contribution of different academic disciplines. Latinists can help to simplify the arena by translating 'inter' as between; 'multi' as many; and 'trans' as across. What everyone is really talking about is simply learning and working together. Multidisciplinary and interprofessional courses are often terms both used to express the coming together of a wider range of health and welfare professionals to further their studies in a context of shared learning. As Hugh Barr (1994) has pointed out, the crucial distinction is that interpro-fessional work relies on interactive learning.

From a terminological quagmire, Table 1.1 seeks to clarify the arena through a selection of key words used to express learning and working together but set out under three headings that distinguish different elements in the arena. Hyphens are another pitfall that are used on a variable basis but have become increasingly discarded.

Any grouping of terms is debatable; alternatives may be considered more appropriate according to the circumstances under view. Furthermore, inter-pretations can differ as 'interprofessional' can mean different things to differ-ent groups of people, even among the professionals themselves who speak different languages that influence both their mode of thought and identity (Pietroni 1992). However, the field is not entirely sublime, as Beattie (1994) has pointed out, when health alliances can become dangerous liaisons. The title of this book has therefore purposely included the word 'collaboration' as

Table 1.1 A selection of key words used variously for interprofessional work to denote learning and working together

Concept-based	Process-based	Agency-based
Interdisciplinary	Teamwork	Interagency
Multidisciplinary	Partnership working	Multi-sectoral
Multiprofessional	Merger	Trans-sectoral
Trans-professional	Joint working/planning	Health alliances
Trans-disciplinary	Collaboration	Confederation
Holistic	Integration	Federation
Generic	Local planning	Consortium
	Coordination	Forum
	Unification	Interinstitutional
	Liaison	Locality groups
	Shared/joint learning	

elements of danger and challenge form part of the overall fabric. Ian Shaw (1994: xi) has also indicated that collaboration can have two meanings: conspiring with the enemy or working in combination with others. By whichever route, three aspects underpin the issues on hand: interpersonal, interprofessional and interagency.

WHO ARE THE PROFESSIONALS?

The title of this book involves two central elements: the first is the place of professionals. Traditionally, a professional person is associated with control of entry to a particular profession; the requirement to undergo a recognised length of training, accredited and, in some cases, licensed, by an acknow-ledged professional body. At the end of training, the professional is recog-nised as having a certain expertise that legitimates practitioner action, usually bound by a code of ethics, although Paul Wilding (1982) has shown that certain professional claims may be problematical. However, increasingly within a context where managers, health and welfare professionals, adminis-trative and reception staff, carers, cared-for and voluntary input are all involved, the term 'interprofessional' begins to lack clarity, other than 'all who seek to work together for the good of the service user'. More recently, semi-professionals (such as health care assistants) further contribute to the many potentially engaged in joint working as well as the evermore significant part to be played by the private sector. By the twenty-first century, however, one point is quite clear: the emphasis has swung significantly behind the importance of upholding the patient/user/customer/client/carer at the centre of interprofessional working.

THE ADVANTAGES AND DISADVANTAGES OF INTERPROFESSIONAL WORK IN PRACTICE

The drawbacks

The second element contained in the book title is to recognise, as reflected in the word 'collaboration', that there can be potentially two sides to the case for working together. In starting with the more negative aspects, this section can then finish on a positive note. Hardy et al (1992) identified, early on, five categories of barrier in joint working and, more problematically, in joint planning across the health and social services:

- *Structural* issues between health and social services, such as service fragmentation, gaps in services and non-coterminosity of boundaries
- *Procedural* matters hindering joint planning through different budgetary and planning cycles and procedures
- *Financial* factors including different funding mechanisms and flows of financial resources as well as administrative and communication costs
- *Status and legitimacy* with differences in legitimacy between elected and appointed agencies wherein local authority responsibilities are firmly based within a democratically elected arena, in contrast to all services appointed and centrally run by the NHS (National Health Service)
- *Professional issues* including problems associated with competitive ideologies and values; professional self-interest; competition for domains; conflicting views about users; as well as differences between specialisms, expertise and skills.

Other commentators have drawn attention to further interprofessional pitfalls such as the different languages and values between professional groups (Pietroni 1992); separate training backgrounds; time-consuming consultation, conflicting professional and organisational boundaries and loyalties; practitioners isolated with little management support; inequalities in status and pay; differing leadership styles; lack of clarity about roles and latent prejudices (Marshall et al 1979; Ovretveit 1990; McGrath 1991). Woodhouse and Pengelly (1991) have further identified psychological and institutionalised defences, while Ovretveit's (1990) report on *Cooperation in Primary Health Care* found that, although health care professionals stated a wish to work more closely together, whenever any significant moves towards true interprofessional working were made, everyone pulled back into uniprofessional groupings.

Loxley (1997: 1) has also pointed out that fundamental differences in 'the division of labour' have developed over the years in the health and welfare services. The perception of doctors as respected professionals has contrasted with the considered limitations of training, knowledge base and autonomy among social workers and nurses who have been regarded as semi-professionals (Etzioni 1969; Hudson 2002).

Throughout the 1990s, the increasing emphasis on teamwork and, subsequently, partnership working has lessened the tensions towards joint working, but further elements have emerged. For example, in November 2001, an occupational therapist shared with me that in one local NHS trust in the UK, while the allied health professions were endeavouring to work together, the underlying challenge was to become 'top dog'. Rather differently, organisational mergers have created a power base difference between a weaker agency or profession that has entered into a territory without acquiring adequate power to defend professional interests.

Meanwhile, from *The Report of the Public Inquiry into Children's Heart Surgery at the Bristol Royal Infirmary 1984–1995* (Kennedy 2001), evidence has emerged of hospital staff, underpinned by a lack of leadership and teamwork, who were dedicated and well motivated but failed to communicate with each other or to work together effectively for the interests of their patients. Central to the recommendations was the need for respect and honesty based on public involvement through patient empowerment and through a three-way partnership: between the professionals themselves; health care professionals and the patient; and between the NHS and the public.

Interprofessional bridge point

Spanning the case against and in favour of interprofessional working, a range of issues cut right across both arenas. For example, the list would include *cultural* and *political* sensitivities; *accountability* – to whom; for what; and how to involve different professions; *patient and user referrals* that can range across different sites and services; and the place of *quality assurance* – who measures what, when and for what purpose, whether with a top-down or bottom-up approach, but wherein an interprofessional value base would need to involve users. The assessment of interprofessional practice can gain from rationalised access to information but any such evaluation has to be set against the likelihood of separate professional inputs working across differing sites and locations. Then again, how far can *risk management* be absorbed by interprofessional working?

The issue of *confidentiality* is also a matter of importance, for example, as to how far access to patient/user records should extend between various professionals. Owens et al (1995: 33) have raised other questions such as what happens to *professional loyalty* when 'solo practice' is no longer the norm? Then again, professional loyalty may be challenged by the organisational requirements of administrative and economic efficiency in possible conflict with the priorities as defined by a profession or the professionals involved. Furthermore, different professions and, indeed, service users may work with varied understandings and hold a differing outlook according to the issues in hand. As a result, to consider the advantages and disadvantages of interprofessional working may begin to appear somewhat simplistic. Nevertheless, in looking now at the case for working together, the picture can at least be clarified with the focus on some positive points.

The positive aspects of interprofessional collaboration

After the catalogue of disadvantages for joint working, an individual might wonder whether there were any advantages. Early on, McGrath's (1991) study valuably assessed both sides of the case in the field of community mental handicap in Wales to show that interprofessional teams led to:

- More efficient use of staff (by enabling specialist staff to concentrate on specialist skills and maximising the potential of unqualified staff)
- Effective service provision (through encouraging overall service planning and goal orientation)
- A more satisfying work environment (through promoting a relevant and supportive service)

McGrath (1991) concluded that the advantages outweighed the acknowledged disadvantages in multidisciplinary work; as a result, coordination in services had improved. Interestingly enough, by the mid-1990s, Rachel Bia (now based at South Bank University) undertook a little mini-run, in the south-east of England, of a repeat format of McGrath's (1991) study, to find that the parents of service users involved with the work of community mental handicap teams did not feel that needs were met by a team at all, but only by individual workers, which draws attention to the potentially differing perspectives of professionals and users.

However, throughout the 1990s and into the twenty-first century, evermore positive aspects of interprofessional working have emerged such as:

- The recognition that what people have in common is more important than the difference, as professionals acknowledge the value of sharing knowledge and expertise
- The response to the growth in the complexity of health and social care provision, with the potential for comprehensive, integrated services
- The recognition of a more satisfying work environment within an arena where professionals can share and support each other

Southill et al (1995) would add that the failure of communications between the different groups of carers and professional groups, patients and clients had prompted attention; there was an increasing awareness of the need to improve the quality of care for patients and clients (memorably termed 'cli-pats'); as well as the potential to improve the effective use of resources. Ann Loxley (1997) has also pointed to the relevance of collective means to underpin mutual interests for agencies and professionals in order to meet individual and community needs. Hudson (2002) has subsequently indicated that an interprofessional approach has also been seen as a positive means to overcome fragmentation.

However, above all, the galvanising force behind interprofessional collaboration has been the perceived need to rationalise resources through coordinating, integrating and merging services, organisations or even some of the professions themselves. The merger movement has been paralleled, in recent years, by banks (Lloyds/TSB), utilities, building societies, universities, engineering and pharmaceutical companies (Kettler 2001), among others, all for the very same reason: rationalisation. What has been achieved by these moves is altogether another, somewhat cloudier, matter. Therefore, set against the drawbacks, by the twenty-first century, collaboration has become a powerful force, spearheaded by the government's modernisation programme to further partnership working across the health and social care services.

The background and outcome of interprofessional policy developments in the UK and abroad are now unfolded for analysis. Due to some differences in structural detail between Northern Ireland, Scotland and Wales, the UK commentary is centred largely on England, but the issues raised have a much wider relevance for interprofessional working.

REFERENCES

Barr, H. (1994) 'NVQs and their implications for inter-professional collaboration', in A. Leathard (ed.), *Going Inter-professional: Working Together for Health and Welfare*, London: Routledge.

Beattie, A. (1994) 'Healthy alliances or dangerous liaisons? The challenge of working together in health promotion', in A. Leathard (ed.), *Going Inter-professional Working Together for Health and Welfare*, London: Routledge.

Etzioni, A. (1969) *The Semi-professions and their Organisation*, New York: The Free Press.

Farrell, M., Schmitt, M. and Heinemann, G. (2001) 'Informal roles and the states of interdisciplinary team development', *Journal of Interprofessional Care* 15 (30), 281–95.

Hardy, B., Turrell, A. and Wistow, G. (eds) (1992) *Innovations in Community Care Management*, Aldershot: Avebury.

Hudson, B. (2002) 'Interprofessionality in health and social care: the Achilles' heel of partnership', *Journal of Interprofessional Care* 16 (1) 7–17.

Kennedy, I. (2001) *The Report of the Public Inquiry into Children's Heart Surgery at the Bristol Royal Infirmary 1984–1995*, July, London: The Stationery Office.

Kettler, H. (2001) *Consolidation and Competition in the Pharmaceutical Industry*, London: OHE.

Loxley, A. (1997) *Collaboration in Health and Welfare: Working with Difference*, London: Jessica Kingsley.

Marshall, M., Preston, M., Scott, E. and Wincott, P. (eds) (1979) *Teamwork For and Against: An Appraisal of Multi-disciplinary Practice*, London: British Association of Social Workers.

McGrath, M. (1991) *Multidisciplinary Teamwork*, Aldershot: Avebury.

Ovretveit, J. (1990) *Cooperation in Primary Health Care*, Uxbridge: Brunel Institute of Organisation and Social Studies.

Owens, P., Carrier, J. and Horder, J. (1995) *Interprofessional Issues in Community and Primary Health Care*, Basingstoke: Macmillan.

Pietroni, P. (1992) 'Towards reflective practice – the languages of health and social care', *Journal of Interprofessional Care* (1) Spring 7–16.

Shaw, I. (1994) *Evaluating Interprofessional Training*, Aldershot: Avebury.

Southill, K., Mackay, L. and Webb, C. (1995) *Interprofessional Relations in Health Care*, London: Edward Arnold.

Wilding, P. (1982) *Professional Power and Social Welfare*, London: Routledge & Kegan Paul.

Woodhouse, D. and Pengelly, P. (1991) *Anxiety and the Dynamics of Collaboration*, Aberdeen: Aberdeen University Press and Tavistock Insititute of Marital Studies.

Chapter 2

Policy overview

Audrey Leathard

SUMMARY

Interprofessional developments in the second half of the twentieth century are reviewed in four phases. The outcome shows how, from tentative and limited beginnings, more particularly involved with teamwork, the momentum speeded up significantly in the 1990s, towards collaborative working between agencies and professions. The challenge for the future is to be able to address constant change and mounting costs while, at the same time, perceive effective ways forward, towards integrated provision that meets the needs of service users.

INTERPROFESSIONAL POLICY DEVELOPMENTS

Phase I   Early initiatives: 1970s–1980s

The background

In 1948, the newly created National Health Service (NHS) inherited the pre-war legacy of a tripartite structure with a clear division between local authority community health and social services, hospital provision and general practice. By 1968, the divisions were reinforced as personal social services became unified under dedicated local authority directorates concerned with the care for community mental handicap, mentally ill, elderly and disabled people among other social care needs (Seebohm Report 1968), but quite separate from the NHS structure and administration of health care provision.

Under the 1974 NHS reorganisation, in order to represent the interests and views of the consumer, although some 200 community health councils were introduced at a 'health district' level to match the local provision of health care, local authorities, meanwhile, lost control of their services for ambulances, public health and their medical officer of health. Therefore, underpinning the professional and boundary divisions that have continued into the twenty-first century, the fundamental disparities between health and social services have been twofold. First, social services are run by local authorities that come under an elected local government structure, whereas health care provision is centrally directed by the Department of Health. Second, while local authority social services are means-tested, the NHS is based on central government financed provision but health care is, in principle, free at the point of use (although availability is a finely argued point) (Leathard 2000).

By the early 1980s, the outcome of cross-boundary working and joint consultative committees (from the mid-1970s) was generally regarded as disappointing (Webb and Wistow 1986; Lewis 1993). As the Audit Commission (1986) pointed out, the professional cultures and forms of accountability differed significantly between health and social services. With a retrospective view some 20 years later, Hudson (2001a) summed up the difficulties with joint approaches in the 1970s, as ministerial ambition, departmental survival and rigid boundaries that have remained to challenge the twenty-first century.

Table 2.1 Phase I   Working together – some
                   early developments: 1970s–1980s

- Teamwork in hospitals
- Mental health teams
- Primary care teams
- 1989 Children Act

Teamwork in hospitals has had a long tradition of working together (Pietroni 1994). However, hospital teamwork has been particularly relevant in surgical teams (Marshall et al 1979) in which each team member is well conversant with the job in hand, seeks to carry out the work with focus, where personal characteristics can thus be overlooked. By the start of the 1990s, Finnegan's (1991) study on collaborative care planning in six West Midlands hospitals showed a significant change in emphasis. A multidisciplinary group set out to assess, implement and evaluate care in collaboration with the patient, but the key issues were to maximise resource use and to ensure planned quality of care (see also Chapter 8 for an analysis of teamwork in hospital bed management policy).

Mental health teams, by the late 1970s, were particularly encouraged by the Department of Health and Social Security to overcome factors that had hindered collaboration between health and social services, such as failures in communication alongside ignorance of the roles, skills and outlooks of other professionals (DHSS 1978). As Kingdon (1992) has pointed out, efficient service provision requires teams and networks to address need; to avoid duplication of effort, pool skills; to share specialist knowledge; to break down stereotypes and to understand the role of other professionals. Key members of mental health teams have included general practitioners, community psychiatric nurses and social workers who, under the 1990 NHS and

Community Care Act, have been further required to assess needs for social care. Team members have increasingly extended to psychologists, psychiatrists, counsellors, occupational therapists and, even more recently, to pharmacists and music/art therapists. Others may also participate in a network of care for individuals, from education, housing, court solicitors, the voluntary and private sectors; in such circumstances, coordination and advocacy are essential (Kingdon 1992).

In order to be effective, the challenge for mental health teams has been not only to be able to provide relevant services and to focus on specific objectives, but also to secure an appropriate team composition to maintain morale and a sense of belonging among staff. In Chapter 15, Tony Leiba discusses subsequent developments in the work of mental health teams.

Primary care teams have similarly become evermore complex, according to the needs of patients and general practice developments. Among the various health and welfare teams that have evolved (e.g. for palliative care, community learning disabilities and for older people) primary care has been in the forefront of team developments over time. Following the reorganisation of general practice in 1967, opportunities for teamwork became a possibility for most professionals involved.

By the mid-1990s, teamwork in general practice-based primary care had become well developed in the UK, but one area of tension still lingered for the general practitioner (GP) in the apparent shift away from the personal doctor who provided first contact, continuing and comprehensive care (Stott 1995). The challenge has been to maintain the continuity in personal care as well as to achieve effective teamwork through shared vision, objectives and protocols, while ensuring adequate resources and cost-effectiveness (West 1994).

Looking back over the last 25 years, teamwork comparisons have been usefully made between the UK and the USA but, on this occasion, more particularly for geriatric assessment teams. Both team compositions and the size of teams have differed between the two: in the USA, a wider variety of disciplines (to include representatives from nursing, psychiatry and psychology, social work, nutrition and dietetics) and larger team numbers (10 or more members) have been more likely to be found than in the UK. In contrast, smaller teams of two to five (which commonly have included at least one general practitioner and a community nurse or health visitor) with fewer core members have been more prevalent in the UK (Douglass 2001).

By the end of the twentieth century in England, the picture continued to move onwards, as primary care teams could include more widely doctors, practice nurses, district nurses, health visitors, practice managers, nurse practitioners, dieticians, receptionists, social workers and midwives (but the latter two not usually based on site). However, in keeping with developments for user involvement by the twenty-first century, for example, a Central Surgery Patient Participation Group has recently been established, as exemplified by my local general practice in Surbiton, Surrey (with their agreement to include this point here) in order to provide a two-way communication between staff and patients, as well as to support the primary care teams in practice to continue the improvement of the service to patients. Some similar earlier developments have also occurred elsewhere; but see also Chapter 9 by Geoffrey Meads on primary care policies more widely from 1997.

The Children Act 1989

In contrast to primary care team developments, the 1989 legislation formed a direct and legal response to an ongoing series of reports and investigations into child abuse cases over the previous 20 years that culminated in the major *Report of the Inquiry into Child Abuse in Cleveland* (Butler Sloss 1988). Two points of general interest have arisen from the initial 1989 legislation. First, in the drive to overcome the lack of interprofessional and interagency coordination between the various groups involved (doctors, health visitors, nurses, social workers, the police, the courts, school welfare officers, teachers, parents and relatives), the Department of Health issued policy guidance in which the title indicated the high priority given to *Working Together: A Guide to Arrangements for Inter-agency Cooperation for the Protection of Children from Abuse* (DoH 1991). Joint policies and procedures were to be established in the working relationships between the social services departments, the police, doctors and community health workers, among others.

Second, equally relevant for interprofessional collaboration, was the setting-up of Area Child Protection Committees to encourage the close liaison of the professionals and agencies for all involved in child protection work. The initiative was funded by social services departments as well as providing funding for training and support for local authority foster parents, voluntary oganisations and social work staff.

Despite strenuous attempts to work together for child protection, the twenty-first century began with, yet again, another case of a child abuse victim and the subsequent death of Victoria Climbie, together with a statutory inquiry into the child protection team responsible for the case (Carvel 2001). One case is clearly not necessarily representative of child protection work as a whole across the country over the last 20 years, but the outcome does reflect some continuing problems (the present-day issues are discussed more fully by Sara Glennie in Chapter 12).

In assessing the nature of the child protection process and the factors that have undermined effective outcomes, Lupton et al (2001) contend that child protection does not fit easily into the health service; collaboration is therefore undermined by the system and by those who operate the arrangements. The role of general practitioners has been less than evident as doctors do not necessarily participate in the child protection networks. In considering whether professionals are working together or pulling part, the way forward is seen through the need to develop collaborative approaches between the NHS and other agencies but, importantly, to be backed by financial incentives (Lupton et al 2001).

Phase 2   Fragmentation and collaboration: 1990–1997

Table 2.2 Phase 2   Fragmentation and collaboration: 1990–1997

- Health alliances:
  1992 *The Health of the Nation* (Secretary of State for Health 1992)
- The internal market:
  1990 National Health Service and Community Care Act

Health alliances

The key government publication on *The Health of the Nation* (Secretary of State for Health 1992) identified joint action within health alliances between health and local authorities, the Health Education Authority, local education authorities and voluntary organisations, in order to develop strategies for health promotion and prevention. By 1993, the Department of Health continued to promote a positive view of *Working Together for Better Health* (Secretary of State for Health 1993) in order to meet the targets set by the Health of the Nation programme. In looking at partnerships for public health in Chapter 10, Alan Beattie considers the wider implications of health alliances.

The internal market

The 1990 National Health Service (NHS) and Community Care Act split health and social care provision between purchasers and providers to create an *internal market*. To curb costs, purchasers were required to assess needs, while providers were intended to compete against each other to secure contracts from the purchasers. To see the overall picture at a glance, Figure 2.1 sets out an overall map of the structure from 1990–97 that shows the clear division between purchasers and providers as well as the division between a centrally run health service, free at the point of use, while the social services, run by local government, accountable to the local electorate, were based on means-tested care especially for older people. The split between purchasers and providers, as well as the competition between the providers themselves, led to fragmentation of services but a collaborative momentum began to build up between the purchasers.

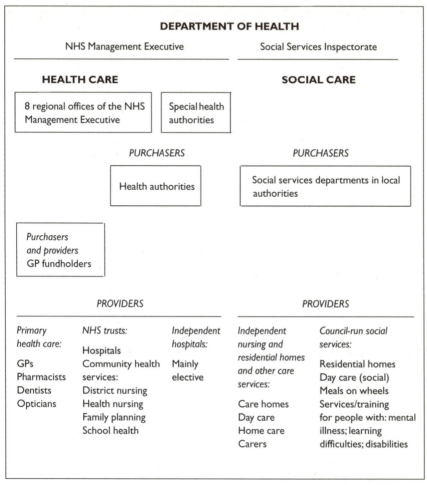

DEPARTMENT OF HEALTH

NHS Management Executive   Social Services Inspectorate

HEALTH CARE   **SOCIAL CARE**

8 regional offices of the NHS   Special health
Management Executive   authorities

PURCHASERS   *PURCHASERS*

Health authorities   Social services departments in local
                                 authorities

*Purchasers
and providers
GP fundholders*

PROVIDERS   *PROVIDERS*

Primary health care:	NHS trusts:	*Independent hospitals:*	*Independent nursing and residential homes and other care services:*	*Council-run social services:*
GPs	Hospitals	Mainly elective		Residential homes
Pharmacists	Community health services:		Care homes	Day care (social)
Dentists	District nursing		Day care	Meals on wheels
Opticians	Health nursing		Home care	Services/training
	Family planning		Carers	for people with: mental
	School health			illness; learning
				difficulties; disabilities

Figure 2.1 The structure of the NHS and community care services in England, 1996.

The purchasers in the internal market

GP fundholders could apply for the status to run their fundholding practices, employ their own staff and to raise funds over and above the NHS monies budgeted for the assessed needs of the fundholding population. Uniquely, GP fundholders were therefore both purchasers for a range of services and service providers. Although the Audit Commission (1996) recorded that 53 per cent of patients were covered by GP fundholding – to rise to 59 per cent by early 1997, GP fundholding remained one of the more controversial aspects of the NHS reforms due to the higher costs incurred than for non-fundholders, the creation of a two-tier service and cream-skimming, among

other factors (Leathard 2000). *District health authorities* now acted as purchasers of hospital care, the *family health service authorities* were responsible
for services provided by GPs, pharmacists, dentists and opticians, while *local
authorities* covered the purchasing of all social services in the community.

The collaborative momentum

With the creation of a purchaser–provider split, collaborative developments
became a driving force to rationalise the purchasing agencies in the internal
market. The fundamental reason was to cut costs by reducing the number of
purchasers and authorities involved. Table 2.3 sets out the sequence of
action.

By early 1997, the number of purchasing bodies had greatly reduced as the
result of mergers and reorganisation. These moves reflected similar merger
developments in the private sector for similar reasons: to curb costs and to
secure service integration but which intended outcomes in the public sector
were not necessarily achieved (Edwards and Passman 1997). With regard to
social care, local authorities largely commissioned care from the voluntary
and private sectors.

Table 2.3 The collaborative momentum: 1991–1997

Regional health authorities (RHAs) were reduced from 14 to 8 by April 1994:

> Under the 1995 Health Authorities Act, the RHAs' functions were taken
> over by eight regional offices of the NHS Executive

District health authorities (DHAs) Harrison's (1992) continuum of purchasing showed how
DHAs started to work together informally, which escalated to 'mergermania':

- Individual DHAs purchasing
- Informal joint purchasing
- Formal joint purchasing
- Consortia or Agencies
- Mergers

Family Health Service Authorities (FHSAs) collaborated with DHAs:

- First informally then formally
- FHSAs and DHAs were then required to integrate by law in April 1996
  under the 1995 Health Authorities Act to become health authorities

Multifunds became established whereby GP fundholders started to work together on
purchasing

Total fund merged and integrated purchasing across health authorities and
holding fundholding practices

The providers in the internal market: primary health care

On the purchaser side, the competition envisaged within the internal market to secure contracts became increasingly unrealisable. The threat to collaborative working thus began to diminish. For a start, by the mid-1990s, the NHS Executive (1995) saw the extension of GP fundholding in policy terms of the provision of a 'primary care-led NHS' with a clear role for the new health authorities to engage in a growing partnership between both to enable health care to become more responsive to the needs and preferences of patients and local people.

Community health services

Meanwhile, a wide range of professionals worked in the community health services – mostly in community nursing, including district nurses, health visitors, community midwives, community psychiatric nurses, nurses for people with learning difficulties, school nurses and community specialist nurses. Indeed, community health services had more in common with 'clans' and 'networks' than markets. Collaborative rather than adversarial relationships were therefore more appropriate between purchasers and providers (Flynn et al 1995).

Hospital provision and mergers

Although initially contracts were competitively sought between hospitals and particular specialties, the need to cut costs, rationalise services and to address financial stability, led hospitals (similarly as with purchasers) to discussions on hospital mergers. NHS trusts leaders began to call for greater collaboration between trusts to enhance services. By the mid-1990s, NHS trust mergers were soaring in order to secure rationalisation, reduce duplication and to ensure survival (Chadda 1996).

Threatened by a financial squeeze, the next step was considered in Andover, Hampshire, to merge a community health care trust with local fundholding practices to create a purchaser–provider hybrid. Such developments were described by Professor Ham as a middle way between old-style NHS planning and outright competition where purchasers and providers were recognising the need to work together as partners as well as to improve the health of patients through 'contestability' (Millar 1996).

Internal market outcomes: joint planning and interagency developments: 1990–97

The NHS internal market itself led health authorities to explore ways in which to cooperate in joint purchasing arrangements in which Ham and

Heginbotham's (1991) early analysis showed that a top-down approach to purchasing together carried high risks; more effective were arrangements in which authorities worked collaboratively on their own initiative, then worked towards joint purchasing.

Overall, little evaluation was undertaken as to the outcome for interprofessional and interagency implications, although evidence was brought together on the effects of the internal market overall (Le Grand et al 1998). However, as Powell (1997: 9) has commented on trying to assess outcomes in terms of a single currency (e.g. collaborative working): different evaluative criteria yield different conclusions.

Coordinating community care plans

Joint planning was set out, under the 1990 NHS and Community Care Act, with the requirement that local authorities published community care plans and laid down a statutory duty to consult with users and a specified range of local agencies (including health authorities, housing departments, the voluntary and private sector as well as informal carers). Wistow et al's (1993) analysis of community care plans showed that a high proportion were joint plans (55 per cent); another 9 per cent were jointly signed; and another 27 per cent were complementary, but the survey revealed the need to clarify the plans as well as the purpose of joint planning. Lewis and Glennerster's (1996: 191) review established that although much effort had been devoted to the obligatory community care plans, the impact had been rather limited with gaps revealed and the inability to meet identified needs.

Hospital discharge

The demands that arose from discharging patients from hospital into the community remained a critical juncture between local authorities, hospitals and social services departments. Under the 1990 legislation, local authorities had been given the responsibility to assess individual need in collaboration with health authority staff. The aims were to empower the service users and their carers as well as to enable people to be cared for in their own homes. However, differences in priorities, organisational styles and cultures between the key agencies in the health and social services had led to a reluctance to work together (Audit Commission 1992). As the voluntary and statutory sectors struggled with the various forms of collaboration required by the 1990s' legislation (Lewis 1993), the assessment of needs introduced complex issues.

Further, the introduction of the new community care arrangements in April 1993 also strengthened the need for joint working between health authorities, GP fundholders and local authorities. The Department of Health (DoH 1995) subsequently sought to clarify the respective responsibilities for continuing care between the NHS and local authorities. Collaboration was considered crucial to ensure effective and integrated delivery of care. By 1997, the long-term care for older people continued to present a major challenge for joint working wherein interprofessional conflicts had arisen over language barriers and different cultures between health and social services but, above all, over the financial difficulties that confronted social services in seeking to cope with the demands that arose from the community care reforms for caring for older people in the community.

Any collaborative momentum, by 1997, had become jeopardised by certain fundamental disjunctions. The internal market turned out to be a quasi-market, but not a conventional market at all (Le Grand and Bartlett 1993), whose perverse incentives had undermined a seamless service (Paton 1995), despite the government's intentions to promote joint working across boundaries (Secretary of State for Health 1996). Next, local authority commissioners were required to place 85 per cent of contracted provision in the voluntary and private sectors, but informal carers actually undertook most of the caring in the community (CNA 1995). Furthermore, the administrative divisions between health and social services remained.

In the spring of 1997, however, with the return of the New Labour government, significant changes were to take place in phase three of the developments of relevance for interprofessional and interagency issues. Table 2.4 places the emphasis on the elements of particular relevance for partnership working, rather than to set out all the details involved with such widespread developments.

Table 2.4 Phase 3   Partnership working: 1997–2000

1997	• *The New NHS: Modern – Dependable* (Secretary of State for Health 1997) planned to replace the internal market with:

Partnership working as the central focus of the new NHS

Primary care groups (PCGs) to have four optional levels of responsibility: from supporting the health authority (HA) in commissioning to becoming established as a free standing body (a primary care trust (PCT) at level 4) accountable to the HA for commissioning care together with the provision of community health services but whose boards were significantly to include a social service nominee and lay member

NHS trusts to provide hospital and community health care; to assess health needs; with a new statutory duty to work in partnership with other NHS organisations and local authorities to shape services and to develop HiMPs

Health improvement programmes (HImPs) to form the basis for a local partnership strategy with NHS trusts, PCGs and local authorities; to identify local population needs; to improve health and health care; and to tackle root causes of ill health

Continued overleaf

Table 2.4 cont.

	Health authorities to give strategic leadership; to identify health needs; to lead local HImP developments; and to work closely with NHS trusts; the PCGs; local authorities; voluntary organisations; and the local community
	NHS Care Direct – a new 24-hour telephone advice line, staffed by nurses, piloted in March 1998, to be extended nation-wide by 2000
1997	• Healthy living centres to improve health and fitness among a target population in the more deprived areas involving a consortium of GP practices; primary health care; community groups; local authorities; health authorities; NHS trusts; voluntary groups; businesses; and schools
1998	• Health action zones (HAZs) to set up 11, then extended to 26, HAZs in areas of pronounced deprivation and poor health; to develop clear targets to tackle entrenched inequalities through partnership working between hospitals, GPs, local authorities, voluntary bodies, local businesses working together to build on successful area regeneration schemes with the potential to advance a public health agenda
1998	• The Social Exclusion Unit to address problems ranging from bad housing and health to education and crime; to bring agencies together with a new commitment to develop policy and plans with central and local government working together with local businesses, voluntary and statutory agencies, which programme was initially to be based on 17 pathfinder districts of deprivation: to develop a new preventive approach together with training of front-line staff among teachers, health visitors, social workers and paediatricians for work in schools and in the home
1998	• *Modernising Social Services* (Secretary of State for Health 1998a): to overhaul the social services to ensure that local authorities, health services and other providers would work together to enable people to lead independent and fulfilling lives
1998	• *Our Healthier Nation* (Secretary of State for Health 1998b) to improve the population's health, that is in the length of people's healthy lives and to improve the health of the worst off in society, based on four priority areas: to reduce the incidence of heart disease and strokes; accidents; cancers; and mental health, through joint working between health and local authorities to implement 'contracts for health' through *healthy schools; healthy workplaces; and healthy neighbourhoods.* Health authorities to establish local arrangements to involve all relevant interests to plan an integrated programme on a partnership basis (NHS Executive 1998)
1999	• *Saving Lives* (Secretary of State for Health 1999) to reduce deaths from heart disease; cancers; suicide; accidents; to help people manage their own illness; to extend the nurse-led NHS Direct telephone helplines; to set up public health observatories to identify and monitor local needs and trends; to be implemented nationally through schools; health centres; the workplace; even shopping centres, to target health inequalities to enable poor people to live longer
1999	• Health Act NHS bodies now had a duty to cooperate with each other and with local authorities; while pooled budgets and resources with 'flexibilities' enabled joint working between health and social services, with delegated commissioning to one lead organisation to pay for an agreed range of services in response to the needs of service users. GP fundholding was to cease to have effect
	• Working together to improve quality (reviewed under no. 4 below): national service frameworks; CHIMP (Commission for Health Improvement); NICE (National Institute for Clinical Excellence); and clinical governance

Phase 3   Partnership working: 1997–2000

From 1997 onwards, the government placed joint working at the centre core of policy. To see the overall picture, Figure 2.2 sets out a map of the NHS wherein local authorities, although still under local government, were embraced within the whole by health improvement programmes.

In reviewing the developments of relevance for collaboration, four key factors stand out.

1 Partnership working

To work in partnership formed the third of the six principles to underpin the new NHS (Secretary of State for Health 1997:11). The intention was to break down the organisational barriers and to forge stronger links with local authorities in order to put the needs of the patient and user at the centre of the care process.

Significantly, a duty was to be placed on local authorities to promote their areas' economic, social and environmental well-being, together with powers to develop partnerships with a range of organisations as well as with the NHS. Hudson (1998) described this type of approach as *programme partnership* that addressed interorganisational fragmentation. Other forms of partnership in the White Paper (Secretary of State for Health 1997: 46) were identified as *professional partnership* when attention was drawn to the importance for staff in NHS trusts to work efficiently and effectively in teams within and cross organisational boundaries. *Administrative partnership* was perceived by Hudson (1998) as the expectation that primary care groups and

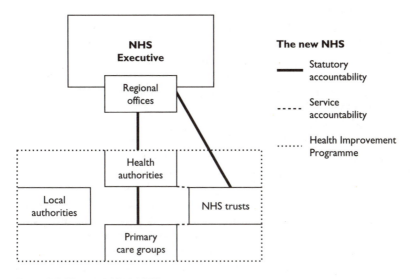

Figure 2.2 The new NHS 1997.

Source: Secretary of State (1997: 21).

social services departments would work closely together, further acknowledged by the recognition given to coterminosity. *Performance partnership* was reflected in the new national performance framework that enabled all management to look at the NHS achievements for the local population as well as the new approach to benchmarking to be driven by the eight regional offices in conjunction with the regional social services inspectorate. Under *governance partnership*, the new NHS sought to make NHS bodies more representative of local communities, which set out to involve a local government presence in NHS governance but no local NHS democratic accountability, in contrast to locally elected local government arrangements.

The importance of *Partnership in Action* (DoH 1998a) was underlined when both the Minister of State and Parliamentary Under-secretary of State for Health respectively drew attention to the need for joint working at three levels:

- *Strategic planning* where agencies needed to use their resources towards the achievement of common goals
- *Service commissioning* to secure services for the local populations
- *Service provision* where the key objectives should be for the user to receive a coherent integrated package of care

By 1999, the Health and Social Care Joint Unit was set up by the Department of Health to take forward the government commitment to build on the partnership agenda to bring health and social services closer together (NHS Executive 1999).

2 Health Act 1999 and pooled funds
A second key feature to underpin partnership working was reflected in the new flexible financial arrangements. Section 31 of the 1999 Health Act gave NHS bodies and local authorities the 'flexibility' to respond effectively to improve services, either by joining up existing services or by developing new coordinated services as well as working with other organisations. The financial 'flexibilities' offered the opportunity for further innovative approaches to user-focused services.

From April 2000, the partnership arrangements were based on pooled funds as well as the delegation of functions such as lead commissioning and integrated provision. Regardless of what contributions NHS bodies or local authorities committed to the pool, the pooled resource could be used on agreed services as set out in the partnership arrangement that gave pooled budgets a unique flexibility, while bounded by agreed aims and outcomes between partners who could be health authorities, primary care trusts and local authorities as well as an NHS trust with the agreement of the health authority (NHS Executive 1999). By April 1999, health and local authorities were also asked to produce joint investment plans for older people as well as for adult mental health services by April 2000.

3 Health improvement, health promotion and health inequalities

Significantly, the acceptance and drive towards collaborative working in health and social care was intended to reach far beyond the provision of health and community care facilities. Health improvement has been seen as a major factor in addressing the root causes of ill health as well as to identify local needs, while seeking to link the structural elements together. Equally important have been the programmes for Health Action Zones as well as the initiatives to address inequalities in health and deprivation (see Table 2.4) by working across a wide variety of agencies and organisations, as well as the voluntary, public and private sectors. The overall purpose was to improve the lives of disadvantaged people and to combat ill health and socio-economic inequalities through relevant groups working together locally.

Health Improvement Programmes (HImPs)

HImPs were intended to provide a local strategy for improving health and health care and to be the means of delivering national targets in each health authority area. The programme was to be led by each health authority, with a main responsibility to draw up a health improvement programme to tackle root causes of ill health and to plan care for patients, but significantly, in consultation with NHS trusts, primary care groups as well as with other primary care professionals (dentists, opticians, and pharmacists), the local social services, the public and other partner organisations.

Therefore, from the start, the HImP programme was to be based on partnership working throughout. Health authorities were to monitor and ensure the delivery of the programme by NHS trusts, primary care groups (PCGs) and others. Health authorities were also required to oversee that the local NHS was working in partnership to coordinate plans for the local workforce. Local education consortia were expected to set up training and education arrangements to provide the relevant skills needed by the hospital and community sectors, as well as by primary and social care. The overall purpose was for health authorities to guarantee that patients would have quicker access to local services. Health authorities would therefore coordinate information and information technology plans across primary care, community health services and secondary care (Secretary of State for Health 1997: 26–7). As Figure 2.2 indicates, HImPs were intended to encompass all aspects of health and social care provision to enable a coordinated whole in the planning and delivery of services.

The HImPs set out to assess:

- The health needs of the local population as well as how the NHS and partner organisations were to meet the most important needs through broader public health programmes
- The health care requirements of the local population together with the

development of local services either directly by the NHS or, where appropriate, jointly with the social services
- The range, location and investment required in local health services to meet the needs of local people

Based on a three-year action plan, the first HImPs were expected to be in place by April 1999. Significantly for partnership working, HImPs were intended to encourage innovative cross-sectoral working that included pooled budgets.

An early appraisal was undertaken by the King's Fund (Arora et al 1999, 2000) to explore the development of some of the first HImPs in London. Welcoming the opportunity to work together, the contributors were largely positive about the HImP initiative. However, six challenges were located with:

- *Work and time overload*
- *Changing roles and responsibilities*
- *The lack of resources*
- *Public involvement and accountability*: the short timescale for the HImP development had limited the extent of public consultation, while local authorities had well-established mechanisms for consultation with local communities, but newly formed PCGs had struggled to consult with constituent practices
- *Measuring progress*: reducing health inequalities was a long-term goal while swifter progress was needed to enable partner organisations to remain signed up
- *Interagency partnerships*: health authorities saw HImPs as part of the public health department, thus marginal to the organisation as a whole, while local authorities and PCGs felt the need to be better equipped with public health skills.

Different cultures and ways of working were also felt to be barriers between the different types of organisations involved. The authors concluded (Arora et al 1999, 2000) that while there was widespread commitment to a health improvement policy, which put an emphasis on partnership, the six challenges needed to be addressed to maintain the enthusiasm, to reduce health inequalities and deliver better health for all.

On reflection, Anna Coote (1999), director of the public health programme at the King's Fund, pointed out that health authorities needed to make sure that the partners involved (PCGs and local authorities) really felt ownership had been shared, even though the process remained the responsibility of health authorities. Then again, doctors had dominated most PCG boards that made it harder for other team members, possibly more attuned to the public health agenda, to exert an influence. Further, no one had addressed how to enable local people, especially marginalised groups, to have an effective voice in developing HImPs, while the problem of user fatigue had started to become evident. Meanwhile, greater flexibility was needed to transfer NHS funds into housing, social services or improving the environment as well as to set up ways to measure local authority contributions to health improvement.

Further studies revealed some similar outcomes, such as the findings from Birmingham University's Health Services Management Centre review of seven HImPs, which showed that although health authorities had tried to involve a wider range of stakeholders, management costs had held back the development of HImPs (Whitfield 1999). Then again, the second largest health authority in the country, Avon, found that to organise a HImP was an immense task, even though the process provided opportunities to bring people together from different organisations as well as to form new partnerships (Ewles 1999). Rather differently, although the government envisaged that HImPs would address areas of inequality in social exclusion, the health authority of relatively affluent Kingston and Richmond (but with deprivation blackspots in Norbiton) showed how partnership working was the key to a successful HImP (Healy 1999).

Subsequently, Abbott and Gillam (2000) pointed out that HImPs had increasingly acquired many differing definitions. Furthermore, a national tracker survey of primary care groups and trusts (Wilkin et al 2001) indicated that although there was evidence that links had been established between PCGs and local government services, the future challenge for multi-agency working was to ensure that performance management concentrated on the population's health rather than on the organisation of health care that remained a central focus of the NHS. However, the future of HImPs was to take a different turn by the start of the twenty-first century with the introduction of a new 'buzzword' and concept: that of 'modernisation' (see Phase 4). By 2002, the Department of Health (Dowse 2001) set out the way forward to reposition HImPs to become Health Improvement and Modernisation Plans (HIMPs) to reflect the importance of bringing together planning for health improvement, including health inequalities, within the modernisation agenda – but a sharp eye is needed to spot the difference in initials on the page.

Importantly, HIMPs were to be underpinned by a process of continuous partnership working to be reviewed (sometimes in part) on an annual basis. HIMPs were to build on existing HImP processes, to be developed in such a way as to reflect a coherent, integrated approach to strategic planning for health improvement, well-being, health care and treatment within the local health system. HIMPs were seen to provide the main strategic planning for all local health systems, to form part of a continuous process of partnership working with key stakeholders, to include health authorities, strategic health authorities (see Phase 4), primary care groups and trusts, NHS trusts, local authorities and local communities. The Department of Health (Dowse 2001: 2) has also suggested that there is 'much to gain by aligning HIMPs with local authorities' community strategies' in order to rationalise partnerships as well as mechanisms and processes for engaging with local communities and the voluntary sector.

From 2002, HIMPs were expected, among other requirements, to take account of national NHS priorities, local modernisation review 'outputs', national service frameworks and national health inequalities targets. HIMPs have to demonstrate where and how priorities, targets and coordinated action for resources are to be placed across local partnerships and planning mechanisms. HIMPs were also to be underpinned by plans to ensure delivery of the local objectives, the financial arrangements and organisational development in which most of the roles and functions of health authorities would devolve to primary care trusts (PCTs).

As the engagement of local people in the previous HImP process had proved variable, the need to create a patient-centred NHS had to be addressed in order to bring in the voices of patients, carers and the public to all levels of the NHS, to enable choice and improvement. The Department of Health (Dowse 2001: 3) envisaged that the approach would build on the local authorities own mechanism for engaging local communities. Only future studies on HIMPs would reveal just how far these proposals would be achieved or would the demands prove excessive for PCTs?

4 Working together for quality

Not until the mid-1990s was the question of quality in health and social care seriously addressed overall. On the one hand, the thrust was to focus on *Working Together: Securing a Quality Workforce for the NHS* (DoH 1998b) through the need to maximise the contribution of the staff. On the other hand, the aim was to build up a responsive, high-quality service consistently in all parts of the country, through breaking down barriers between organisations to provide integrated services by pulling together the right teams to meet the needs of users.

The performance of health and social services was to be monitored through new evidence-based *national service frameworks*, from 1998, initially for mental health services and services for older people, but increasingly for other groups who needed special care. The national service frameworks were intended to bring together the best evidence of clinical and cost-effectiveness for major care areas and disease groups. Significantly for joint working, the NHS executive was to work with the professions and service users to determine the best ways to provide consistency in the availability and quality of services (Secretary of State for Health 1997: 18, 57).

External inspection was to be applied to social care through the Social Services Inspectorate, joint reviews with the Audit Commission and, to health care, by the new *Commission for Health Improvement* (CHIMP). Directly responsible to the Health Secretary, CHIMP was to undertake service reviews; to support and oversee the quality of clinical services at local level; to undertake regular inspections of NHS trusts; to assess their local arrangements for clinical governance and to monitor local progress in implementing national service frameworks. All these initiatives reflected pathways towards working together for quality.

By April 1999, the *National Institute for Clinical Excellence* (NICE) was established, as a special health authority. The purpose was to provide national guidance to the NHS on cost-effectiveness and quality standards, in order to bring together a programme of evidence-based national service frameworks, clinical guidelines and national clinical audits so as to achieve best clinical practice (DoH 1998c).

Furthermore, NHS trusts had a legal duty under the Health Act 1999 to ensure quality, complemented by a new framework of *clinical governance* for which the chief executive would be ultimately accountable. Clinical governance applied equally to primary, community health care and the acute sector to ensure that clinical standards were met; to see that quality was complemented by the national service frameworks in the developments for particular specialties; and to oversee that the processes were in place to ensure continuous improvement, backed by the now statutory duty for quality. Quality had become a top priority for all NHS trusts and PCGs and PCTs based on a partnership between the government and the health professions.

Overall, the claim in *The New NHS* (Secretary of State for Health 1997: 63) was to achieve improvements in standards and performance by working together, by comparing performance and sharing best practice, not by financial competition. A King's Fund policy review of the new NHS (Gillam 1998) concluded that success in the mechanisms for monitoring and managing clinical performance would hinge on adequate resourcing of the structures and systems.

The Care Standards Act 2000 also marked further developments to underpin quality in care. A National Care Standards Commission was to make provision for the registration, inspection and regulation of a range of services that included children's homes, independent hospitals, care homes, domiciliary care agencies, fostering agencies and voluntary adoption agencies. A General Social Care Council and Care Council for Wales was also to make provision for the registration, regulation and training of social care workers.

By the end of the twentieth century, the main parts of the quality assurance programme were gaining increasing momentum. As a result, the impact on health and social care provision furthered working together for quality, more particularly between services and professionals but, in the light of the Bristol enquiry, on occasions with less involvement from patients and users (Kennedy 2001). Nevertheless, the Health Act 1999 had placed quality and partnership as a statutory duty to ensure that NHS bodies cooperated with each other and with local authorities to secure and advance the health and welfare of the people of England and Wales.

Outcomes for joint working by 2000

Between 1997 to 2000 the moves towards interprofessional and interagency working had been both significant and considerable. A further step still remained: integration. However by 1998, social services chiefs backed Department of Health officials in opposition to integrated health and social services organisations. The Association of Directors of Social Services ruled out the idea of extending the Northern Ireland model of integrated health and social care services. The view held was that social services would have much to lose with the fear that community care services would be down-graded; nor did social services favour having to absorb a dominant medical model of helping, but preferred to remain with a social model. Furthermore, the differing legislative and funding regimes of the two sectors limited opportunities to share resources effectively, while social services also wanted to see their current lines of democratic accountability upheld (*Health Service Journal* 1998).

By the turn of the twentieth century, however, the pressure to move towards joint working could not be ignored by health and local authorities who now considered that shared boundaries did help, as did the health improvement programmes and community strategies that brought agencies together. Further, the national service frameworks had aided clarification of roles, responsibilities and areas for joint action. Nevertheless, tensions remained between nationally determined priorities and local priorities; health authorities investing a disproportionate amount in the acute sector at the expense of local community health services; and a lack of local democracy in the governance of the NHS (Shifrin 2000). So the question for the twenty-first century was: for how long could the structural divisions remain?

Phase 4   Collaborating towards integration: 2000 onwards

By the twenty-first century, an avalanche of change was now being intro-duced to further integrated provision with modernisation as a key factor at the leading edge.

MODERNISATION

By October 1999, Alan Milburn had replaced Frank Dobson as Secretary of State for Health, with the continued pledge to modernise the NHS. By June 2000, with a promised national plan for health, Mr Milburn stated that vari-ation in performance had little to do with lack of money and resources but everything to do with lack of modernisation: 'We need a cultural change to break through the old demarcation barriers between doctors, nurses and

Table 2.5 Phase 4   Collaborating towards integration: 2000 onwards

2000	• *The NHS Plan* (Secretary of State for Health 2000): the NHS and social services to work together; to pool resources; to develop an NHS concordat with the private sector; new care trusts to commission health and social care in a single organisation; to involve the views of patients through their involvement on local health services; patients' surveys; and forums
	• Intermediate care to enable older people to lead more independent lives supported by health authorities; primary care groups; hospitals; and local authorities, all working together with a collaborative response from GPs, nurses, care workers and social workers
	• Community pharmacies to implement a pharmacy national plan jointly with health authorities and primary care organisations
	• Patients' councils to be created as umbrella bodies, grouping together patients' forums to have a comprehensive overview of a local health economy to include primary care and an independent advocacy service whose role would be to make reports to health and local authorities
	• Independent Patient Advocacy and Liaison Services (PALs) to support patients' complaints but to be commissioned by the local health authority ('Advocacy' was subsequently changed to 'Advice')
2001	• Health and Social Care Act to give the government powers to direct local authorities, health authorities and health care organisations to pool their budgets especially where services are failing
	• Care trusts confirmed by law
	• A modernisation programme: NHS Modernisation Agency (2001)
	• Integrated care pathways: to make explicit the most appropriate care for a patient group based on the available evidence and consensus of best practice with a multidisciplinary approach to the care pathway
	• One-stop health and social care services: a single care network to assess needs with staff working alongside each other with a primary and community health care team as part of single network
	• Walk-in (drop-in) centres: to extend access to primary care, staffed by nurses, some administrative staff and some have GPs on site; but the service is payable, not free at the point of use.
	• NHS Direct and Care Direct to work jointly as a one-stop approach to information by telephone round the clock
	• 28 Strategic health authorities to replace health authorities; to lead strategic development of the local health services; to manage the performance of primary care and hospital trusts on the basis of local accountability agreements; primary care trusts to become lead NHS organisation; to assess needs including general, dental and optical needs; to plan health services; improve health; and to forge new partnership working with local government and local communities; changes starting from April 2002 (DoH 2001a)
	• Private concordats
2001/02	• NHS Reform and Healthcare Professionals' Bill: NHS funding to allow ministers to channel money directly to GP-led primary care groups/ trusts; Commission for Health Improvement to be an independent body to report to Parliament; new measures for patient and public involvement

physiotherapists' (White and Carvel 2000). The modernisation agenda had therefore placed interprofessional matters centre stage. Six modernisation action teams were set up in June 2000, as a consultation exercise, one of which featured partnership working.

The NHS Modernisation Agency

In April 2001, the NHS Modernisation Agency was set up to coordinate management and leadership development as well as, significantly, to coordinate work to modernise services to meet the needs and convenience of patients. Among the joint working intentions were collaborative projects for cancer services, coronary heart disease; and primary care; to create effective working relationships at local, regional and national levels; to challenge traditional boundaries between agencies, professions and teams by working together, sharing success and learning from each other, in order to bring about change and initiatives to aid service improvements, clinical governance and learning (NHS Modernisation Agency 2001).

A new Leadership Centre for Health was set up at the Modernisation Agency, to break down the stereotypes of different professional groups and to link leadership with improved patient care (Shifrin 2001a). The modernisation agenda was therefore perceived as part of the widespread pressure on staff to meet new demands (Donnelly 2001a). By November 2001, the Modernisation Agency had had a limited impact on the general public as the launch was overshadowed by the Health Secretary's announcement at the same time of a wholescale restructuring of the NHS (Donnelly 2001b).

A Modernisation Board was to lead the changes, under the NHS Plan (Secretary of State for Health 2000), to be headed by the Health Secretary, advised by leading figures from the royal colleges, clinical staff, managers and patients. However by 2001, partnership working had become a central feature overall. Therefore the key issues for collaboration are now drawn out from the overall developments at the turn of the century regarding care trusts; intermediate care; the place of users; and private concordats. The proposals for strategic health authorities form part of the overall conclusion.

1 Care trusts

Care trusts represented the most crucial development for integration whereby health and social services could form into one organisation (a new level of PCT), by common agreement from April 2002, to provide closer integration to commission and deliver health and social care (Figure 2.3).

One aim was to prevent older people from falling into the cracks between the two services (Secretary of State for Health 2000). However, the main purpose was to provide a vehicle to modernise both health and social care as well as to ensure integrated services to focus on the needs of patients and

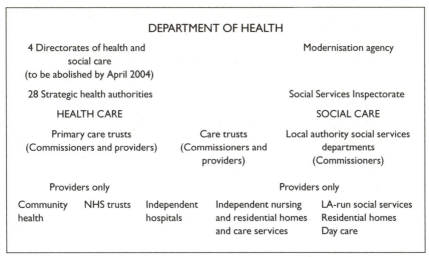

DEPARTMENT OF HEALTH

4 Directorates of health and social care
(to be abolished by April 2004)

Modernisation agency

28 Strategic health authorities

Social Services Inspectorate

HEALTH CARE

SOCIAL CARE

Primary care trusts
(Commissioners and providers)

Care trusts
(Commissioners and providers)

Local authority social services departments
(Commissioners)

Providers only

Providers only

Community health

NHS trusts

Independent hospitals

Independent nursing and residential homes and care services

LA-run social services
Residential homes
Day care

Figure 2.3 The structure of the health and social care services in England from 2002.

users. Care trusts were not intended to be a take-over either by the NHS or by local government but to lead to improvements in the quality of service delivery, by mutual arrangements, although the 1999 Health Act financial flexibilities would continue. Care trusts could be formed by application to the Secretary of State for Health by a PCG or PCT or by a local council (DoH 2001b). The future was now set for the integration of services after over half a century of division.

2 Intermediate care

Backed by an investment of £900 million, by 2003/4 intermediate care was intended to allow older people to lead more independent lives through rapid response teams of GPs, users, care workers, social workers and therapists, to provide emergency home care to curb hospital admissions. The interprofessional element was also evident in the proposals for integrated home care teams. As Hudson (2001b) pointed out, delivering partnership had become a political necessity, but intermediate care was the first real test and crucial to the NHS Plan. However, the early delivery of the proposals tended to remain more a concept than a reality.

Subsequent Department of Health (DoH 2001c) guidance put a six-week limit on an episode of care which, especially for older people, might be insufficient for longer recovery periods. Significantly for integration, the guidance emphasised that intermediate care was only one component of a wider system that should form an integrated part of a seamless continuum of services linking health promotion, preventive services, primary care, community health services, social care and support for carers.

Nevertheless, from the Anchor Trust, John Belcher (2001) commented that intermediate care should not ignore the role of housing. Further concerns have arisen over a funding shortfall for intermediate services that have loomed after most of the new money, about £500 million, which had been allocated to local authorities without being ring-fenced (Stephenson 2001).

Despite the various issues raised, some schemes have become well established. For example, in Thameside and Glossop, Portsmouth, and Sheffield, an important aspect of the intermediate care developments has been the development of multidisciplinary teams where health and social services staff work together to deliver patient care for rehabilitation work. In discussing these developments, Laurent (2001) has pointed out that little evaluation has taken place on the model introduced, nor has there been any evidence that added benefits have accrued. Nevertheless, further reports from Sheffield have shown how intermediate care services are helping to keep older people out of hospital, as social services and health professionals as well as local voluntary organisations work together with older people. The intention is to map ways of reversing the historic trend of low investment in community health services, home support and recuperation services as well as to avoid an overspend on general and acute hospital care (George 2001).

3   The place of patients and service users
By 2001, the government was seeking to abolish Community Health Councils (CHCs) which had, since 1974, been one limited way for patients to make their views known and for action to be taken. The NHS Plan (Secretary of State for Health 2000) heralded alternatives, such as patients' councils, forums and Patient Advocacy (later Advice) Liaison Services (PALS) (see Table 2.5) A new patient protection strategy (DoH 2001d) set out an additional independent advocacy service to support complaints. After the government's defeated attempts to try to abolish the CHCs, under the NHS Reform and Health Care Professions Bill in November 2001, CHCs were given an extra year's allocation of money for 2002/3. Meanwhile, the staff-only Voice organisations had attracted widespread criticism, as campaigners highlighted the absence of lay members' involvement above individual trust level together with a lack of coordination across local health economies. The grouping together of local patients' forums of lay members was likely to be one mechanism for the future (Shifrin 2001b). Overall, in health care, patient involvement had become complex, subject to change, without any particularly clear outcomes (see Chapter 24 for subsequent developments).

In contrast, user involvement has been altogether more positive in the social services. Government emphasis has been placed on the requirement for social services departments to work closely with service users in planning, developing, evaluating and monitoring services and their outcomes. In partnership working, the context is developing more broadly to include closer working together with housing, health and the social services. Some innovative strategies are also being developed across the country, such as funding service users to provide their own services, for example, through a group or through direct payments. Turner and Balloch (2001) have also drawn attention to the Wiltshire and Swindon Users' Network that promotes a membership organisation of service users to be involved in the planning, delivery and evaluation of services. More problematical is just how far users of social services feel empowered to work in partnership with professionals.

In comparing the two arenas for service users, patient involvement with health care provision is set within a medicalised approach based on changing and somewhat complex arrangements. While partnership arrangements might suggest that user involvement should work more closely together across health and social services, user organisations in the social services might prefer to remain within their own more developed arrangements that better suit their context and needs. The challenge will come when fully integrated, partnership-based, services have taken over from a dual pathway for health and social care.

4 Private concordats

Meanwhile, the most significant collaborative development in the fourth phase of developments has been the opening up of public–private partnerships whereby the public sector pays for health care treatment from the private sector. In comparison with the third phase from 1997–2000, the policy emphasis started to shift from encouraging joint working between the NHS and social services towards enabling joint NHS and private sector arrangements. With a national commitment to a publicly funded health and social care system, public–private partnerships have stirred up much controversy.

On the positive side, there are those who argue in favour, such as Karen Bryson et al (2001) who have claimed that in east Surrey, where health needs could not be met through the NHS facilities available locally, cooperation with private hospitals has been beneficial. From January to March 2001, some 1,000 people were taken off the NHS waiting lists; prices were comparable, sometimes cheaper than the NHS; patient satisfaction seemed high; the quality of care was good; but the programme had been carefully constructed through the health authorities' legal advisers to secure a tight contract.

Wider developments were also announced by the Health Secretary in December 2001, when an agreement in principle had been reached to allow the private sector to run and manage an acute diagnosis and treatment centre exclusively for NHS patients whose care would be paid by the taxpayer. The move was consistent with the concordat between the NHS and the private sector as part of a 10-year NHS plan to revitalise the health care system in order to raise standards to the European Union level (White 2001).

Dr Tim Evans of the Independent Healthcare Assocation (ICA) also felt the developments were good news as the capacity of the ICA was big enough to make a difference without the charge that the NHS was to become privatised. More widely, the government had already agreed to one million NHS operations being conducted in the private sector during the present parliament, while the intention was for some 300,000 NHS operations to be carried out annually in the private sector before 2010, out of an annual total of five to six million (Smith and Waterhouse 2001). Even more widely, the Prime Minister threw his weight behind a plan, for people waiting more than six months for surgery, to have the opportunity to obtain free (is NHS-funded) treatment abroad (Carvel and White 2001). The extent of public–private concordats began to appear endless. However, in the light of the first survey of the £100 million programme, from the National Audit Office (2001), the government considered that 80 of the first 100 private finance initiative (PFI) projects delivered a good service or better value for money than conventional funding (Hencke 2001).

As the patients set off for NHS operations abroad, the first 10 people from southern England, to travel by Eurostar for free treatment in Lille, northern France, welcomed the opportunity. Some hundreds more were expected to follow over the months to come (Carvel 2002a). However, as Berman and Higgins (2002) have pointed out, although the better educated and more informed patients were most likely to benefit, the private–public concordat would encourage comparisons between health services in the UK and other countries that could offer a test bed of new ideas from countries sharing the deeply held belief that universality and solidarity are essential elements of health care provision.

Meanwhile, the drawbacks of a public–private concordat are considerable. The problematical issues include:

- Transferring NHS staff to private companies with disagreements over the conditions of work
- A furious reaction from the public service unions that reflects both workplace anxiety and opposition to private sector involvement on principle
- Markets undermining universality by limiting the public sector's ability to pool the costs of expensive patients and areas of care across society as a whole
- Considerable administrative costs to the NHS as corporations demand a high price when governments seek to offload responsibility for universal health care (Pollock 2001)
- Practical dilemmas with regard to regulation, accountability, safeguards and even partnership working itself, with the temptation to under-regulate to encourage market entry
- The place of contractual relations may not follow the legal form when the public sector is tempted to forgo penalty entitlements for poor performance (Pollock et al 2001)

Despite the concerns, the Health Secretary slapped down Labour party unrest about growing private sector involvement in the NHS by announcing a further commitment to partnership involving commercial firms to run pathology services and modernising GP surgeries (Carvel 2002b). More plans reflected the government's determination to raise standards by allowing charities and the private sector to take over NHS hospitals that failed to meet new standards. Some five hospitals, given three months to show standards had been raised, were expected to be candidates (Watt 2002: 9). The public–private concordat was also likely to extend beyond the provision of health care to include the possibility that the private sector would also contribute to the cost of training hospital doctors (Wintour 2002). Overall, the Health Secretary's view was that the NHS was the last great nationalised industry where patients were expected to be grateful for whatever treatment they received, but the model was untenable for the twenty-first century (Watt 2002: 9).

Finally, while fears have been expressed that the public–private concordat could well lead to the privatisation of the NHS, Joan Higgins (2001) has warned that the more likely outcome could be the nationalisation of private medicine. Warning signs could already be seen: the uneven spread of private facilities across the country that leads to the undermining of partnership working; the Commission for Health Improvement has authority to monitor private hospitals treating NHS patients, whereby the private sector is subject to the NHS complaints' procedure; and, significantly, as NHS waiting lists reduce, so will the demand for private medical insurance that has already begun to occur (Collinson 2001).

Conclusion

Over the four phases of interprofessional and interagency collaboraton, from a limited start, the momentum has built up over the years to achieve significant joint working between the health and social services, the voluntary and private sectors, which has extended to housing and education, more particularly in the field of health promotion and social exclusion. By the turn of the twentieth century, a picture of public sector partnerships was moving apace to implement new initiatives across the work of NHS trusts, PCTs and PCGs as well as local authorities, which has involved local boards, committees, task force and modernisation programmes. The pattern was also to involve patients, users and customers.

By the start of the twenty-first century, public–private concordats have increasingly played a part in health care but less so in social care, where private residential and nursing homes continue on a means-tested basis. The idea of public–private concordats for social care could only be relevant once the government finally accepts fully publicly funded personal care that is intended for Scotland.

The introduction of 28 Strategic Health Authorities (SHAs) from 2002 (see Figure 2.3), to lead on strategic developments, while the former health authorities were to be disbanded, underlines a major issue in the NHS: constant change. SHAs are intended to cover a population of some 1.5 million people to be coterminous with an aggregate of local authorities, but the reorganisation required will be extensive.

Then again, PCGs are to merge; PCGs and PCTs are to cover more than 100,000 people to generate cost savings or improvements in performance. With the intention to make a difference to the provision and commissioning of health services, PCGs and PCTs are required to develop local health improvement priorities; set standards for service provision; improve patient services; to extend their role to cover general dental, pharmaceutical and optical services; as well as to inherit many functions from the disbanded health authorities such as needs assessment and, importantly, partnership working with local government. The government's proposals for change, set out under *Shifting the Balance of Power within the NHS: Securing Delivery* (DoH 2001a), raise some fundamental issues on delivery: the immense expectations placed on PCTs; the speed with which changes are to be carried forward; the impact on the ability to deliver the programme; and the lack of any real evidence to show that the proposals are what the NHS needs (Walshe and Smith 2001).

Meanwhile, the Prime Minister announced on 19 March 2001 that the government would invest £25 million over three years to establish up to 30 teaching PCTs in disadvantaged and underprivileged areas to be used to build up career and educational opportunities; to act as resource centres; and to work with universities and other local health organisations (DoH 2001e). Overall, Wilkin et al (2001) have questioned whether larger PCGs and PCTs will generate any significant cost savings or improvements in performance or whether bigger is likely to be better. Bosna and Higgins (2002) have also warned that PCTs are chronically short of staff with little evidence of workforce planning for the future as they struggle to get on top of the widening new agenda.

These latest changes underline a key point in interprofessional developments: no sooner has one initiative taken place than the programme is overtaken by new structures and events. Therefore, in policy terms, little has been evaluated over time to assess the benefits or otherwise of joint working with the exception of specific projects such as HiMPs (Arora et al 1999, 2000) and HAZs (Judge 1999). Few exercises have been undertaken to calculate cost benefits, although more recently, the public–private concordats have been engaged in financial audits. Nor has much evidence-based practice been assembled to evaluate the effectiveness and outcomes of interagency developments, but working together in teams has been more widely evaluated (see conclusion in Chapter 7 on models).

Even the present context of interprofessional and interagency working may be changed and modified again as proposals are discussed for a new kind of service altogether – put forward by the NHS Confederation. The suggestions call for the involvement of local networks of consultants, GPs, nurses and therapists, to provide diagnosis and treatment outside hospitals. Pharmacists could also be given a wider role in the treatment of chronic conditions with the overall intention of providing care and treatment outside hospitals (Carvel 2002b) – to which might be added that such a community programme could also include the support and involvement of social and community workers. Constant change is likely to be a key factor in the twenty-first century, while partnership working will have to find a method of measurement and outcome assessment overall to ensure user effectiveness.

So while collaborative endeavours and joint working have become increasingly established across health and social care, anomalies remain outstanding on costs and structure. The differences continue between a centrally run health service, which is free at the point of use, while social care is, to a greater extent, means-tested but with the social services based within democratically run local authorities. The field is complex, buffeted by professional and sectional interests. Care trusts have sought to move around the complexities by creating a more integrated approach. Should all health and social services be fully integrated? How far should housing provision be included? Where should integration begin and end? A final question for the future of interprofessional collaboration might be: just how long can the impediments caused by these fundamental disjunctions remain?

REFERENCES

Abbott, S. and Gillam, S. (2000) 'Health without a care', *Health Service Journal* 110 (5629) 32.

Arora, S., Davies, A. and Thompson, S. (1999) *Developing Health Improvement Programmes: Learning from the First Year*, London: King's Fund.

Arora, S., Davies, A. and Thompson, S. (2000) 'Developing health improvement programmes: challenges for a new millennium', *Journal of Interprofessional Care* 14 (1) 9–18.

Audit Commission (1986) *Making a Reality of Community Care*, London: HMSO.

Audit Commission (1992) *The Community Revolution: Personal Social Services and Community Care*, London: HMSO.

Audit Commission (1996) *What the Doctor Ordered: A Study of GP Fundholders in England and Wales*, London: Audit Commission.

Belcher, J. (2001) 'Defining moments', *Health Service Journal* 111 (5749) 32.

Berman, P. and Higgins, J. (2002) 'Worlds apart', *Health Service Journal* 112 (5787) 24–6.

Bosna, T. and Higgins, J. (2002) 'No can do', *Health Service Journal* 112 (5793) 26–7.

Bryson, K., Williams, E. and Bell, C. (2001) 'Public pain, private gain', *Health Service Journal* 111 (5771) 24–5.

Butler Sloss, E. (1988) *Report of the Inquiry into Child Abuse in Cleveland 1987*, Cm. 413, London: HMSO.

Carvel, J. (2001) 'Climbie inquiry to prosecute witness', *The Guardian*, 4 December, 13.

Carvel, J. (2002a) 'First patients ready for NHS ops abroad', *The Guardian*, 11 January, 8.

Carvel, J. (2002b) 'Milburn hails more private links for NHS', *The Guardian*, 10 January, 7.

Carvel, J. and White, M. (2001) 'Heart patients "guinea pigs" in health drive', *The Guardian*, 7 December, 14.

Chadda, D. (1996) 'Welsh chorus', *Health Service Journal* 106 (5518) 8.

CNA (Carers National Association) (1995) *Better Tomorrow*, London: Carers National Association.

Collinson, P. (2001) 'Private medical cover is in crisis', *The Guardian (Money)*, 8 June, 5.

Coote, A. (1999) 'Divisions no longer add up', *Health Service Journal* 109 (5662) 18–19.

DHSS (Department of Health and Social Security) (1978) *Collaboration in Community Care – A Discussion Document*, Personal Social Services Council and Central Health Services Council, London: HMSO.

DoH (Department of Health) (1991) *Working Together: A Guide to Arrangements for Inter-agency Cooperation for the Protection of Children from Abuse*, London: Department of Health.

DoH (1995) *NHS Responsibilities for Meeting Continuing Health Care Needs*, London: Department of Health.

DoH (1998a) *Partnership in Action: New Opportunities for Joint Working between Health and Social Services*, London: Department of Health.

DoH (1998b) *Working Together: Securing a Quality Workforce for the NHS*, London: Department of Health.

DoH (1998c) *A First Class Service: Quality in the new NHS*, London, Department of Health.

DoH (2001a) *Shifting the Balance of Power within the NHS: Securing Delivery*, July, London: Department of Health.

DoH (2001b) *Care Trusts: Emerging Framework* (http//www.doh.gov.uk).

DoH (2001c) *Intermediate Care*, HSC 2001/01: LAC (2001)1, London: Department of Health.

DoH (2001d) *Assuring the Quality of Medical Practice: Implementing 'Supporting Doctors, Protecting Patients'*, London: Department of Health.

DoH (2001e) *Teaching PCTs*, London: Department of Health (http://www.doh.gov.uk/pricare/teachingpcts.htm).

Donnelly, L. (2001a) 'Tears for fears', *Health Service Journal* 101 (5778) 12–13.

Donnelly, L. (2001b) 'Inside the labyrinth', *Health Service Journal* 111 (5783) 14–15.

Douglass, C. (2001) 'The development and evolution of geriatric assessment teams over the past 25 years: a cross-cultural comparison of the US and the UK', *Journal of Interprofessional Care* 15 (3) 267–80.

Dowse, C. (2001) 'Health Improvement and Modernisation Plans (HIMPs): Requirements for 2002', Leeds: Department of Health.

Edwards, N. and Passman, D. (1997) 'All mixed up', *Health Service Journal* 107 (5557) 30–31.

Ewles, L. (1999) 'Avon calling', *Health Service Journal* 109 (5660) 24–5.

Finnegan, E. (1991) *Collaborative Care Planning*, West Midlands Health Region: Resource Management Support Unit.

Flynn, R., Pickard, S. and Williams, G. (1995) 'Contracts and the quasi-market in community health services', *Journal of Social Policy* 24, Part 4, October, 529–50.

George, M. (2001) 'Quick thinking', *The Guardian (Society)*, 5 December, 92.

Gillam, S. (1998) 'Clinical governance', in R. Klein (ed.) *Implementing the White Paper: Pitfalls and Opportunities: A King's Fund Policy Paper*, London: King's Fund.

Ham, C. and Heginbotham, C. (1991) *Purchasing Together*, London: King's Fund Institute.

Harrison, A. (1992) *Health Care UK 1991*, London: King's Fund Institute.

Health Service Journal (1998) 'Social services chiefs oppose integration', 108 (5595) 6.

Healy, P. (1999) 'Equal to the task', *Health Service Journal* 109 (5646) 6–7.

Hencke, D. (2001) 'Public services benefit from private sector money', *The Guardian*, 29 November, 26.

Higgins, J. (2001) 'Let's drink to that', *Health Service Journal* 111 (5737) 22–4.

Hudson, B. (1998) 'Take your partners', *Health Service Journal* 108 (5590) 30–31.

Hudson, B. (2001a) 'Trapped in a wicked web', *Health Service Journal* 111 (5783) 18.

Hudson, B. (2001b) 'No more piggy in the middle', *Health Service Journal* 111 (5749) 20.

Judge, K. (1999) 'National evaluation of health action zones', in A. Bebbington and K. Judge (eds), *PSSRU Bulletin*, Canterbury: Personal Social Services Research Unit.

Kennedy, I. (2001) *Report of the Public Inquiry into Children's Heart Surgery at the Bristol Royal Infirmary 1984–1995*, July, London: The Stationery Office.

Kingdon, D. (1992) 'Interprofessional collaboration in mental health', *Journal of Interprofessional Care* 6 (2) Summer 141–7.

Laurent, C. (2001) 'Independence way', *Health Service Journal* 111 (5751) 22–23.

Leathard, A. (2000) *Health Care Provision: Past, Present and into the 21st Century*, 2nd edn. Cheltenham: Nelson Thornes.

Le Grand, J. and Bartlett, W. (eds) (1993) *Quasi-markets and Social Policy*, London: Macmillan.

Le Grand, J., Mays, N. and Mulligan, J. (1998) *Learning from the NHS Internal Market: A Review of the Evidence*, London: King's Fund.

Lewis, J. (1993) 'Community care: policy imperatives, joint planning and enabling authorities', *Journal of Interprofessional Care* (7) Spring, 7–14.

Lewis, J. and Glennerster, H. (1996) *Implementing the New Community Care*, Buckingham: Open University Press.

Lupton, C., North, N. and Khan, P. (2001) *Working Together or Pulling Apart? The National Health Service and Child Protection Networks*, Bristol: The Policy Press.

Marshall, M., Preston, M., Scott, E. and Wincott, P. (eds) (1979) *Teamwork For and Against: An Appraisal of Multi-disciplinary Practice*, London: British Association of Social Workers.

Millar, B. (1996) 'The facts of life', *Health Service Journal* 106 (5588) 16.

National Audit Office (2001) *Managing the Relationships to Secure a Successful Partnership*, London: The Stationery Office.

NHS Executive (1995) *Developing NHS Purchasing and GP Fundholding: Towards a Primary-care Led NHS*, Leeds: Department of Health.

NHS Executive (1998) *The new NHS – Modern and Dependable: Implementing the new NHS and our Healthier Nation*, HSC 1998/021, Leeds: Department of Health.

NHS Executive (1999) http://www.doh.gov.uk/jointunit/about.htm

NHS Modernisation Agency (2001) *Introducing the Agency*, London: Department of Health.

Paton, C. (1995) 'Present dangers and future threats: some perverse incentives in the NHS reforms', *British Medical Journal* 310 (1) 1245–8.

Pietroni, P. (1994) 'Inter-professional teamwork: its history and developments in hospitals, general practice and community care', in A. Leathard (ed.), *Going Inter-Professional: Working Together for Health and Welfare*, London: Routledge.

Pollock, A. (2001) 'Privateers on the march', *The Guardian*, 11 December, 14.

Pollock, A., Shaoul, J. and Rowland, D. (2001) *A Response to the IPPR Commission on Public–Private Partnerships*, Health Policy and Health Services Research Unit, London: University College.

Powell, M. (1997) *Evaluating the National Health Service*, Buckingham: Open University Press.

Secretary of State for Health (1992) *The Health of the Nation: A Strategy of Health for England*, Cm. 1986, London: HMSO.

Secretary of State for Health (1993) *Working Together for Better Health*, London: Department of Health.

Secretary of State for Health (1996) *The National Health Service: A Service with Ambitions*, Cm. 3425, November, London: The Stationery Office.

Secretary of State for Health (1997) *The new NHS: Modern – Dependable,* Cm. 3807, London: The Stationery Office.

Secretary of State for Health (1998a) *Modernising Social Services: Promoting independence, Improving protection, Raising standards*, Cm. 4169, London: The Stationery Office.

Secretary of State for Health (1998b) *Our Healthier Nation: A Contract for Health,* A Consultation Paper, Cm. 3852, London: The Stationery Office.

Secretary of State for Health (1999) *Saving Lives: Our Healthier Nation*, London: Department of Health.

Secretary of State for Health (2000) *The NHS Plan: A plan for investment, a plan for reform*, London: The Stationery Office.

Seebohm Report (1968) *Report of the Committee on Local Authority and Allied Personal Social Services*, Cmnd. 3703, London: HMSO.

Shifrin, T. (2000) 'More than just a drag', *Health Service Journal* 110 (5727) 14.

Shifrin, T. (2001a) 'New leadership head to target stereotypes', *Health Service Journal* 111 (5752) 4.

Shifrin, T. (2001b) 'Blears raises "Voices" in bid to replace CHCs', *Health Service Journal* 111 (5771) 5.

Smith, D. and Waterhouse, R. (2001) 'New Labour's quack cure for the NHS', *The Sunday Times*, 9 December, 8.

Stephenson, P. (2001) 'Funding shortfall as intermediate care loses out to local pressures', *Health Service Journal* 111 (5739) 6–7.

Stott, N. (1995) 'Personal care and teamwork: implications for the general practice-based primary health care team', *Journal of Interprofessional Care* 9 (2) 95–9.

Turner, M. and Balloch, S, (2001) 'Partnership between service users and statutory social services', in S. Balloch and M. Taylor (eds), *Partnership Working Policy and Practice*, Bristol: The Policy Press.

Walshe, K. and Smith, J. (2001) 'Drowning, not waving', *Health Service Journal* 111 (5768) 12–13.

Watt, N. (2002) 'Milburn to give top hospitals power to run own affairs', *The Guardian*, 15 January, 9.

Webb, A. and Wistow, G. (1986) *Planning, Need and Scarcity: Essays on the Welfare State*, London: Allen & Unwin.

West, M. (1994) *Effective Teamwork*, Leicester: BPS Books.

White, M. (2001) 'NHS to pay for private health treatment', *The Guardian*, 4 December, 1.

White, M. and Carvel, J. (2000) 'PM returns with call for change in NHS culture', *The Guardian*, 6 June, 3.

Whitfield, L. (1999) 'Cost pressures bring threat to HImP work', *Health Service Journal* 109 (5653) 4.

Wilkin, D., Bojke, C. and Gravelle, H. (2001) *Is Bigger Better for Primary Care Groups and Trusts?* Communications Unit, Manchester: National Primary Care Research and Development Centre.

Wintour, P. (2002) 'Milburn may look to private cash for doctor training', *The Guardian*, 7 January, 6.

Wistow, G., Hardy, B. and Leedham, I. (1993) 'Planning blight', *Health Service Journal* 103 (5430) 22–4.

Chapter 3

Management and interprofessional collaboration

Charles Engel and Elin Gursky

SUMMARY

Why should management be concerned with interprofessional collaboration? Is it enough for management merely to expect collaboration to be implemented? This chapter sets out to explore some of the pressures that bear on practising professionals, who might well see collaboration as yet one more call on their time and energy. The roles of management in this context are thus worthy of some attention.

The challenges that face every health care system are discussed in relation to those who are entrusted with its management. The consideration of different models of health care form the environment in which the managers' roles are discussed. These include the management of collaboration and the related management of expertise.

Still on this wider canvas, the chapter sketches the important tasks that are involved in managing the vision that illuminates major organisational change. This is followed by a closer look at what managers may be able to encourage and implement at the local level.

Will management take up the challenge and plan for real and sustained collaboration, including some quite fundamental research? Will management not only expect collaboration, but also foster a culture that facilitates, recognises and rewards collaboration?

INTRODUCTION – CHALLENGES FOR HEALTH CARE IN THE TWENTY-FIRST CENTURY

The dawn of the new millennium and naissance of the twenty-first century heralded unprecedented progress towards improving the health of populations. Methods to detect and diagnose diseases in early and intervenable stages, vaccines to prevent, eradicate or control diseases, bioengineered joints, gene-based therapies, implants to resyncopate organ systems, and technologies to improve food, water safety and sanitation have afforded many global citizens a longer and better quality of life than ever before. Despite this powerful potential of health care, the challenges of health disparities and access remain conspicuous for many within both the developed and developing world. Remnants from decades of industrial and military growth continue to compromise health status in the forms of toxic waste, non-potable water, shifts in the balance of ecology and gaps in social justice. These effects on health are only recently being appreciated as risk factors associated with poor fetal health (i.e. low birth weight, adverse gestational outcomes and birth defects) and diseases that result from long-term exposures, such as certain cancers and respiratory diseases.

Higher standards of living have not necessarily improved population health status, as seen in the correlation between diet, substance abuse and other negative behaviours with the increased incidence in obesity, diabetes and cardiorespiratory diseases.

Many of today's health problems, either acute or chronic, defy remediation through traditional 'one-stop, one-shot' medical approaches. Rather, they require interventions that target behaviour and lifestyle changes such as diet, exercise and smoking cessation and other risk reduction strategies. Behaviour modification, health education, as well as empowering and enlisting patient responsibility within the wellness-attaining process are essential components for improving the health of populations and reducing increasing fiscal strains on health care. So, too, is the necessity of building health systems that focus their efforts on health prevention rather than disease intervention, and that redirect their resources to early identification and deterrence of reversible conditions to avoid chronic, life-threatening and costly illnesses.

Health delivery models that merely dispense curative and therapeutic interventions for individuals must be replaced by solutions that focus on the root causes, not just the symptoms, of the illnesses within populations. A readiness to invest in new approaches will be essential to reverse the economic and social vulnerabilities that decrease the health status of populations and increase the burden placed on health care resources. An increasingly complex and smaller globe, in which wealth and profit are juxtaposed with an acknowledgement of health care as a social good, will increasingly confront the ethically and politically tenuous balance between assuring that populations benefit from the most sophisticated medical and pharmaceutical advances, while concomitantly containing health care expenditures.

The health care systems of today are unlikely to be able to address the health care needs of tomorrow. New health systems will require paradigms of collaboration and partnership within and outside the traditional rubric of health care, as well as a redeployment of assets. To maximise finite resources, health care managers will need the leadership skills and competences to inspire innovation from their workforce, facilitate respect for the mission of the organisation, integrate multiple professional proficiencies and engender appreciation for the value of health as an investment in society's economic and cultural future.

PROFESSIONAL PRACTICE AND STRESS

There can be little doubt that the care of our fellow human beings, often anxious, in discomfort, in distress, handicapped, frequently confused and perhaps even aggressive, is not an easy task. Indeed, such care, practised on a daily basis, can become quite seriously stressful (Myerson 1997). There are no admissible shortcuts; there is little that can be done to save time and labour; health and social care constitute labour intensive occupations.

Systems of delivery of care are in a constant state of flux, subject to numerous extrinsic influences that challenge the individual practitioner to adapt to change and to participate in the management of change. In most countries health and social care, public and private, employ rather more people than the manufacturing and service industries. What, then, are some of the factors that affect all who are involved in these caring occupations? What, therefore, is the challenge for managers who are responsible for ensuring that their professional colleagues are enabled to function effectively and can be retained to continue to contribute their expertise and experience within these occupations?

Some extrinsic influences

Perhaps the most fundamental factor may be the constant conflict between the demands of curing, dealing with problems and caring, not only for individuals (Coulter and Cleary 2001), but also for communities (Spencer 2001). While the literature is replete with papers on the quality of care (Blendon et al 2001) and on evidence-based practice (Sackett and Rosenberg 1995), there is a relative dearth of information devoted to the interplay between quality of care and quality of cure. It is the more remarkable that the 11th Postgraduate Paediatric Course in the Philippines (October 2001) was concerned with 'the compassionate paediatrician in the context of current technological advances' (Christobal 2001).

A better educated public is increasingly less tolerant of professional paternalism and expects to be involved in decisions that relate to their perceived or actual problems. This trend is supported by ready access to professional information, not necessarily peer reviewed, via the media and the Internet. Excessive expectations are perhaps also due to the populism of the media and their frequent 'beating the gun'. Individuals expect to be free from pain, disability and discomfort and to be able to look forward to an extended life span. However, continuing advances in science and technology, that underpin such expectations, have also opened Pandora's box with a plethora of new ethical dilemmas. At the same time the treasure chest, whether public or private, is not bottomless. Finite funding confronts any prospect of unlimited technological application. Indeed, even a scientific and technological status quo would not allay the present and predictable shortage of doctors, nurses, therapists and other carers in countries with near full employment and with a wider choice of perhaps less demanding training and careers. This shortage may come to play a greater role still, as the demographic shift (WHO 1996, 1998) comes to intensify the competition between industry, commerce and the professions for a shrinking number of young people in an ageing society.

Some consequences

Contrary to professional expectations, equity of access to health and social care and, indeed, to absolute quality (e.g. expensive, new 'wonder drugs') have to be 'rationed' in one way or another (WHO 1999). In many countries, in particular in the developing world, globalisation tends to encourage health care for profit that may exclude the majority of the population. The conflict between increasing demand and finite resources in industrial countries has led to a sharper focus on accountability (Donabedian 1981) and recertification (Hewson 1991; Irvine 2001).

Thus, the resulting ethical dilemmas, combined with the pressures for enhanced accountability and productivity, inhibit job satisfaction and generate additional stress. It is unlikely that organisational emphasis on technical productivity, with little recognition of time and effort devoted to *caring*, will help to redress the balance between curing and caring. This is especially serious, as professionals and their managers face the demands of an ageing population with multiple problems, the appearance of new diseases, the rapid spread of infections, due to mass air travel and migration, and a continuing increase in the number of chemotherapeutic resistant organisms (WHO 1996). The daily working environment is further complicated by language barriers, cultural diversity and change in social climate. The general public has lost much of its traditional respect for the professions, and legal commercialism tends to encourage claims for financial compensation for alleged mistakes and/or misconduct. Little wonder that altruism can be displaced by cynicism and defensive practice.

In addition, professionals no longer enjoy the security of defined, traditional roles. Across the world there is a progressive change from practice-based training to university-based education for the professions of nursing, therapy and social work. The law, too, is changing to expect the assumption of responsibilities and tasks that used to be reserved for registered medical practitioners. Why, then, in this turmoil of pressures and changes, should individual practitioners be expected to, or want to, collaborate with each other?

AIMS OF INTERPROFESSIONAL COLLABORATION

There is an extensive literature on this subject, ranging from the views of individual professionals (Leathard 1994) to documents from health authorities (NHS Executive 1997) and international agencies (WHO Study Group 1987). The aims relate to benefits for patients, clients and support for carers; avoidance of stress and improved job satisfaction for professionals; and improved efficiency of health and social care.

Patients, clients and their carers benefit from inclusion as 'members of the team'. They need to be assured that their personal circumstances, feelings and preferences are acknowledged and acted upon. Collaboration with patients, clients and carers can thus lead to informed consent and informed compliance with mutually agreed interventions. Consideration of the psychosocial, as well as the biological/material aspects of care (Engel 1980) are thus of fundamental importance for interprofessional collaboration with patients, clients and carers. Collaboration between professionals is fostered by an appreciation of each other's expert contributions, agreement on the aims and goals in relation to a patient or client and agreed distribution of roles and related tasks in the context of an agreed programme of action.

Particular satisfaction for professionals, patients, clients and carers will flow from an active sharing of information. This, in turn, is dependent on mutual trust, an interpersonal relationship that demands time and effort for its development and maintenance.

There is one more important, though not universally recognised, need for interprofessional collaboration. This relates to the *management of change*, not only change within and between the professions, but also change for the socio-economic-environmental well-being of patients, clients and carers. The latter aim relates to the *advocational* role of the caring professions. So, for example, Watt (1996) emphasised the inverse relationship between health and poverty and suggested that 'doctors should renounce their silence and start to speak up about the wider aspects and implications of poverty and deprivation'. No doubt, all the professions would acknowledge this responsibility for advocacy on behalf of their patients, clients and their carers. The influence of a single professional would clearly be increased materially through an alliance with colleagues. Collaboration by two or more professions would surely potentiate their power for intersectoral advocacy.

There is perhaps a wider, societal responsibility that involves all professions, not only the health professions, in the management of change. Continuing expansion of the world's population (Potts 2000), coupled with the influences of advancing technology and globalisation, lead to overuse of irreplaceable raw materials, as well as pollution of air, water and soil (Brundtland 1987; World Commission on Health and Environment 1992; McMichael et al 1996). This constellation influences a continuing growth of the many who exist near or below subsistence level and growing nationalism associated with political and religious extremism. Resulting mass migrations create social destabilisation. This less than happy scenario would counsel that all professions should combine for *intersectoral collaboration* with governments. The aim would be to support governments in addressing these intricate and interrelated causes and effects (Engel 2000).

MANAGING COLLABORATION

Appropriate management practices will balance professional independence with professional interdependence; to recognise the value of each member's skills and to magnify these skills many times through the skills of other professionals. Many strategies may be brought to bear that perfect this equilibrium, through rigorously maintained schedules of cross-professional discussions, to health outcome-inspired projects, and to the aligning of values through joint research activities that seek to compare the relative successes of a variety of health intervention strategies (Muller et al. 2001).

Another constructive management tool is found through assessing an organisation's reporting relationships and chain-of-command structures. A management structure, for example, that reflects an administratively top-heavy, vertical and multi-layered hierarchy may reveal that there are limited opportunities for mid- and senior-level managers to gain direct knowledge of what is occurring on the 'front lines', and for professionals to collaborate with one another. This structure may impede timely intervention on potential (and avoidable) problems, the integration of skills and the seamless delivery of health services.

Conversely, a horizontally assembled organisation encourages, even demands, collaboration across the panoply of professional talents. Unlike the traditional health care model where the 'control' is a single point at the top of a pyramid, a bottom-up approach enlists the diversity of collective expertise and shared decision-making (Anderson 1998; Drucker 1998; Glouberman and Mintzerg 2001). At the outset this approach may appear to run contrary to the traditional chain-of-command model that has long defined medical care. Managers may perceive this alternative model to be a threat to their administrative authority. Physicians, who historically have functioned in a command-control relationship with subordinate medical staff, may query such an arrangement as an impediment to clinical efforts. However, this approach is not merely the repositioning of the organisational pyramid; it is the repositioning of health care itself. It is recognising that the model of *how* care is delivered reflects *what* is delivered; it can support the opportunity to shift from a framework of disease intervention to one of health promotion.

Collaborative models can promote the development of teams. This is a useful strategy for focusing a diverse spectrum of professionals towards specific problems or concerns. For example, traditional health care delivery mechanisms have been structured according to departments of expertise such as nursing, housekeeping and dietary and nutrition. When re-formed not within but across specialties, retitled perhaps as patient management teams, the wide matrix of skills and training can enhance the effectiveness of patient care. Good patient outcomes reflect this team dynamic, and both the patient and the workforce benefit.

The burden and challenges of management to facilitate these structures for collaboration is great. Managers must be evermore prescient in learning from the people they manage, so that they may both lead and follow others. Their knowledge base must include not only the schooled tenets of management, but also the emotional capacity to change and to implement change. The application of emotional intelligence will become an essential part of sensitive human resources management (Goleman 1996).

Whether managers of service units, support personnel or human resources, a health care organisation will only be as effective as its willingness to facilitate collaboration among, and provide needed support to, their health care professionals. A fully collaborative model does not exclude those in the uppermost rungs. Building effective health care systems, not merely assuring the delivery of health care services, must be the priority of senior leaders and policy-makers. They must demonstrate their support and will by espousing a full understanding of the mission, and by providing active participation in the process of recrafting strategies to promote good health. The most dedicated and skilled workforce cannot compensate for absentee governance, or for those whose responsibilities distance them from a full appreciation of the importance of improving the health status of a population and the difficulties associated with delivering their health care. As new health care crises occur, as they most definitely will, senior leadership must facilitate the reprioritisation of efforts and recognise the ramifications of taking on new problems with existing resources (Allen 2000). Improved health care systems and the health status of populations will occur only when those possessing authority in health care come to enjoy equal partnership with those possessing power over health care.

Crises in health and the emergence of new diseases will be two of the defining issues of this new century. As resources continue to be strained and the workforce is challenged, new collaborations and partnerships will be forged within and outside the health care sector. The importance of quality of housing, access to transportation, as well as security of employment and income, will increasingly be recognised as critical contributing factors affecting the levels of health or illness of a society (Cribb 2000). Models of teamwork, collaboration and partnership will be extended beyond the health sector and across a wide spectrum of other stakeholders, including government agencies and non-governmental organisations, industry, academia and even grass roots coalitions.

MANAGING EXPERTISE

The dilemmas facing health care organisations include obtaining and retaining a workforce whose skills are equal to evolving practice standards, technological advances and disease symptomatology. Another predicament is that of dealing with members of a health labour force whose older skills are now of limited use (Taylor 1999). In both instances the most effective answer is found when the organisation itself invests in the career growth and retraining of the workforce (Department of Health 2001). In most cases the expenses associated with retraining today's workforce for tomorrow's skills are less than those associated with advertising, interviewing, recruiting, hiring and orienting new staff. This tactic also reduces the burden on the rest of the organisation, which is subjected to increased workloads and unmet patient needs during the recruitment process. Providing opportunities for professional growth is one of the best incentives for the worker. It is also one of the best investments for the organisation. In a changing world, where salaries and benefits may appear more attractive in other sectors, health care stands to benefit most from the cohort of enthusiastic and dedicated professionals who recognise an industry that invests in its workforce, an industry that is committed to a social good.

Training and reskilling the health care workforce does not ensure excellence. It is, rather, the ability of management to make the best possible use of professional knowledge that presents the most difficult challenge and is, in fact, a defining hallmark of the organisation's quality of excellence (Quinn et al 1996).

The ability to harness the intellectual treasure depends on many of the issues reviewed above. It requires that the professional works in an environment that imparts challenges and provides new technologies. It taps into the professional's talents as well as the professional's creativity and innovation. It respects skill-specific egocentricity but demonstrates how successful collaboration augments the application of this expertise.

Managers have unique responsibilities. They translate the wider perspective of senior administration to lower levels within the organisation and assure that senior administration is apprised of staff concerns, potential problems and suggested strategies. They must be the impartial arbiters of bidirectional information and honest brokers of the organisation's mission. In assuming responsibility for the stewardship of the resources in their charge, managers must retrain their own skills and be subjected to appropriate oversight and performance evaluation by more senior managers and also the staff complements under their charge. It cannot be overstated that the ultimate success of an organisation rests in large part with the level of excellence derived from its managers.

MANAGING THE MISSION

Over the past two decades, escalating health care costs and tightening economies, coupled with increasing demand, have strained the health care sector, resulting in such strategies as restricted and delayed patient access to services. These often draconian-appearing tactics have eroded professional morale and consumer confidence. Additionally, rather than saving money, these strategies have weakened health care organisations, driven away talent and contributed to falling health status indicators.

It is not surprising that opportunities to affect change in many health care systems may engender scepticism and doubt among both the providers and the users, promulgated by the belief that these efforts are fiscally rather than socially driven. For change to be successful, therefore, all parties must become involved stakeholders as architects and assessors of the new product (Daake and Anthony 2000).

It is only after the vision and mission of the health care organisation are shaped that the appropriate number and breadth of skills across the workforce, the operational strategies, and the requirements for non-human resources can be appreciated. It is also from this starting point that management can facilitate discussion regarding the appropriate measures of organisational effectiveness.

Older and traditional health delivery models, which see their mission as one of providing as much care to as many individuals as possible, may look to counts of services, budget overrides, the ratio of staff work units to patient volume, the number of immunisations administered, or the usage of consumable supplies (i.e. bandages and pills) to assess its efforts. In essence the question proffered is, 'How much does it cost to deliver health care services to a defined group of people?'

In a health care paradigm, which is directed through more enlightened management, the mission and measurement evolve consistent with the commitment to improve health status rather than delivering services, indexed according to standardised medical codes. The measurement is not an 'accounting' of goods and service units but 'accountability' for the improved health status of populations. The mission-related question becomes one of, 'What are the costs associated with reducing (some risk factor) within a group of people?'

In this second health care paradigm, efforts would focus on high-risk individuals and, for example, the opportunities for successful hypertension intervention through medical, behavioural and lifestyle changes. Through this alignment of mission and strategy, society achieves a reduction in the population rate of adverse cardiovascular-related outcomes and, over time, a lessening burden on health care costs and resources associated with such outcomes as stroke, paralysis, ongoing rehabilitation, physiotherapy and supportive care.

The process of building consensus around the organisation's mission and vision is a difficult one for managers, as they must assure inclusion of those at the most senior, decision-making levels and those at the provider level within the community. Without sufficient 'political will', the most expert of health care providers will be unable to meet the health needs of their communities. Without sufficient community input, the organisation may deliver quality care but fail in its efforts to improve health status.

EPILOGUE

What are the competencies that are essential for effective collaboration? Which of these competencies are needed for collaboration quite generally, and which additional competencies are required for specific tasks, situations or circumstances? For example, the challenges faced at an interprofessional case conference must surely differ from those encountered during a joint home visit.

If managers were to encourage and facilitate investigations for the identification of such competencies, their evident interest and support would contribute to a greater awareness of collaboration as an integral part of everyday professional life. Such an approach would help to focus research and development towards more effective educational interventions in the development of the requisite skills. Further managerial initiatives could then concentrate on sustainable continuing professional development of more advanced aspects of interprofessional collaboration and appropriate role modelling.

Overt organisational and administrative arrangements will be desirable, so that busy professionals can devote appropriate time and attention to working with each other and with their managers. Above all, management should devise ways and means for official recognition and suitable reward for consistent interprofessional collaboration that is not only acceptable, but also effective and efficient.

These changes in the working environment would facilitate trust, that essential prerequisite for a relaxed and effective working relationship between managers and their professional colleagues. Perhaps some expenditure on joint staff rooms for more informal interaction between managers and their colleagues might pay handsome dividends.

Once interprofessional collaboration is not only an expected, but also a *facilitated* part of professional practice, both managers and practitioners will recognise the need for perfecting their requisite skills. The further development of these competencies can then become an accepted, integral part of continuing professional education for all members of the caring professions, including their managerial colleagues.

ACKNOWLEDGEMENT

We wish to extend our sincere thanks to Dr George Dorros of the World Health Organization for his invaluable guidance and advice throughout the development of this chapter.

REFERENCES

Allen, I. (2000) 'Challenges to the health services: the professions', *British Medical Journal* 320 1533–5.

Anderson, S. (1998) 'How healthcare organizations can achieve true integration', *Healthcare Financial Management* February 31–4.

Blendon, R., Schoen, C., Donelan, K., Osborn, R., Des Roches, C., Scoles, K., Davis, K., Binns, K. and Zapert, K. (2001) 'Physicians' views on quality care: a five-country comparison', *Health Affairs* 20 (3) 233–43.

Brundtland, G. (1987) *Our Common Future*, New York: United Nations.

Christobal, F. (2001) Personal communication.

Coulter, A. and Cleary, P. (2001) 'Patients' experiences with hospital care in five countries', *Health Affairs* 20 (3) 244–52.

Cribb, A. (2000) 'The diffusion of the health agenda and the fundamental need for partnership in medical education', *Medical Education* 34, 916–20.

Daake, D. and Anthony, W. (2000) 'Understanding stakeholder power and influence gap in health care organization: an empirical study', *Health Care Management Review* 25, 94–107.

Department of Health (2001) *Shifting the Balance of Power: Securing Delivery – Human Resources Framework*, London: Department of Health.

Donabedian, A. (1981) 'Advantages and limitations of explicit criteria for assessing the quality of health care', *Millbank Memorial Fund Quarterly – Health and Society* 59 (1) 99–106.

Drucker, P. (1998) 'Management's Paradigms', *Forbes* 5 October 153–77.

Engel, C. (2000) 'Health professions education for adapting to change and for participating in managing change', *Education for Health* 13 (1) 37–44.

Engel, G. (1980) 'The clinical application of the biopsychosocial model', *American Journal of Psychiatry* 137, 535–44.

Glouberman, S. and Mintzerg, H. (2001) 'Managing the care of health and the cure of disease – Part II: Integration', *Health Care Management Review* 26 (1) 70–84.

Goleman, D. (1996) *Emotional Intelligence*, London: Bloomsbury Publishing.

Hewson, A. (1991) 'Continuing medical education in obstetrics and gynaecology: the challenge of the nineties', *Australian and New Zealand Journal of Obstetrics and Gynaecology* 31 (3) 249–53.

Irvine, Sir D. (2001) 'The changing relationship between the public and the medical profession', *Journal of the Royal Society of Medicine* 94, 162–9.

Leathard, A. (ed.) (1994) *Going Inter-Professional: Working Together for Health and Welfare*, London: Routledge.

McMichael, A., Haines, A., Slooff, R. and Kovatz, S. (eds) (1996) *Climate Change and Human Health*, Geneva: World Health Organization.

Muller, J., Shore, W., Martin, P., Levine, M., Harvey, H., Kelly, P., McCarty, S., Szarek, J. and Veitia, M. (2001) 'What we learn about interdisciplinary collaboration in institutions', *Academic Medicine* 76 (4) S55–S60.

Myerson, S. (1997) 'Seven women G.P.'s perceptions of their stresses and the impact of these on their private and professional lives', *Journal of Management in Medicine* 11 (1) 8–14.

NHS (National Health Service Executive) (1997) *Education and Training Planning Guidance*, NHS Executive Letter EL (97) 58, Leeds: Department of Health.

Potts, M. (2000) 'The most pressing issue', *Journal of the Royal Society of Medicine* 93 (1) 1–2.

Quinn, J., Anderson, P. and Finkelstein, S. (1996) 'Making the most of the best', *Harvard Business Review* March–April 71–80.

Sackett, D. and Rosenberg, W. (1995) 'The need for evidence-based medicine', *Journal of the Royal Society of Medicine* 88 (11) 620–24.

Spencer, H. (2001) 'The changing field of academic public health', *Academic Medicine* 76 (5) 400–401.

Taylor, R. (1999) 'Partnerships or power struggle? The "Crown" review of prescribing', *British Journal of General Practice* 49, 340–41.

Watt, G. (1996) 'All together now: why social deprivation matters to everyone', *British Medical Journal* 312, 1026–31.

World Commission on Health and Environment (1992) *Our Planet, Our Health*, Geneva: World Health Organization.

WHO (World Health Organization) Study Group (1987) *Learning Together to Work Together for Health: The Team Approach*, Report of a Study Group on Multiprofessional Education, Geneva: World Health Organization.

WHO (1996) *World Health Report, 1996*, Geneva: World Health Organization.

WHO (1998) *World Health Report, 1998*, Geneva: World Health Organization.

WHO (1999) *World Health Report, 1999*, Geneva: World Health Organization.

Chapter 4

Going round in circles?

Identifying interprofessional dynamics in Australian health and social welfare

Richard Hugman

SUMMARY

Although considerable attention has been paid to promoting interprofessional developments in Australian health and social welfare, recent evidence suggests that the boundaries between professions have reformed rather than reduced. The policy context of economic rationalism, with a subsequent emphasis on the managerial restructuring of organisation and practice, must be understood as the circumstances to which the professions have responded. The persistence of some strong professional boundaries can be seen as plausible in these circumstances, even though there is conflicting evidence about the benefits for service users.

INTRODUCTION

Beattie (1995) describes the health professions as 'tribes'. Using this metaphor, derived from social anthropology, his analysis of the relationships between the health professions considers the nature of interactions between these groups to be analogous to 'tribal conflict' (Beattie 1995: 11). Underlying this concept is the structuralist notion that cultural categories operate through processes of classification and separation (Beattie 1995: 17; see also Traynor 2000). From such a perspective, the development of professions can be seen as a process of struggle over the classification and separation of occupational categories (defined in terms of knowledge, skill, values and claims to the object of these attributes, that is the clientele). In this context interprofessionalism is highly dangerous as it introduces ambiguity and threatens the existing order. This concept of interprofessional relationships as an arena of boundary maintenance will be used here to examine the contemporary situation in Australia. Of particular interest is the way in which the relationships between the different occupational groups in the health and social welfare fields can be seen as living up to the goals of interprofessional collaboration.

The 1990s saw two major trends in the organisation of the health profes-sions in Australia (Boyce 2001). The first trend was towards greater interpro-fessional integration and the second has been a reversal of the direction of change with a re-emergence of professional boundaries. A similar pattern can be seen in the arena of social welfare (or human services).[1] This chapter looks at the reasons for the shifting direction of change and considers the implica-tions for interprofessional relations in Australian health and social welfare. It also examines the place within such developments of the assumption that interprofessional collaboration is of itself a desirable goal.

POLICY AND ORGANISATION

During the 1990s health and social welfare policy in Australia has followed a path of response and adaptation to the processes of 'economic rationalism' (Hancock 1999).[2] The primary underlying concern has been that of cost containment in the context of an ageing population and continuing develop-ments in high-technology acute health interventions (McCallum 1997). In social welfare the ageing population is also an important factor, alongside the implications of social restructuring for changes in the family, employment, education and so on (which in turn are connected to the processes of global-isation) (Hugman 1998). The outcome for policy is similar to that in health, with a continuing focus on reducing costs. While the primary intention is to reduce government expenditure and hence the level of taxation, with the objective of achieving global economic competitiveness, the impact on health and social welfare is not always a literal reduction in the number of dollars allocated in annual budgets. The concern with costs is also expressed in a demand that 'productivity' increases, in the form of gains in efficiency and effectiveness through the development of new practices on the part of the professionals and others whose work produces health and social welfare services.

Changes in practices take a number of different forms. They may be devel-opments of new techniques and interventions at the individual level of service provision. However, this discussion focuses on the broader level of the organ-isation of practice, as the middle range in which macro-level policy is articu-lated with care provided to service users. At this middle range there are three particular initiatives that must be understood in the context of economic rationalism and which have implications for the way in which interprofes-sional dynamics are being developed: 'case-mix'; 'case management' (and other forms of 'managed care') and 'new public management'. These are discussed in turn.

Case-mix

Case-mix is primarily a mechanism for the funding of health services in relation to outcomes (Lange and Cheek 1997; Lin and Druckett 1997). In this sense it 'is a health information and funding system' (Draper 1999: 140). So, case-mix is a management tool, intended to control expenditure by standard-ising costs and achieving equity between services based on a comparison of the activity required to achieve outcomes for health service users. The impact of case-mix on the professions whose work creates these services has been to require each one to be clearer about the way in which it contributes to the overall pattern of care provided (Diers 1999). As a consequence, this approach to the economic rationalisation of health and social welfare has emphasised each profession as a separate occupational entity. This has occurred for two reasons. First, the very process (as well as the complexity of the Australian approach to case-mix) has forced each profession to focus on itself separately from other professions, and for managers to examine each profession as discrete alternatives (Diers 1999: 62, 65). Second, and following from the first point, it has created a dynamic in which each profession is encouraged to regard the others as potential competitors (Brandis 2000: 65). The growing enthusiasm for 'evidenced-based practice' can be seen as deriv-ing as much from a concern to be able to argue for the contribution of particular professions as it can be seen as stemming from a detached pursuit of scientific inquiry (Traynor 2000; see also Diers 1999 and Astley and Wake-Dyster 2001).[3]

Managed care

Case management was, in its early days, a way of rethinking practice rather than a device for rationalising health and social welfare provision. The 'case' in that sense was the set of needs and responses relating to a particular service user (whether this was an individual or a family) (Remenyi 1997; see also Raiff and Shore 1993). However, in the Australian context, while some practi-tioners continue to assert this view, for the most part case management has come to be seen as part of the wider domain of 'managed care' (Draper 1999: 139). This area includes not only case-mix, but also 'purchaser/provider models' (Hugman 1998; Muetzelfeldt 1999) and 'coordinated care' (Battersby et al 2001). The key element that separates these other approaches from case-mix is the extent to which they combine new ways of understanding profes-sional practices with the organisational structures required for the economic rationalisation of health and social welfare services.

These forms of managed care are focused at the clinical level, in the inter-action between the professional practitioner and the service user. Common features of case management, the purchaser role and coordinated care are that a 'key' professional establishes the areas of need with the service user and works to put together and manage a 'package of care' (Remenyi 1997; Muet-zelfeldt 1999; Battersby et al 2001). Considered from the central concerns of this chapter, a major defining difference between these practices is clearly not *what* is done but *who* has the key role in the process. Indeed, the major differences between case management and coordinated care appear to be twofold. The first dimension is the source of funds, which tend to be pro-gramme-specific in the former and combine federal and state resources in the latter. (For Battersby et al 2001: 172, a primary reason for the development of coordinated care is to access federal funding.) The second dimension con-cerns the managing or coordinative role, which is usually held by an allied health professional in the former and a general medical practitioner in the latter. Case management developed out of social work (McDonald 1999: 21) and has now become a site for the assertion of a generic skill base, in which allied health, nursing, psychology and social work are held to be equally plausible professional backgrounds. In contrast, from this perspective, coordinated care represents an assertion of control by one profession (medi-cine, in the form of general practitioners) over managed care, rather than a new set of practices (Battersby et al 2001: 173). Having said this, the object-ives remain the same: to enhance or increase the effectiveness of service deliv-ery while maintaining or reducing costs. These practices have developed because the lack of integration, particularly between professions and agen-cies, has long been identified as a potential source of difficulty in achieving service efficiency and effectiveness (Raiff and Shore 1993; Remenyi 1997; Draper 1999).

New public management

Organising health and human services in Australia, as in the UK, the USA and other western countries, has proved to be a never-ending puzzle (Hug-man 1991; Boyce 1997; Hancock 1999). These are highly contested areas, in which agreement on any aspect of human need is very hard to reach, if not impossible (Doyal and Gough 1991). In the last decade there has been a shift in western countries away from the institutional model that had dominated in the middle and later part of the twentieth century, with the growth of what has come to be known as New Public Management (NPM) (Pollitt 1993; Hancock 1999; Boyce 2001). The features of NPM are summarised by Hancock (1999: 50) as:

- Managing public services in the same way as private business
- A move from accountability through process to accountability for results
- Emphasis on generic management rather than discipline expertise
- Devolution of control under strict accounting systems
- Separation of 'core' and 'peripheral' functions
- Separation of policy-making from the provision of services

- Marketisation (including privatisation, contractualism and 'competitiveness')
- An emphasis on quantifiable economic definitions of efficiency

Despite having begun to emerge in the 1980s and now being the dominant, orthodox ethos in health and social welfare, the term 'new' continues to be applied to NPM.

There are several implications for the health and social welfare professions arising from the impact of NPM. These may be grouped roughly in two main ways: patterns of employment and the content of work. First, there is the change in patterns of employment, often referred to as 'post-Fordism' (Hoggett 1994). This includes the break-up of large institutions, 'contracting-out' and so on. It is the organisational form of which NPM is the practice. Second, the impact on the content of work can be seen in the increasingly prescribed areas that form the mandates for clinical practice (and often as a corollary limit the right of professionals to engage in policy debate unless specifically employed in a 'policy' position).[4] NPM provides both the vehicle and the rationale for the restructuring of health and social welfare, in which the underlying goal has been to limit the power of professionals and to increase control by the state in order to exert control over public expenditure (Hancock 1999).

Organisation and difference

To a large extent, the impact of case-mix, managed care and NPM in Australia on the caring professions has varied according to the location and size of agencies. There are differences, for example, between state and non-government services, and within these services between federal, state and local levels. As McDonald (1999) notes, the history of community-based social welfare services in Australia has been marked by a diversity of organisation, with a relatively large non-government sector. Interprofessional dynamics in such organisations at times differ markedly from the large formal organisations of hospitals and government departments. In the community sector, as it is also known, there has been evidence of a particular challenge to professional boundaries that has been less evident in the larger agencies. This is the phenomenon of the 'generic worker' (or, perhaps more accurately, the 'generic position'). In some instances the reality of 'genericism' might mean that several professional backgrounds will be seen as equally plausible for the same job (e.g. case management) (Brandis 2000: 65). However, in other circumstances it may be the case that a job is regarded as equally appropriate for someone with a para-professional or ancillary level of training in competition with someone who has a professional qualification (McDonald 1999: 21). Interprofessionalism in this context can be seen, at least potentially, also to include the drawing of knowledge and skills from existing professions and their application in new ways by workers whose training and orientation lies outside the existing professions.

There is no evidence that the changes in interprofessional structures arising from the policy and organisational developments of the last decade are now fixed. They remain open to debate and to the actions of the different professional stakeholders. So, to consider where interprofessional dynamics are moving, this discussion now looks at some of the practice issues raised by these changes in policy and organisation.

PULLING IN BOTH DIRECTIONS?

The discussion so far has emphasised two apparently countervailing forces. On the one hand, there is a questioning of existing professional boundaries, in the form of a recognition that there is a considerable overlap between professions in the skills that they bring to designated tasks. On the other hand, the professions are resistant to the perceived erosion of the important distinctiveness that each brings to the provision of services. To understand how this tension is played out, it is necessary to look at each aspect in turn.

Genericism and professionalism

The idea of the 'generic worker' can be understood in several different ways. At one extreme of a continuum, there is the identification of an overlap in those activities or services to which several professions may be seen as making a plausible contribution. For example, there are several professions that incorporate counselling as part of their range of practices. These include some allied health (especially occupational therapy), nursing, psychology and social work. The same professions also practise in case management. However, each profession continues to exert its own identity and practitioners may explicitly claim to undertake these roles in a distinctive way (Brandis 2000; Griffin 2001). This is a limited form of genericism.

At the other end of the continuum is full genericism. No examples are evident in the recent discussions in Australia, although some projects do work with a great deal of flexibility (Lengyel and Bartlett 2000). Empirical examples are reported by research in the UK, where community nurses and social workers appear to be positive about a more thorough sharing of knowledge, skills and identity as generic practitioners (Brown et al 2000; Fowler et al 2000). Reasons given include that the sharing of knowledge and skills is mutually beneficial and that service users are provided with the best service according to their needs (rather than as a consequence of professional boundaries). In contrast, reports from similar community-based services indicate that while a full genericism may have been applied to specific jobs it has not permeated more widely across services (e.g. Bain 1995; Lengyel and

Bartlett 2000; Wilson et al 2000). The services may be generic, but within them the difference between professions is regarded as important for the maintenance and development of quality services and appropriate responses to service users' needs.

As a consequence, community-based services can also be experienced as providing the basis for an *enhanced* sense of separate professional identity, precisely because of the interprofessional dynamics that are experienced (Adamson and Harris 1996; see also Brown et al 2000). It is noticeable that these studies focus on nursing, including mental health nursing. The explanation offered is that the interprofessional slant of community-based services provides the basis for nurses to assert their skills and knowledge in settings where they experience less hierarchical subordination from medicine than they do in hospital settings (Adamson and Harris 1996: 77; see also Brown et al 2000: 426). It is noticeable that the community-based teams described in the literature are, effectively, 'allied health teams' in the same sense as that described by Boyce (2001). However, such teams report improved relationships with other health providers, especially general medical practitioners, than when working in single profession defined settings (Bain 1995; Lengyel and Bartlett 2000).

Professionalism *versus* genericism

What is happening in Australia is that the reality of the 'generic worker' has been seen as *de*professionalising rather than *inter*professionalising (Hugman 1998: 117–20). Indeed, there is evidence in the community sector in particular that the proportion of recognised professionals employed is in decline, in favour of para-professionals trained on shorter degree programmes or in the further education sector (McDonald 1999: 21). Such a shift is seen largely as a consequence of 'genericism' undermining the professionalisation of community services. This has further encouraged the response on the part of the professions to emphasise *multi*professional approaches over the more thorough integration and flexibility implied by the idea of *inter*professionalism (see also Leathard 1994).

A particular example of this tendency can be seen in the development of allied health in the health services. Boyce (1997, 2001) notes that from the late 1980s to the middle 1990s there have been three major types of organisational development for allied health in Australia (Boyce 2001: 24). These are:

- The 'traditional (classical) medical model' in which each profession was separately managed and reported to a medical director
- The 'allied health division model', the core feature of which is the coming together of profession-managed departments under a director who is a member of an allied health profession
- The 'unit dispersement model' in which individual professionals are

dispersed through clinical units (clinical supervision and consultation replaces profession-specific management; management is undertaken by the medical director of the unit)

Boyce (2001: 24) also records that the third of these, the 'unit dispersement model', was fiercely contested by allied health groups as a major threat to professional identity. This model has not developed as widely as the other two models, which between them represent almost all of the structures identified (with the 'classical medical model' the most common, at 56 of the 107 units surveyed) (Boyce 2001: 32). However, a further model has also emerged in the late 1990s in a small number of locations (6 of 107 units surveyed) (Boyce 2001: 27):

• The 'integrated decentralisation model' in which profession-specific departmental management reporting to a director of allied health is retained, but in which the service is provided to clinical units through a team-based pattern of internal service agreements to provide 'allied health packages of care'

Boyce (2001) notes that the 'integrated decentralisation model' has only developed out of the 'division of allied health model' and not from the other two. There are two reasons for this development. The first is that 'integrated decentralisation' of this kind requires an interprofessional identification rather than the maintenance of professional separatism. Drawing on the same anthropological metaphor employed above, this is seen as a move from 'tribes' to an 'allied health "nation"' (Boyce 2001: 31). The second factor that links to 'integrated decentralisation' with 'division of allied health' is that the other two models are those in which medicine dominates the relationships between the professions. As Boyce notes

[there is] mounting evidence of the development of the relationships *between* allied health professions that has been argued elsewhere as representing a shift from the traditional understanding of allied health as 'allied to medicine' toward a position of 'allied to each other'.
(Boyce 2001: 32, emphasis original)

As has already been noted above, this development applies across the community health services as well as hospitals (Lengyel and Bartlett 2000; Wilson et al 2000). The interesting feature of the phenomenon of 'allied health' is the extent to which it simultaneously represents both a degree of interprofessionalism, while at the same time embodying difference and a sense of separate identities for the professions that constitute 'allied health'. It is in this sense that the metaphor of a 'nation' made up of 'tribes' seems quite apt (Boyce 2001: 31). The other point to notice is that the idea is quite flexible, and at times embraces all the health professions that are not medicine (Adamson and Harris 1996; Boyce 1997, 2001; Brandis 2000; Griffin 2001; Van Eyk et al. 2001). One 'tribe' only (medicine) remains completely outside this particular 'nation', a point that emerges more clearly when allied health studies are compared with those undertaken from a medical perspective (see Battersby et al 2001: 174).[5] Yet within the 'nation' the separate 'tribes' also maintain their boundaries (and, indeed, to take the metaphor to its limit, there continue to be skirmishes over disputed territory). What is important, however, is to note that multiprofessionalism appears to be preferred to a more fully developed interprofessionalism (Leathard 1994), precisely because the former is understood to be built on a clearer differentiation between the professions.

GOING ROUND IN CIRCLES?

The process that has been identified in this chapter is one in which the degree and form of interprofessional collaboration in Australian health and social welfare has been shown to have been shaped by the policy context of the late twentieth century. Moves to create greater flexibility or to reduce boundaries have been met with a reassertion of the distinctive natures of each of the separate professions, *as the basis for collaboration*.

So, does this mean that rather than breaking out of previous closed circles, or integrating existing professional circles, the health and social welfare professions are simply 'going round in circles'? Recent discussions of 'interprofessional' education may appear to suggest that this is the case, in so far as each focuses on what a particular profession can gain from and contribute to education undertaken jointly with others (Patford 2001; see also Fowler et al 2000). Yet education can only be part of a strategy, given the extent to which the post-educational experience continues to be a very powerful force on the constant development of professional knowledge, skills and identity. Defensive 'tribalism' may be an entirely understandable response in the context of the rapid changes that have followed from the economic rationalisation of health and social welfare policy and organisation. To characterise it as 'fear of change' (Battersby et al 2001: 173) may be partially correct, but such fear may be reality-based (like fear of heights or fear of poisonous snakes). In other words, it may be the *impact* of a *particular* change that is feared, rather than the process of changing in itself. Boyce et al (2000) provide an example of allied health professionals willing to embrace change (in this case becoming more 'entrepreneurial' in their approach to an internal quasi-market in health services as a way of extending their services). The important point is that the changes were perceived by the professionals as improving their capacity to provide better allied health services to patients rather than reinforcing the existing power of other professions.

Ultimately, the strongest argument for interprofessional collaboration in health and social welfare is the expected improvement of services to the users of those services (Greenwell 1995). Many of the recent contributions to the debate about these issues in Australia have identified the importance of such an outcome (e.g. Rowan 1998; Lengyel and Bartlett 2000; Wilson et al 2000; Battersby et al 2001). However, the very definition of service users' perspectives depends on what questions are asked, and there are differences between these studies that appear to reflect underlying professional perspectives. What is happening in Australia has parallels in other countries, including the UK and the USA (e.g. Rowan 1998; Diers, 1999; Muetzelfeldt 1999; Patford 2001). In Australia, as elsewhere, the same question is yet to be addressed. This is to ask 'what are the incentives for any of the health and social welfare professions to move beyond their "tribal" circles?' when the very understanding of the benefit for service users is seen differently from within these separate perspectives (and attempts to weaken boundaries have been experienced as a collusion with the attack on professionalism *per se* from economic rationalism). Until that question is addressed we may expect the 'tribal' circles to remain strong and hence to risk continuing to 'go round in circles'.

ACKNOWLEDGEMENT

I should like to thank Tracey Crawcor for research assistance in the preparation of material for this chapter.

NOTES

1 An international readership may find some confusion in the differing use of terms. Here, the term 'social welfare' is used synonymously with 'human services' and not, as in the USA, to mean income support. I am aware that this will not be agreeable to everyone in the Australian context (e.g. O'Connor 2000), but it avoids the ambiguities that 'health' is also a 'human' service. The alternative of 'social services' has no foundation across Australia. Also, in Australia 'allied health' refers to dietetics, orthotics, occupational therapy, optometry, physiotherapy, podiatry, radiography and speech pathology (Adamson and Harris 1996; Rowan 1998); in many health services it may include pharmacy, psychology and social work, but this is not found in every instance (Astley and Wake-Dyster 2001). Normally nursing is not included in allied health, as it might be in the USA – one notable exception is Battersby et al (2001: 174). A particular feature of this latter study is its categorisation of participants into 'medicine' (two categories: 'general practitioners' and 'specialists'), 'all other health professionals' (one category: here called 'allied health') and 'all other' (one category: including patients, managers and academics).

2 'Economic rationalism' is the Australian term coined by Pusey (1991) to describe the political-economic ideas and practices that elsewhere are known as 'the New Right' or 'neo-liberalism' (or, more nationally specific, as 'Thatcherism' or 'Reaganomics'). Quite simply, Pusey intended the term to convey the dynamic of social

policy that is driven by an economic rationale. It has had a profound impact on the direction and pace of development in health and social welfare (Hancock 1999; McDonald and Jones 2000).

3 Traynor (2000) refers to the same structuralist social anthropological concepts as does Beattie (1995), noting the emphasis on categorisation and separation as the means to achieve 'the good' (seen as 'purity' of theory and practice in relation to a given profession). I return to this point later in the chapter.

4 I have discussed this aspect of the post-Fordist welfare regime elsewhere (see Hugman 1998: 117–20).

5 In this sense it could be argued that nothing much changes, and that the interprofessionalism of 'allied health' is a further strategy of 'usurpation' in the struggle for professionalisation (Hugman 1991: chapter 4). It must also be noted that this separation of 'medicine and the rest' continues to be a division characterised by gender and social class differences (Hugman 1991; Adamson and Harris 1996; Lange and Cheek 1997; Griffin 2001). It is the occupations traditionally regarded as 'women's professions' and with a more diverse social class base that are working more closely together.

REFERENCES

Adamson, B. J. and Harris, L. (1996) 'Health personnel: perceived differences in professional relationships and work role', *Australian Health Review* 19 (3) 66–80.

Astley, J. and Wake-Dyster, W. (2001) 'Evidence-based priority setting', *Australian Health Review* 24 (2) 32–9.

Bain, J. (1995) 'Best practice in community health', *Working Together to Build Healthy Rural Communities*, proceedings of the Rural Health Conference, Perth, WA: Rural Health Reference Group.

Battersby, M., McDonald, P., Pearce, R., Tolchard, B. and Allen, K. (2001) 'The changing attitudes of health professionals and consumers towards co-ordinated health care trials – SA HealthPlus', *Australian Health Review* 24 (2) 172–8.

Beattie, A. (1995) 'War and peace among the health tribes', in K. Soothill, L. Mackay and C. Webb (eds), *Interprofessional Relations in Health Care*, London: Edward Arnold.

Boyce, R. (1997) 'Health sector reform and professional power, autonomy and culture: the case of Australian allied health professions', in R. Hugman, M. Peelo and K. Soothill (eds), *Concepts of Care: Developments in Health and Social Welfare*, London: Arnold.

Boyce, R. (2001) 'Organisational governance structures in allied health services: a decade of change', *Australian Health Review* 24 (1) 22–36.

Boyce, R., Shepherd, N. and Mickan, S. (2000) 'Restructuring professional culture: the impact of "enterprising" management ideologies and entrepreneurship on public sector professionals', paper presented to the International Sociology Association Conference *State, Political Power and Professional Structures*, Lisbon, 13–15 September.

Brandis, S. (2000) 'The Australian Health Care Agreement 1998–2003: implications and strategic directions for occupational therapists', *Australian Occupational Therapy Journal* 47, 62–68.

Brown, B., Crawford, P. and Darongkamas, J. (2000) 'Blurred roles and permeable boundaries: the experience of multidisciplinary working in community mental health', *Health and Social Care in the Community* 8 (6) 425–35.

Diers, D. (1999) 'Casemix and nursing', *Australian Health Review* 22 (2) 56–68.

Doyal, L. and Gough, I. (1991) *A Theory of Human Need*, Basingstoke: Macmillan.

Draper, M. (1999) 'Casemix: financing hospital services', in L. Hancock (ed.), *Health Policy in the Market State*, St Leonards, NSW: Allen & Unwin.

Fowler, P., Hannigan, B. and Northway, R. (2000) 'Community nurses and social workers learning together: a report of an interprofessional education initiative in South Wales', *Health and Social Care in the Community* 8 (3) 186–91.

Greenwell, J. (1995) 'Patients and professionals', in K. Soothill, L. Mackay and C. Webb (eds), *Interprofessional Relations in Health Care*, London: Edward Arnold.

Griffin, S. (2001) 'Occupational therapists and the concept of power: a review of the literature', *Australian Occupational Therapy Journal* 48, 24–34.

Hancock, L. (1999) 'Health, public sector restructuring and the market state', in L. Hancock (ed.), *Health Policy in the Market State*, St Leonards, NSW: Allen & Unwin.

Hoggett, P. (1994) 'The modernization of the UK welfare state', in R. Burrows and B. Loader (eds), *Towards a Post-Fordist Welfare State?* London: Routledge.

Hugman, R. (1991) *Power in Caring Professions*, London: Macmillan.

Hugman, R. (1998) *Social Welfare and Social Value*, Basingstoke: Macmillan.

Lange, A. and Cheek, J. (1997) 'Health policy and the nursing profession', *International Journal of Nursing Practice* 3 (1) 2–9.

Leathard, A. (1994) 'Inter-professional developments in Britain', in A. Leathard (ed.), *Going Inter-Professional: Working Together for Health and Welfare*, London: Routledge.

Lengyel, C. and Bartlett, J. (2000) 'Successfully integrating community health and rehabilitation: a new model linking primary care services', paper presented to the *International Primary Health Care Conference*, Melbourne: Southern Health Care Network.

Lin, V. and Druckett, S. (1997) 'Structural interests and organisational dimensions of health system reform', in H. Gardner (ed.), *Health Policy in Australia*, Melbourne: Oxford University Press.

McCallum, J. (1997) 'Health and ageing', in A. Brorowski, S. Encel and E. Ozanne (eds), *Ageing and Social Policy in Australia*, Melbourne: Oxford University Press.

McDonald, C. (1999) 'Human service professionals in the community services industry', *Australian Social Work* 52 (1) 17–25.

McDonald, C. and Jones, A. (2000) 'Reconstructing and reconceptualising social work in the emerging milieu', *Australian Social Work* 53 (3) 3–11.

Muetzelfeldt, M. (1999) 'Contracting out in the health sector', in L. Hancock (ed.), *Health Policy in the Market State*, St Leonards, NSW: Allen & Unwin.

O'Connor, I. (2000) 'Mission, evidence and outcomes: building a future for social work', *Australian Social Work* 53 (3) 17–18.

Patford, J. (2001) 'Educating for cross-disciplinary collaboration: present trends and future possibilities', *Australian Social Work* 54 (3) 73–82.

Pollitt, C. (1993) *Managerialism and the Public Services*, 2nd edn., Oxford: Blackwell.

Pusey, M. (1991) *Economic Rationalism in Canberra*, Cambridge: Cambridge University Press.

Raiff, N. and Shore, B. (1993) *Advanced Case Management*, Newbury Park: Sage Publications.

Remenyi, A. (1997) 'Policy determinants and developments in rehabilitation', in H. Gardner (ed.), *Health Policy in Australia*, Melbourne: Oxford University Press.

Rowan, S. (1998) 'Provider and consumer perceptions of allied health service needs', *Australian Health Review* 21 (1) 88–97.

Traynor, M. (2000) 'Purity, conversion and the evidence based movements', *Health* 4 (2) 139–58.

Van Eyk, H., Baum, F. and Houghton, G. (2001) 'Coping with health care reform', *Australian Health Review* 24 (2) 202–206.

Wilson, K. with Chaplin, R., Howard, J. and Slater, C. (2000) *Integration, Innovation, Congruence and Community: A Positive Response to Demographic and Social Complexity*, Melbourne: Inner South Community Health Service.

Chapter 5

Some ethical issues arising from interprofessional working

Andrew Wall

SUMMARY

Professional practice is not sacrosanct. Professions are challenged from within by the need to change practice in the light of scientific developments. They are challenged by other professions seeking to extend their own practice. An increasingly knowledgeable public now require a clearer account of what professionals do. Finally, the government and managers, working on their behalf, are holding professions to account more rigorously than ever before. This chapter explores the ethical consequences of these challenges.

ETHICAL ISSUES

Ethics can be seen as some sort of insurance cover that not only validates a profession but also protects it from unjust criticism. This limited view is scarcely adequate at any time and even less so now that health care professions are facing increasing challenges. Pressures arise from changes in policy such as *The NHS Plan* (Secretary of State for Health 2000), which requires more interprofessional working, from a more discriminating public, from more demanding patients. Within the professions themselves, there are demands to extend areas of practice. New occupational groups are seeking admission to professional status.

It is therefore important to be clear about the ethical obligations facing professional groups. But before discussing that, there has to be some understanding as to what ethics are. Students from the health care professions are often somewhat bemused by more philosophical definitions but quickly warm to the idea that ethics are needed to manage the relationships between people who are unequal. They understand immediately that a health care professional and his or her patient are separated by unequal knowledge and the expertise they hold puts the professional at an advantage. Extending this concept, they see that the employee needs protection from the potentially abusing employer; the citizen needs protection from the power of the state. The question shifts from what *are* ethics to what are ethics *for*?

This practical approach may have its limitations because it implies that unless ethics are in some way useful, they are not needed. The 'grand' issues such as justice, who shall live and who shall die, what is right, may be left high and dry with no principles to support them. Practical examples may reduce the philosophical debate to an exercise in decision-making, the flavour of which is slightly enhanced with a light ethical sauce. Such an empirical approach can lead to relativist arguments that end up with the view that ethics are so determined by context and circumstance as to be almost impossible to codify or standardise. Every situation is different so every action will depend on the present situation.

At the very least, this is clearly unhelpful. Professionals need to have some agreement as to what defines their professionalism, much as their client/patient needs to know what those definitions mean to them. Without this neither party is protected. The answer to the question as to what are ethics for becomes clearer. Professionals need to agree standards of conduct within which they are able to work knowing that providing they do not infringe these standards they are protected from accusations of wrong doing. Clients/patients need to understand what these standards are so they can understand what to expect.

There is now a need to redefine some of those standards. Government policies, such as *The NHS Plan* (Secretary of State for Health 2000), envisage more flexibility in working, which in itself appears to be friendly to the patients' interests. Why pass a patient from hand to hand if by a little adjustment the same person could look after them? This is not, of course, just a matter of protecting patients' interests. The professions themselves have reasons for altering the boundaries of their practice. Most obviously nurses are increasingly claiming tasks (at a simple level, the taking of blood; at a more complex level, screening patients) that have been habitually undertaken by doctors. But just how far should such changes be allowed before they lead both patient and professional into a no man's land where neither is entirely clear of what is to be expected?

More fluent care of patients and the consequential need to redefine boundaries of professional practice are two reasons for redefining ethical standards. A third is that exerted by citizens and their mouthpiece, the media. Distrust has developed between the professions and the public generally. Both Conservative and Labour governments have tended to promote a more questioning approach. Their motives would appear to be estimable in that they wish the public to be better educated and more discriminating in their relationship to the professionals. But it is also evident that it has been the wish of both Parties to remove some of the traditional power of the professions. Some would say that they have been altogether too successful in this. It is scarcely helpful to imply that all GPs (general practitioners) left to their own devices will show a Shipman tendency or indeed that James Wisheart, the Bristol children's cardiac surgeon, was callously unconcerned with the patients he had spent years developing new techniques to help. Nevertheless, such examples have shown that things can go wrong, people can do the wrong things and that all potential patients are made uneasy by this. There has to be a way of putting professionals to the test that is not punitive.

CODES

The most obvious way of securing ethical practice is by regulation. Revised codes of conduct are continually being discussed by the clinical professions. Even managers have devised their own code (IHM 2001) which influenced the government's own code in 2002. The government has attempted through *The Patient's Charter* (DoH 1991) to set standards expected of the NHS as a whole. But it is a truism that codes of conduct are not self-fulfilling; things go wrong and people act badly even though they are signed up to the code. Their value is that the codes provide an explicit benchmark of expected conduct against which it is possible to establish whether an individual has acted appropriately or not. The public may wish codes to go even further but this is unrealistic. If codes cannot guarantee good conduct, what can?

Principles such as those most often quoted of justice, beneficence, non-maleficence and autonomy (Beauchamp and Childress 1994) are usually cited as the most useful and manageable. But as has been pointed out (Fisher and Gormally 2001), these principles need considerable analysis in themselves to establish exactly what the difference is between doing the right thing (beneficence) and not doing the wrong thing (non-maleficence). The principles are resounding but again scarcely self-fulfilling. They at least provide a way of thinking about these matters. And it is by this process that we begin to get to the nub of the problem. Tensions arise between one principle and another and between seemingly absolute principles and practice. Although not all philosophers will agree, ethics for clinicians and managers in a health setting cannot be laid down on tablets of stone; they always need to be explored within the context of practice. How is this best done?

It may be useful to explore the issue by returning to the idea that ethics are required to manage the differences between people: individual to individual, individual to group and group to group. This requires us to examine the following relationships in the context of interprofessional conduct: clinician and patient, clinician and clinician, clinician and profession, clinician and manager and clinician and public. The changing obligations brought about by changing interprofessional boundaries will become clearer, it is hoped, in the process.

Clinician and patient

In some respects, this is the easiest discussion. Traditionally, the relationship has been characterised by a moral obligation on the part of the clinician. This requires that the clinician endeavours to do the patient good, not knowingly wishing to harm him or her and above all to respect his or her individuality, his or her autonomy. Confidentiality is an outcome of these principles, as is being truthful.

Once applied to real situations problems arise. So what is the nature of good; are we referring to the intention, the process or the outcome? Is the clinician allowed to do a little harm to secure a greater good? How far should information about the patient be shared with others if it is in the patient's interest to do so? Is it right to tell the patient the truth if the knowledge may be potentially harmful? Does not failing to tell them the whole truth abuse their 'personhood' by treating them as incompetent to handle that truth?

None of these dilemmas have changed nor do they change intrinsically with changing professional boundaries. Nevertheless, a changing context may make them even more difficult to address.

The one-to-one relationship of clinician to his or her patient is at least a simple relationship; the two face each other alone. But within this relationship the interests of others may arise. The patient may wish to consider the implications of his or her illness on others. Indeed, in some cultures it would be considered appropriate for the clinician to address the nearest of kin rather than the patient particularly if the news is bad.

Clinician to clinician

The situation becomes more complicated when more than one clinician is involved. If they are of the same kind – doctor to doctor – at least they share a similar way of looking at things, but when they are two clinicians of different kinds, they need to be sure not only that they understand each other's language but also that they are happy sharing information. Their comparative professional status can become an issue.

Although attempts have been made to secure the flapping flysheet by broad statements declaring the fundamentals of each profession's *raison d'être*, in practical situations it is not possible to be so dogmatic. So Kitson's (1988) proposal that '. . . rather than emulate the medical goal of getting the patient better, the nurse ought to focus on caring for the person who is sick and helping him to feel better' now seems unnecessarily limiting on the nursing role.

But the nurse has a point; can clinicians relate satisfactorily to one another if their practice overlaps? What exactly is the difference between the nurse practitioner and junior doctor in an accident and emergency department, the social worker and health visitor in matters of child protection, the social worker and community psychiatric nurse, the occupational therapist and the physiotherapist in the head injury rehabilitation unit and so on? Even managers may have seemed to usurp clinical responsibilities by establishing alternative ways of living for people with learning disabilities.

Shifting boundaries can also be an excuse to 'dump' unpalatable or boring bits of professional work on others. Notorious, as an example, is the insistence that the management of challenging behaviour is a behaviour disorder rather than a manifestation of mental illness. Psychiatrists leave nurses and their managers to sort the matter out.

Another problem of interprofessional relationships is the relative status of each team member. Traditionally, doctors have been dominant and initially the law accepted that what was done to patients was the doctors' responsibility even if they had not administered the particular treatment. That position has long since changed but where is the boundary now? Obviously a person in training cannot be expected to carry the same responsibility as a fully qualified person. So how does that place a senior house officer, who is fully registered but is still in training or, indeed, a senior newly qualified and registered nurse, whose experience is as yet limited?

The habitual way of sorting out these problems is the catch-all concept of 'teamworking'. If we all work together there will be no problem. This is naïve. At worst it can lead to gross inefficiency or the 'tyranny of the unstructured group' where it is no longer clear who is in charge of what. An example from my own experience was when the principal clinical psychologist in a team, responsible for resettling people with learning disabilities in the community, failed to turn up to a crucial discussion because she was in town at an estate agents looking for suitable housing for the clients. Her justification was that as a member of the team she was sharing in the work. But her expertise was being wasted; she was doing a job a much less qualified and less well-paid person could have done.

Teamwork then has to be examined carefully; it is not a universal panacea. It is not good enough to say, 'If we all work as a team with the patient's interests paramount, we will be seen as acting ethically'. Instead ethical practice requires that each person's role is understood and accepted. Where professions are pushing at the boundaries of their practice as in nursing in primary care, this may not be easy to establish.

One way into agreement as to ethical practice is the establishment of clinical governance. Clinical governance is a great deal more than the government's latest slogan. One of the definitions of professional practice is having the ability, and indeed duty, to reflect on practice. Clinical governance systemises that reflection in a team setting. Its introduction into the NHS is arguably very late although some aspects have long been with us such as the confidential enquiry into maternal deaths.

It is difficult to establish without doubt what is good and what is bad practice. At the extreme, team members may feel that a fellow professional is acting unethically and may have to decide between keeping the integrity of the team or whistleblowing. But in a well-regulated team it should not be necessary to resort to such action. I can remember a heated discussion in a maternity liaison committee, which in many respects undertook what we now call clinical governance, as to whether transfers in labour from community obstetric units to the consultant unit at the DGH (District General Hospital) were a suitable index of good or bad practice. Even when it was agreed to be appropriate, there was further discussion as to what would constitute a suitable rate. One unit 24 miles from the centre argued that 17 per cent transfers in early labour was an index of good practice because it showed that the GP, obstetrician and attending midwife were responding quickly to potential difficulties. The majority did not agree and felt that 5 per cent should be the benchmark. What was apparent to the non-clinical managers in that committee was that a great deal of discussion in a trusting climate was needed to establish satisfactory interprofessional relationships, which were in themselves necessary to establish good practice aimed at safeguarding the patient's interests.

Clinician and profession

Professional regalia are a symbol of their good faith. Despite this, professions have begun to lose their benevolent aura. As stated above, the attacks from government, the media and the public themselves have not, in this writer's view, been necessarily in the ultimate interests of patients. Nevertheless, the professions themselves have not always acted wisely. The general dissatisfaction with the General Medical Council has demonstrated that secrecy and exclusiveness have corrupted some professional standards.

Other professional groups have fought internecine battles under their professional flag. Midwives, while claiming accurately enough, a different professional history from nurses, have continually voiced their desire to be seen as separate from the nursing profession. They were corralled under the Nurses, Midwives and Health Visitors Act 1979, but have fretted ever since. Their major concern is that the natural function of childbirth has tended to become unduly medicalised and that non-midwife nurses fail to recognise adequately the particular needs of the mother.

It could be argued that much of the professional ethic is insufficiently grounded in clinical practice. The very titles of the Royal Colleges of this and that obscure the fact that the professional is primarily there to serve patients and clients and scarcely needs the historical trimmings and arcane committee structures. What purpose do they serve in satisfying patients' needs?

Not that this is to underestimate the importance for the members of a profession to feel part of a highly esteemed group of people. Professional pride is not just a regrettable manifestation of self-importance; it establishes that the obligations of the profession are more than the simple contract between clinician and doctor; it reinforces an overall sense of identity that feeds altruism and the desire to do good to fellow citizens. Fundamentally, it helps establish the trust that is an essential ingredient of the patient–clinician relationship.

If this is so, how do the new groups of practitioners develop into professionals? There certainly is a well-recognised process. First, the groups of practitioners establish some degree of exclusive practice and then they set up unique training for that practice from which they can control entry to the group. Once this is recognised, they can set rules of practice, the infringement of which leads to exclusion. The pursuit of professional recognition takes time. This will be conditioned by how readily kindred professions accept the emerging professional group. It is not altogether clear why osteopathy and chiropractics have had an easier ride than aspects of psychotherapy or herbalism except that the practice of the former are perhaps more tangible than the latter.

State registration is the official seal on professional status and gaining that relies in some degree on political acumen. Nevertheless, it is a useful rite of passage that allows the emerging professions themselves, other professions and the public more generally to accept that practice has been accredited.

The newer professional groups have also been valuable in helping the more established to revise their views about what they are doing. So physiotherapists have enriched their own practice by extending their work into new forms of manipulation and into acupuncture. GPs faced with intractable symptoms in some of their patients are now more prepared to look at psychological aspects of illness and recognise that other types of intervention and support may be appropriate.

From this discussion, we can see that professions' natural conservative instincts are challenged by interprofessional practice and that can often be in the patients' best interests.

Clinicians and managers

Clinicians are likely to have a more troubled relationship with managers who may be seen as enemies of professional status. Indeed, many of the policy initiatives since the Griffiths Report (1983) seem to have been aimed at pushing the interests of the managers at the expense of the clinician. It is now the case that top managers are seen as being accountable for clinical practice even though the large majority of them have no clinical training. This relationship seems therefore to threaten patients' interests and to denigrate the idea of professional status. If this is the case ethics seem to have been affronted.

Fundamental is the accusation that managers are not themselves professional. Anyone can become a manager and clinicians might be excused from feeling that at times anyone has! But this is to downgrade the sense of responsibility that most health service managers have habitually brought to their role (Wall 2001). The problem in philosophical terms is the tension between the managers' innate inclination to rehearse a utilitarian approach that aims to maximise benefit to the majority and the clinicians' inclination to maximise benefit to the individual. This has become even more complicated for the manager who, while attempting to maximise the common good, has now also to recognise the demands of the consumer and his or her supposed right to choice.

The context for much of the discussion between managers and clinicians will be the appropriate use of resources given that in any health system they will be limited. Professionals, who fail at least to acknowledge that resources are always limited in one way or other, are abdicating from at least one aspect of ethical practice. Promoting the interests of one patient, knowing that this will potentially threaten the interests of another, is in any terms unethical. It must be seen as a quibble when a consultant refuses to show any concern for patients on a list waiting to be assessed on the grounds that until they themselves have seen the patient, they cannot feel any responsibility for them. Nevertheless, their dilemmas can also be appreciated: they can scarcely be expected to worry about every potential patient while at the same time giving adequate attention to the patient in front of them. The way out of this is for both managers and clinicians to recognise that although they could be considered as coming from opposite philosophical poles, they are bound to meet in the middle on common ground. Within this common ground claims of professional superiority over the managers are unhelpful in resolving problems as to which patient should have what. For clinicians not to engage in these discussions is to be unprofessional and may appear as merely luddite.

Clinicians, managers and the public

Following this discussion, it is now possible to see interprofessional behaviour as being united by a common concern for the welfare of patients. But what about those who have yet to become patients, the general public? How can their expectations be met? What if they are unreasonable? How can the professionals and the managers respond ethically to unrealistic demands?

Accountability would seem to be the key concept here, but accountability for what and to whom? For both clinicians and managers, accountability could be said to be graduated. Professionals feel that their prime duty is to the individual patient in front of them with their responsibility to the population less important. Managers reverse this order. But both share a responsibility for acting fairly in the patients' interests and not primarily in their own. Here the original virtues of bureaucracy are worth reviving. It has become customary to use the term 'bureaucracy' in a pejorative manner. It is worth attempting to rehabilitate the more creditable aspects of that concept. Bureaucracy was originally used as a principle to govern public organisations whose concern was to be fair and disinterested (in its proper meaning) creating a suitable distance between demands and their satisfaction, a distance allowing proper consideration of the issues and free from undue or corrupt influence.

Professional status is a help to this manner of working because professionals have rules indicating that they are not to be unduly influenced by inducements, material or psychological. This may of course be more difficult when it is in the interests of an emerging professional group to harness the pressures for users to endorse their claims to professional recognition.

Despite this, what the public presumably needs is expert opinion and it may be that the recognition of expertise has in some respects become a casualty of both the increased democratic involvement and its pernicious side effect, consumerism. In this situation expertise is not sufficiently valued and what the patient wants gains ascendancy over what the patient needs.

The resolution of this potential tension requires professionals to demonstrate not only that they have appropriate expertise but that they are prepared to demonstrate how they can best use it. Fundamental to that use is judgement and the public in their turn need to appreciate that judgement, like trust, has to be accepted not as a fact but as a value. Judgement and trust cannot be proved, but their absence can certainly be recognised by the consequences.

CONCLUSION

Interprofessional working has required us to think more deeply about the ethical basis for professional practice. Would it help to prepare a pan professional code of conduct to assure the public that whoever the clinician was, their aims were the same?

The answer must be 'no'. Such a code would be generalised to such an extent that it would suffer from the platitudes found in many an organisation's mission statement which I have described elsewhere as being 30 words not necessarily in the same order but of which 20 are common. This is not to deny that mission statements have their uses principally in the discussion that leads up to their formation. Similarly, professionals constantly need to assess their own ethical position to demonstrate that they are meeting appropriate standards that are in the interests of their patients. For each profession these will need to be expressed in a different manner.

Even if there is no reason why interprofessional working should be more difficult, there are dangers resulting from crossovers of practice – managers making clinical decisions, clinicians making managerial decisions and also one profession usurping the function of another without agreement – may have unethical consequences. This in turn may lead to the degrading of not only patient/client well-being but also the quality of a caring service in society as a whole.

Ethical interprofessional working requires first a sure sense of professional identity rooted in practice. Second, while accepting that professionals are acting as servants to their patients and clients, they only fulfil their purpose adequately if they use all their expertise in the process. This expertise is not just technical but also has 'the nature of artistry' (Fish and Coles 1998), which perceives more than mere outcomes, and can make patterns, develop concepts and assess uncertainties. Ultimately, experience and wisdom, harnessed to imagination, ensure that professional practice is constantly renewed with patients' interests paramount.

REFERENCES

Beauchamp, T. and Childress, J. (1994) *Principles of Biomedical Ethics*, 4th edn., Oxford: Oxford University Press.

DoH (Department of Health) (1991) *The Patient's Charter*, London: Department of Health.

Fish, D. and Coles, C (1998) *Developing Professional Judgement in Health Care*, Oxford: Butterworth-Heinemann.

Fisher, A. and Gormally, L. (eds) (2001) *Healthcare Allocation: an Ethical Framework for Public Policy*, London: The Lincacre Centre.

Griffiths Report (1983) *NHS Management Inquiry*, London: Department of Health and Social Security.

IHM (Institute of Healthcare Management) (2001) *The IHM Management Code*, London: IHM.

Kitson, A. (1988) 'On the concept of nursing care' in G. Fairburn and S. Fairburn (eds), *Ethical Issues in Caring*, Aldershot: Avebury.

Secretary of State for Health (2000) *The NHS Plan: A Plan for Investment: A Plan for Reform*, London: The Stationery Office.

Wall, A. (2001) *Being a Health Service Manager – Expectations and Experience*, London: Nuffield Trust.

Chapter 6

New forms of technology, new forms of collaboration?

Scott Reeves and Della Freeth

SUMMARY

Traditionally, much intraprofessional and interprofessional collaboration in health and social care has been based on simultaneous face-to-face inter-action. The use of information technology presents staff with a number of opportunities to engage with new forms of collaboration. The particular advantage of these technologies is that they can overcome the need to share the same physical space and time for collaborative activities. This chapter examines the issues surrounding the policy and practice of these technologies in supporting collaboration within health and social care settings.

INTRODUCTION

The past decade has witnessed a phenomenal expansion in the use of infor-mation technology for both work and leisure purposes. Growing economies of scale within the information technology industry have meant that com-puter and telecommunications technologies have become more affordable. This expansion of technology has led to the development of several forms of electronic communication. All have potential for improving collaboration in health and social care.

This chapter initially describes the traditional construction of collabor-ation and some of the difficulties associated with this model. It goes on to discuss how information technology transcends these difficulties to create novel forms of collaboration. Examples are given of effective collaboration that is aided by harnessing the potential of information technology. A gloss-ary is provided at the end of the chapter for terms that may be unfamiliar.

CONVENTIONAL COLLABORATION

Traditionally, collaboration (whether formal or informal) has centred on sharing the same physical space to interact in the planning, undertaking or reviewing of joint activities. Examples include Reeves et al (1999), Williams and Laungani (1999) and Molyneux (2001). Common formats for traditional collaboration include ward rounds, patient review meetings, multidisciplinary case conferences and interprofessional planning groups. These formats work well if all the relevant people are able to attend and they are able to make valued contributions. However, such meetings are a resource-hungry form of collaboration.

The demands of managing caseloads in different locations often restrict time for staff to meet. Differing work patterns also create difficulties in meeting with colleagues. Restricted interaction, regardless of whether the restriction is in time or quality, often causes interprofessional collaboration to become problematic. Allen (1997) provides a useful example of the difficulties practitioners face in trying to work together. In a study of doctor–nurse relations, Allen (1997) found that the temporal–spatial organisation of work in hospitals meant that doctors and nurses shared only a small amount of time together. This lack of shared time and space restricted opportunities for doctor–nurse negotiation and agreement over patient care.

Traditional collaboration is also limited by its resource requirements and the willingness of participants to prioritise this activity over other calls on their attention. For example, in her study of teamwork, Cott (1998) revealed that collaboration was often hindered by a lack of formal mechanisms for information-sharing between professionals and support workers. This shortfall often resulted in poor communication between these multidisciplinary team members.

Where meeting together is not possible synchronous (or real-time) collaboration can be conducted by telephone. This interaction is usually limited to a one-to-one exchange of concerns and advice, or one-to-one discussion and planning. However, much collaboration at a distance is asynchronous (or time-delayed), occurring through the written word, for example, shared patient notes, letters between primary and secondary care and reports between health and social care. Effective collaboration for the benefit of patients or clients relies on the timely exchange of accurate, pertinent information. Time lags can reduce the effectiveness of care and waste resources in the form of duplicated effort or inappropriate interventions.

If we want to improve collaboration, we need to look at ways of increasing the efficiency of collaboration and also the means of enhancing enthusiasm for this activity. The next section of the chapter examines the potential of information technology in this area.

INFORMATION TECHNOLOGY

The rapid development of accessible, reliable and user-friendly information technology offers improvements to traditional collaboration and makes new approaches possible. Many platforms for the exchange of information such as the Internet, email, video-conferencing and telephone-conferencing are well-established aids to collaboration. However, provision of access to these technologies from health and social care settings is, as yet, patchy. Nevertheless, they offer possibilities to enhance collaboration at any distance: local, regional, national or international. These new forms of technology also permit many-to-many interaction.

The use of information technology can help to overcome the time–space problems normally associated with collaboration within health and social care settings. These technologies can offer an 'electronic bridge' to ensure that practitioners can communicate either synchronously and asynchronously. Rapid responses are possible and the barriers to collaboration encountered when individuals or agencies do not work the same hours lessen. Collaboration across the world's time zones becomes straightforward. As a result, information technology can be an effective vehicle for sharing good practice and managing risk.

Recent policies have increasingly recognised and embraced the potential of information technology. For example, the NHS Information Authority (1999: 17) states that new technology will assist staff to 'manage information effectively by helping them to share information across professional boundaries', which goes on to assert that the use of information technology will ultimately enhance collaboration across the service: between clinics, hospitals, departments and professions. In turn, it is hoped that this will lead to the development of shared interprofessional objectives, standardised documentation and an overall consensus on joint working practices.

Government policies have outlined a range of technological developments designed to support health and social care staff in their work. Some of these are described in the next part of the chapter. However, these policies tend to overlook a range of cultural, organisational and individual tensions associated with employing new forms of technology within these settings. We return to these issues later.

Technologies that support communication between practitioners can change the way people work together. The intention is that this improves patient/client care and working lives. However, it should be remembered that the use of technological innovations involves losses as well as gains. Coiera and Tombs (1998) provide a useful example of the complexity of employing information technology in a care setting. In their evaluation of the impact of a hospital bleep system (technology designed to overcome problems with contacting staff working in different locations), they found that bleeps created an 'interruptive workplace' for many doctors. Regular bleeping from nurses and other care staff meant that doctors' work was frequently inter-rupted. To cope, doctors often ignored the bleeps to focus on the completion of their work. Typically, this led to repeated bleeping and increased frustra-tion by the staff waiting for medical input. This experience serves as a useful reminder that the introduction of technology in care settings requires careful cost–benefit evaluation.

Let us term 'collaboration' which is primarily facilitated by information technology, 'e-collaboration'. E-collaboration is multifaceted and growing rapidly. There are a number of basic requirements for successful e-collaboration, most importantly: policy commitment, organisational sup-port, ethical considerations, staff development and attention to cultural factors. These requirements are considered in the next section.

Policy commitment

Harnessing the potential of information technology to support the work of health and social care practitioners requires cultural shifts and reallocation of resources. These changes are made much easier if there is firm national or regional policy commitment. The case of the UK will serve as a good example. In a series of policy documents (that we expect to continue), the government has outlined its vision of information technology supporting the work of health and social care staff (e.g. Department of Health 1998, 2000, 2001; NHS Executive 1998). At the heart of these policy papers is the belief that the use of new technologies will assist professionals, often located in geographically disparate locations, to work closer together in a more seamless fashion.

Building on the existing use of email and web technologies within the NHS, these policies outline some exciting new possibilities for interprofes-sional collaboration between National Health Service (NHS) staff. Informa-tion technology therefore has a central role in 'bridging gaps in language, communication, values, knowledge, and skills that often exist in the NHS' (Department of Health 1998: section 2.2a). In essence, the government's plan is to create a national information technology system that practitioners can effectively employ to support their collaborative work. In particular, informa-tion technology will help ensure practitioners' work is better coordinated to meet the demands placed on the NHS by an ageing population.

Implementing policy through the use of new technology

Current NHS policies anticipate that four different forms of technology will contribute towards more effective collaboration: NHSnet, electronic patient records, National Electronic Library for Health and NHS Digital. Each of these technologies is briefly outlined below.

NHSnet

The recently established NHSnet is an Intranet that staff can access from their computers. Its aim is to provide staff with the facility to communicate and share patient information more effectively and efficiently, while safeguarding confidentiality. When this system becomes fully operational, it will be possible for staff working in any care setting to obtain or transmit patient information, prescriptions and test results (e.g. X-ray images).

Electronic patient records

By 2005 it is expected that electronic patient records (EPRs) will be created for every NHS patient: pilots are well under way. EPRs will be stored in a database, accessible via the NHSnet. Staff will be able to access, read and update patient information from any networked computer with ease. Collaboration with patients and clients could also be improved since they will be able to check and add to fields within their own EPR.

National Electronic Library for Health

The National Electronic Library for Health (NeLH) aims to provide NHS staff with the latest on-line research evidence. An important part of the NeLH will be the creation of a National Virtual Classroom. This resource will be accessible to all NHS staff via the NHSnet to provide them with a range of audio-visual reference and learning materials that they may use individually or collaboratively.

NHS Digital

NHS Digital is a programme of pilot projects that is exploring the potential uses of digital media, such as digital television, to access and share information between practitioners. The advantage of using digital technology is that it will overcome the current problems (i.e. poor quality data) related to using analogue technology.

Organisational support

The introduction of new forms of technology demands considerable investment: comprehensive needs analyses, the allocation of resources, thoughtful purchasing, technical assistance, champions to promote cultural change, staff development, ongoing maintenance and systems development. Therefore, support from both strategic and operational management is a fundamental requirement.

Managers at all levels need to ensure that staff can access and make effective use of any technology that is introduced into their workplace. This is not easy, given the heavy and unpredictable workloads that many clinical staff regularly face (Annandale et al 1999). Simply installing information technology is not sufficient to ensure that it will be used to support care delivery or work-related learning (Freeth 2000). Practitioners need time and support to develop confidence and expertise with new technologies. Some protected time, carefully tailored staff development or 'trouble-shooting' assistance can help here. Making the systems as 'user-friendly' as possible is important.

Once practitioners become confident with information technology, they are likely to innovate, push existing provision to its limits, ask for more sophisticated technologies, greater capacity and faster processing. The anticipation of such demands need to be addressed in strategic planning. However, the technology to support collaboration does not always need to be 'all singing and all dancing', nor the newest and the best on the market. For example, telephone-conferencing technology has been available for many years. It is relatively inexpensive and reliable.

Ethical considerations

The use of information technology to store and exchange personal clinical information between health and social care staff raises three important ethical considerations: confidentiality, consent and safety.

Great attention must be paid to the security of electronically stored and transmitted patient/client information. We must ensure that confidential information is protected from computer hackers who deliberately infiltrate computer systems, inadvertent access by inappropriate parties and possible misuse by staff. Passwords, encryption and digital signatures are all examples of electronic safeguards, but they need to be sophisticated and constantly updated. A recent study of fraud and abuse of information technologies (Audit Commission 1998) found that hackers have affected around half of all public sector organisations in the UK, thus vigilance and the ongoing development of protective mechanisms are essential.

Encouragingly, the tension between maintaining ethical requirements for confidentiality and the ease/speed of using information technology is gradually being resolved. Recent developments in encryption technology (e.g. Young et al 2001) have meant that more secure and speedy systems are being tested in a number of health and social care settings.

When it is easy for practitioners and agencies to share information, the enthusiasm for collaboration can result in overlooking the ethical requirement for consent. Attention needs to be paid to the type of consent that has been given by clients and patients, and to future consent requirements as information systems become more powerful and sophisticated.

The use of back-up copies of electronic information, stored at different locations, makes electronic information less susceptible to loss than paper records in events such as fire or flood. However, corruption of information can occur during the transmission, copying and storage of electronic information. The systems used need to be as reliable as possible. Checking mechanisms need to be developed to detect emergent errors. Reliability is also vital in the general running of safe information technology systems. If practitioners cannot swiftly access reliable information, due to the poor reliability of the system, patient/client safety will be compromised. Such 'down time' must be kept to a minimum through high quality system design and maintenance.

Cultural factors

If new technology is to become integrated into practice, staff need to alter their traditional patterns of working together. This change requires a shift in culture. As with any cultural shift, it can be both daunting and empowering.

Rheingold (1994) discusses the future development of a 'virtual community' where discussions, debates and joint problem-solving can all be supported by a range of technologies. As a result, conventional forms of interaction will alter. For example, high status staff, who traditionally dominate face-to-face meetings, will be 'no more visible than those who would remain silent or say little in a face-to-face meeting but say a lot via computer mediated communication' (Rheingold 1994: 63). For Rheingold, a 'virtual community' will result in people being judged more by their contributions to debate and less by their disability, race, gender, age, terms of employment or professional status. Of course, e-communication opens up new opportunities for fraud and safeguards must be put in place.

The type of debate that occurs through information technology is different from the interaction in face-to-face meetings. Synchronous, technology-based 'conversations' can be difficult to chair; simultaneous contributions are difficult to manage and prevent. Aspects of body language that moderate face-to-face communication may be imperfectly projected or absent, depending on the technology used. Participants may be unsettled by the technology and this will affect their contributions.

Asynchronous, technology-based 'conversations' may be characterised by more considered responses than is normal in face-to-face discussion. Such conversations are also characterised by the interwoven development of several threads of conversation caused by the time delays of responding and the parallel working of participants. In face-to-face discussion, participants do not expect to make all the points that occur to them. Participants expect threads to be handled sequentially rather than in parallel; some of the things that are said may make no impact on the debate and simply disappear. In contrast, for participants of technology-based discussion, there is often an expectation that every point they make is given a response and that all contributions remain in an archive. Technology-based communication is different to face-to-face communication and we must recognise it as such. People will need to develop new skills.

Many health and social care staff have become confident with email, often initially through home use. Once the technology has been mastered the cultural change in communication should not be so huge: communicating by email has similarities with sending postcards. Email is a 'push' technology: when you send a message it is delivered into the mailboxes of the intended recipients. Receipt of your message is passive, just like a traditional postal service. On the other hand, computer-conferencing and bulletin boards are 'pull' technologies. You post messages to intended recipients that they must obtain (or pull) from the computer conference or bulletin board. This is a cultural shift for senders and receivers. E-collaboration utilising different forms of technology will feel different; there will be different demands on participants and different cultural norms derived from the strengths and weaknesses of the particular technology.

Individuals who lead e-collaboration initiatives need to be aware of cultural factors when selecting and combining technologies. These individuals should identify and support differing levels of confidence, experience and expertise among participants. A shift in culture can be made more acceptable if key enthusiasts are identified within the work environment. Typically, there are a small number of enthusiasts for any new venture who can act as catalysts for change among their peers by acting as role models and by providing informal peer support during any transition period. Input from an e-moderator can greatly aid newcomers' transitions to e-collaboration or e-learning (Salmon 2000).

The full power of technology will not be harnessed and used creatively to forge new collaborations and improve the quality of care unless practitioners develop trust and confidence in new technologies. Motivation is important, too. Before installing new technology we need to pose the question: does this technology allow people to do new and exciting things, or is it just a complicated and inconvenient way of addressing old tasks?

Staff development

Whereas many young children are growing up routinely using different forms of information technology, a significant proportion of the current health and social care workforce were introduced to new technology in their adult lives. The workforce contains enormous variation in levels of information technology literacy. Therefore, any programme of staff development needs to be targeted: programmes should offer novice, intermediate and advanced sessions. The training needs to be focused on individuals' current work-related needs and aspirations, while making practitioners aware of possibilities they had not imagined. A good model is awareness-raising from champions, followed by self-directed learning with easy access to practical assistance from an encouraging individual who is an expert in the use of technology. Staff turnover, current skill levels and rapidly developing technologies require an acceptance that staff development will be an ongoing need for the foreseeable future.

EXAMPLES OF E-COLLABORATION

This part of the chapter provides examples of how synchronous (real-time) and asynchronous (time-delayed) technologies have been harnessed to support collaboration between health and social care practitioners in a variety of service delivery settings.

Synchronous technologies

Harrison et al (1996) describe how the use of e-conferencing technology supported real-time patient consultations between primary care and secondary care staff. Three different types of technology were employed to facilitate this form of e-collaboration: networked computers, telephone handsets and video cameras. At a mutually convenient time for staff and patients, a joint 'teleconsultation' was conducted. After overcoming some early problems due to technical failure (loss of sound and/or vision), it was found that these teleconferenced consultations adequately assisted care staff in their joint work. In particular, it was felt that the use of this real-time audio-visual technology may have an important benefit in improving communication between primary and secondary care.

Similar examples of the use of e-conferencing technology include Pham and Yearwood (2000) who describe the use of this technology to enable health care staff located in distant locations across the USA to share data in order to agree care decisions. Also, Wootton (2001) reports on the use of e-conferencing technology to support the work of nurse practitioners running a minor injuries unit when interacting with doctors (based at a nearby accident and emergency department) for their advice around complex treatments.

Asynchronous technologies

Young et al (2001) describe the development of a network that has connected staff working in primary, secondary and tertiary care settings. Using Internet technology, these authors outline how this system has provided a reliable, secure and inexpensive system of sharing patient information between staff based in these different care sectors. It was found that the previous paper-based system of communication between these staff relied on an annual review of patients. However, this method of communication was inflexible, slow and unreliable: patient information was quickly out of date; data needed to be retyped when passed between staff. To overcome the high costs of setting up an Intranet system, the Internet was used. This technology was considered to have a number of advantages, including ease of access (it only requires a computer linked to an existing telephone line) and little additional training needs (most staff had good prior knowledge of using the Internet). However, the Internet can be a relatively insecure means of transmitting information. Therefore, the authors describe how they established a secure encryption system to ensure that patient information could be safely shared between staff. Overall, it was felt that this system was effective in supporting interprofessional collaboration.

Similar examples are offered by other authors such as Bookman et al (1998) who report on an initiative that used an electronic database containing information on clinical protocols accessed through Internet software that offered an effective system for sharing information. Polley et al (1996) also describe the use of e-conferencing technology for staff based in two countries (Australia and Canada) that helped develop an interprofessional course for medical, nursing and social work students.

Combining technologies

Synchronous and asynchronous technologies can be combined to support e-collaboration. For example Wootton (2001) describes an initiative based in Finland that combined real-time interactive e-conferencing technology between clinicians with an asynchronous electronic patient referral system. These technologies were found to facilitate good communication between staff located in acute and primary care settings. In particular, staff found these newer forms of electronic communication more efficient and effective than traditional face-to-face consultations and the paper-based referral system. Patel et al (1999) describe a similar initiative that employed email and electronic-conferencing technology to overcome the traditional temporal–spatial problems related to hospital-based collaboration.

EVIDENCE AND EVALUATION

Evaluation of e-collaboration is in its infancy. As a result, there is little reliable evidence in the cost-effectiveness of using information technology within health and social care settings. Currently, most research tends to be restricted to small-scale feasibility studies. For example, findings from a recent systematic review of patient satisfaction with telemedicine (Mair and Whitton 2000) revealed that of the 32 studies in this review, most used simple survey tools with small convenience samples of patients. In drawing their conclusions,

Mair and Whitton (2000) pointed out that these methodological deficiencies mean that the impact of information technology cannot yet be fully appreciated.

Encouragingly, more rigorous studies are emerging. Wootton et al (2000) describe a multi-centre trial comparing the use of video-conferencing technology to facilitate consultations between primary and secondary care staff. Findings from this research revealed that it was clinically effective to employ information technology to support primary–secondary interaction. However, due to the short distance between clinics, the use of information technology was not considered cost-effective. However, Wooton et al (2000) argued that cost-effectiveness could be achieved if the participating clinics were located at a greater distance from one another.

Although the use of information technology does appear to offer a number of advantages for staff working in different care settings, until a systematic programme of evaluation is undertaken, there will be a continuing uncertainty regarding the actual costs and benefits of employing information technology to support the work of staff based in health and social care settings.

CONCLUDING COMMENTS

Collaboration is essentially a social process that needs to take place in an environment where people can share resources, communicate and provide mutual support. Technology will never obviate the need for traditional forms of interaction, but new forms of technology offer opportunities for new forms of collaboration.

This chapter considered the issues surrounding the use of information technology for supporting collaboration within health and social care settings. One particular advantage of information technology is its ability to offer an electronic bridge to overcome the temporal–spatial difficulties associated with traditional forms of collaboration. Nevertheless, several policy, managerial, ethical, cultural and educational issues need to be considered when employing technology within health and social care. Careful consideration is needed to ensure that new forms of technology are well evaluated in terms of their costs and benefits.

ACKNOWLEDGEMENT

We are grateful to David Morgan, independent information technology consultant, for sharing his technical expertise during the development of this chapter.

GLOSSARY

Audio-conferencing takes place over the telephone by simultaneously connecting the different group members to allow real-time communication.

Bulletin boards provide either public or private discussion forums for groups of similarly interested individuals. They offer an asynchronous form of communication whereby emails are sent to a particular bulletin board and stored until the other group members access and reply to them. Bulletin boards can also contain archives of previous group messages to enable new group members to review prior discussions and debates. Bulletin boards need an e-moderator.

Computer-based conferencing (sometimes termed 'computer-mediated communication' or 'telematics') is a text-based conference where communication takes place via computers connected together via an Intranet or the Internet. This type of conference can be held in real-time, where the group simultaneously interact through their computers in an electronic dialogue. Or the conference can be undertaken by use of asynchronous communication, where messages are sent around group members over a number of days or weeks.

Computer hackers are individuals who break into electronic networks to disrupt systems and/or obtain information.

Digital signatures are used to verify the source of electronic information and to ensure that it has not been tampered with.

E-conferencing facilitates communication when it is difficult for members of a group to meet in the same geographical location. There are three types of technology that can be employed for e-conferencing purposes: computer-based-conferencing, audio-conferencing and video-conferencing.

Electronic databases are pieces of computer software that allow the user to store, search and selectively retrieve hundreds of thousands of pieces of information in a summarised form.

Electronic network is any number of connected computers. Networking computers allows information to pass between individuals. Connections are usually made by computer cables and telephone lines.

Email is the primary method of computer-based asynchronous communication with billions of email messages being sent every day. Emails are produced, sent and received from computer to computer. All messages are stored on a server until they are obtained by the user to read on their computer. As messages are held on a server they can be accessed (through the use of a password) from any computer in the world that is connected to the Internet.

E-moderator preside over a computer conference in a similar fashion to a chair presiding over a meeting. E-moderators help individuals access, navigate and make good use of a bulletin board. They challenge inappropriate use, offer tips to the less experienced and set an example of good use. Periodically, an e-moderator must summarise and archive contributions so that new or returning participants can cope with the volume of information generated by this form of technology.

Encryption is used to alter the contents of electronic data so that it becomes unreadable to unauthorised users. Encryption 'keys' are used to encrypt and decrypt data. Without the key data is effectively locked. Therefore, when encryption is used to safeguard data the key must also be kept safe.

Internet is a world-wide electronic network that allows users to communicate with one another and access audio-visual information.

Intranet is an electronic network that has been set up within an organisation to communicate and share information between members. People outside the organisation cannot gain access. One Intranet can be connected to another to allow communication between different organisations.

On-line is when individuals are connected to the Internet, either through email or the web.

Server is a central computer system that facilitates Internet and Intranet communication. It stores outgoing and incoming information.

Software are the applications, programmes or codes that the computer needs to function. For example, email software needs to be installed on a computer before emails can be created or received.

Video-conferencing is currently the most sophisticated and expensive form of e-conferencing. Through the use of video pictures and sound, group members can simultaneously interact both verbally and visually. The cost of video-conferencing is falling with the availability of digital technology.

The web (sometimes called the world wide web) is the main method for accessing electronic information from the Internet. Information on the web is displayed in the form of electronically created web pages. These pages can contain a range of textual, audio and visual information.

REFERENCES

Allen, D. (1997) 'The nursing-medical boundary: a negotiated order?', *Sociology of Health and Illness* 19, 498–520.

Annandale, E., Clark, J. and Allen, E. (1999) 'Interprofessional working: an ethnographic case study of emergency health care', *Journal of Interprofessional Care* 13 (2) 139–50.

Audit Commission (1998) *Ghost in the Machine: An Analysis of IT Fraud and Abuse*, London: The Stationery Office.

Bookman, M., McLaughlin, L., Burgess, S. and Wolfenden, A. (1998) 'Web-based resources for clinical protocol management', *Oncology* 12, 352–5.

Coiera, E. and Tombs, V. (1998) 'Communication behaviours in a hospital setting: an observational study', *British Medical Journal* 316, 673–76.

Cott, C. (1998) 'Structure and meaning in multidisciplinary teamwork', *Sociology of Health and Illness* 20, 848–73.

Department of Health (1998) *Working Together with Health Information: A Partnership Strategy for Education, Training and Development*, Leeds: NHS Executive.

Department of Health (2000) *Implementing Information for Health – IM&T for Primary Care Groups/Trusts* (December Bulletin), London: Department of Health.

Department of Health (2001) *Building the Information Core: Implementing the NHS Plan*, London: Department of Health.

Freeth, D. (2000) *Evaluation of Doctors' Responses to the Provision of On-line Library Material in Clinical Areas*, Research Report 17, London, St Bartholomew School of Nursing and Midwifery: City University.

Harrison, R., Clayton, W. and Wallace, P. (1996) 'Can telemedicine be used to improve communication between primary and secondary care?', *British Medical Journal* 313, 1377–80.

Mair, F. and Whitton, P. (2000) 'Systematic review of studies of patient satisfaction with telemedicine', *British Medical Journal* 320, 1517–20.

Molyneux, J. (2001) 'Interprofessional teamworking: what makes teams work well', *Journal of Interprofessional Care* 15, 29–36.

NHS Executive (1998) *Information for Health*, Leeds: NHSE.

NHS Information Authority (1999) *Information for Practice: The National Information Management Agenda and You*, Bristol: NHS Information Authority.

Patel, V., Kaufman, D., Allen, V., Shortlife, E., Cimino, J. and Greenes, R. (1999) 'Toward a framework for computer mediated collaborative design in medical informatics', *Methods for Informatics in Medicine* 38, 158–76.

Pham, B. and Yearwood, J. (2000) 'Delivery and interactive processing of visual data for a co-operative telemedicine environment', *Telemedicine Journal* 6, 261–8.

Polley, F., Humphreys, J., Grogan, H., Hegney, D., Knight, S., Nichols, A. and Veitch, C. (1996) 'Fostering multidisciplinary research and approaches to rural health issues: the concept of an international summer institute', *Australian Journal of Rural Health* 4, 80–88.

Reeves, S., Meyer, J., Glynn, M. and Bridges, J. (1999) 'Co-ordination of interprofessional health care teams in a general and emergency directorate', *Advancing Clinical Practice* 3, 49–59.

Rheingold, H. (1994) *The Virtual Community: Surfing the Internet*, London: Minerva.

Salmon, G. (2000) *E-moderating: The Key to Teaching and Learning Online*, London: Kogan Page.

Williams, G. and Laungani, P. (1999) 'Analysis of teamwork in an NHS community trust: an empirical study', *Journal of Interprofessional Care* 13 (1) 19–28.

Wootton, R. (2001) 'Telemedicine', *British Medical Journal* 323, 557–60.

Wootton, R., Bloomer, S., Corbett, R., Eedy, S., Hicks, N., Lotery, H., Mathews, C., Paisley, J., Steele, K. and Loane, M. (2000) 'Multicentre randomised control trial comparing real time teledermatology with conventional outpatient dermatological care: societal cost–benefit analysis', *British Medical Journal* 320, 1252–6.

Young, A., Chadwick, D. and New, J. (2001) 'Providing secure remote access to legacy healthcare applications', *Computing and Control Engineering Journal* 12, 148–56.

Chapter 7

Models for interprofessional collaboration

Audrey Leathard

SUMMARY

The purpose of a model is initially set out with interprofessional collaboration mathematically justified. Models for collaborative grading, collaborative working and interprofessional consultation are presented. A selection of models are then discussed for professions and organisations working together towards integration followed by an action map for health needs assessment. Models for user empowerment, user-centred approaches and change conclude the review. The place of evaluation is considered, followed by an overall compendium for effective teamworking.

THE PURPOSE OF MODELS

In bringing together various models for display and analysis, the purpose is fourfold. First, the possibility of comparable application is useful whereby other fields of interprofessional practice can then be compared and possibly applied. From comparison, new approaches can be considered for different arenas. The model on mergers, to be shown later, provides a neat example for application.

A second opportunity is for a model to display a manageable context of how professionals or sectors can work together effectively, or otherwise, within an interagency context. In this chapter, subsequent models on interprofessional practice provide some useful examples.

A third, rather different, purpose can be to indicate ways forward for change and innovation as well as to show the need for professions and organisations to change over time. A significant model to demonstrate the effects of change is the Sigmoid Curve that is presented as the final model in the sequence.

The fourth factor is probably the most important in that a model can provide a basis for evaluation to enable the context to be applied and assessed over time. The following presentation of models does not necessarily seek to expand on all four points in each illustration but rather to open up a vision of possibilities in different ways of working together. Overall, in answer to the question, why bother with interprofessional collaboration, the sequence on models starts with a mathematical justification.

THE ADDITIVE AND MULTIPLICATIVE EFFECTS MODELS

Don Rawson (1994) has creatively argued that two distinct versions of the effects of interprofessional work are possible. Under the *additive effects model*, each profession adds its own particular contribution where interprofessional practice is defined as the sum of the professional perspectives. No one group controls the area in total but contributions from each of the professional groups involved must be taken into account and this is best achieved when professions work together. However under the *multiplicative effects model*, combined, integrated efforts can achieve more than is possible simply by adding contributions. Interprofessional work can thus generate new potential and enhance the input of individuals whereby professionals thus working together can produce a magic between groups. The multiplicative effects model thus underpins collaborative potential in the belief that the whole can become greater than the sum of the parts.

Expressed mathematically, the *additive effects model* reflects a lower score, for example: $2 + 2 + 2 + 2 + 2 = 10$, which achieves less than *multiplicative effects*: $2 \times 2 \times 2 \times 2 \times 2 = 32$. The outcome suggests a nice mathematical justification to support interprofessional collaboration.

MODELS FOR PROFESSIONALS WORKING TOGETHER

This section starts by setting out a taxonomy of collaboration, based on collaborative grading, which shows how far professionals were working together in the early 1990s. Other models are then considered on different ways of approaching interprofessional practice and teamworking.

Collaborative grading

In one of the first studies on *Interprofessional Collaboration in Primary Health Care Organisations*, Gregson et al (1991, 1992) developed indices for the degree of collaboration between district nurses, general practitioners and health visitors in a stratified random sample of 20 district health authorities in England. Table 7.1 displays the outcome: a taxonomy of collaboration adapted from work by Armitage (1983) on joint working in primary health care.

Table 7.1 A taxonomy of collaboration

I No direct communication	Members who never meet, talk or write to each other
2 Formal, brief communication	Members who encounter or correspond but do not interact meaningfully
3 Regular communication and consultation	Members whose encounters or correspondence include the transference of information
4 High level of joint working	Members who act on that information sympathetically, participate in general patterns of joint working; subscribe to the same general objectives as others on a one-to-one basis in the same organisation
5 Multidisciplinary working	Involvement of all workers in a primary health care setting

Source: Gregson et al (1992).

By the early 1990s, the results showed a relatively low level of joint working between doctors and nurses (24 per cent) and an even lower score for doctors and health visitors working together (8 per cent). At the highest level of collaboration – multidisciplinary working – for both groups, the scores were the same and minimal in both cases (3 per cent). Gregson et al (1992) concluded overall that only 27 per cent of general practitioners and district nurses with patients in common and 11 per cent of general practitioners and health visitors 'collaborated'. While valuable in providing a useful grading approach, one problem is to perceive what actually counts as collaboration across the rating elements. The five terms used in the model can be interpreted differently in a span of potential collaboration. However, by the early twenty-first century, if a similar study were to be conducted in the UK, the 'collaborative' elements, however interpreted, would undoubtedly achieve a higher score but the arena has become more complex as other professional groups have increasingly worked in primary health care teams. Further, from 2002, with the development of care trusts between health and social care services, a sixth level could now usefully be introduced under 'integration'.

Models of interprofessional collaboration

In the light of the White Paper *The new NHS* (Secretary of State for Health 1997), the New Labour government outlined a strategy of joint working underpinned by a partnership approach at the front line. In this context, Hudson (1998) pins down collaboration under four different models of joint working (Table 7.2) that span lower to higher levels of collaborative involvement.

At the lower level of collaboration, *communication* can vary from simply giving information or, with a little more structure, can lead to formal

Table 7.2 Models of interprofessional collaboration

• Communication	Interactions are confined to the exchange of information
• Coordination	Individuals remain in separate organisations and locations but develop formal ways of working across boundaries
• Co-location	Members of different professions are physically located alongside each other
• Commissioning	Professionals with a commissioning remit develop a shared approach to the activity

Source: Hudson (1998: 26–7).

agreements between primary care practices and social services. *Coordination* can cover various forms of shared assessment and joint provision. *Co-location* has generally referred to social services staff based in a general practice from which evaluated arrangements have usually been favourable. However, *commissioning* can include not only the three previous elements, but also a higher level of collaboration where joint commissioning takes place between primary health care practices and social services departments. However, as Hudson (1998: 26–7) points out, what is also needed is a strategy of planning for joint working where health and social care needs are held together. Meanwhile, partnership prospects can be challenged by professional and cultural barriers, different perceptions of costs and benefits, as well as different patterns of employment, accountability and decision-making.

A model for interprofessional consultation

From a background of psychiatry and psychotherapy, Steinberg (1989) sets out to consider the ways and means of how professionals and patients can work together based on the viewpoint that interprofessional consultation is one form of collaborative work. While good consultation is likely to be educational, consultation uniquely provides a joint method of enquiry into the 'fundamental nature of problems and ways of responding to them' (Steinberg 1989: 14). Consultation can therefore provide new approaches to understanding problems and innovative management strategies. Consultation can equally demonstrate where an institution or organisation is failing and where training, staffing or supervision are inadequate. The categories in Table 7.3 reflect the wide arena in which consultative work can operate.

From the model presented, Steinberg (1989: 23) argues that consultation, through the various mechanisms suggested, may be the most appropriate way to bring people together with different skills and experience. Although perceived essentially as a teaching and learning experience based on shared appraisal, the model also points a way forward, more widely, for professionals to work together effectively in practice.

Table 7.3 Categories of consultative work

1 The circumstances under which undertaken	• Single *ad-hoc* consultation: both urgent and non-urgent • Planned consultations: either a series or indefinite
2 The overall aim	• Primarily problem-solving, with training as a secondary benefit • Primarily training, with problem-solving as an additional benefit
3 The focus of the work	• Client-centred; consultee-centred; work-centred
4 The people involved	• Individual • Group: open or closed
5 Continuing reappraisal at a more informal level: circularity in consultation	• What are the facts of the situation? • Who is involved? • What are the feelings? • How does the situation look now?

Source: Modified from Steinberg (1989: 23, 65).

Models for interprofessional practice

In a consideration of how groups of professionals can work together, Don Rawson (1994) has devised a mapping of sets in Figure 7.1.

The model of sets can be applied to various fields of interprofessional practice to elucidate what aspects of the sets are working well and where problems need to be addressed. As Rawson (1994: 43) points out, the inter-section of different types of professional work is likely to blur tasks and responsibilities that can lead some professionals involved to try to recreate their own specialisms and work relationships. A further challenge to joint working is the likelihood that different groups in the health and welfare professions may well be at different levels of development in working practices. Levels of expertise, job descriptions and standard operating procedures can well influence who gives way and on what issues.

Nevertheless, as constant changes occur in the structure of the services for

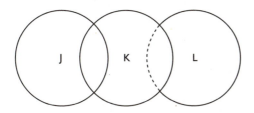

Figure 7.1 Sets with permeable and impermeable boundaries: J = General Medicine; K = Community Medicine; L = Health Education.

Source: Rawson (1994: 43). Reproduced by kind permission of Brunner-Routledge.

health and social care, Figure 7.1 demonstrates the possibility that some boundaries may dissolve (denoted by a dotted line) whereupon professional responsibilities may be transferred, shared or absorbed by one group. As applied hypothetically to Figure 7.1, health education work may become eclipsed by community medicine, which then has the potential to take over or assimilate the field. As boundaries become impermeable, so professionals have to reach an agreement over work sharing and involvement that is mutually acceptable or agree to differ. As Rawson (1994: 44) points out, to survive intact professions, which are overshadowed by more powerful rivals, have to make their professional concerns functionally dissimilar. One alternative model for the professions is to uphold a new common purpose to realign, assimilate or meld the older occupational groupings into an interprofessional engagement and outlook. A more ambitious model is to dissolve boundaries through seamless care which, in theory, is the intention behind the integration of health and social care provision for care trusts in the future.

Models for teamwork

Teamwork can, however, represent one effective way for professionals to work together. From many in this field, three models have been selected that reflect some interesting aspects of interprofessional practice; Chapter 8 later looks at teamworking in more detail.

First, the place of the individual in a team is nicely illustrated (Figure 7.2)

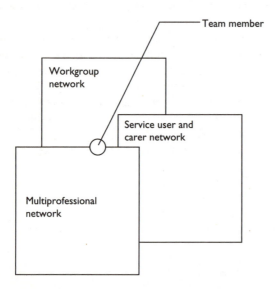

Figure 7.2 Three interlocking networks in multiprofessional teamwork.

Source: Payne, M. (2000: 127) *Teamwork in Multiprofessional Care*, London: Macmillan Press. Reproduced with permission of Palgrave Macmillan.

by Malcolm Payne (2000: 127). A team member, more particularly working within the field of health and social care, is essentially placed at the centre of three interlocking networks involving the workgroup, user and carer, as well as the multiprofessional team network which connects the relevant professionals to the team member, the carer and service user. An important aspect of effective teamwork is usually regarded as based on meeting the individual needs of team members and respecting their contributions (Payne 2000: 114). Key factors in building up teamwork include respect for professional identity, clearly agreed goals and the acceptance of each individual member (see also the conclusion to this chapter).

Second, the role of team members has been widely analysed in seeking to define a successful team. Table 7.4 brings together some of the ideas set out by Belbin (1981) from a management training background, alongside a somewhat corresponding but more simplified analysis from Parker (1990). Belbin's (1981) argument is that, to be effective, teams need leaders, shapers and other useful members; in other words without the inclusion of the contributors (Table 7.4) the team becomes unbalanced and functions less well.

However, as Payne (2000: 122) comments on acknowledging the influence of Belbin's work, the labels for people and the roles of groups may change over time nor is the full complexity of the roles of team members necessarily reflected. Further, Belbin's work is based on management teams that may not necessarily relate to interprofessional practice. However, Belbin's ideas do provide a context in which to understand teamwork and are a useful introduction to teams and their roles.

Third, applied to interprofessional working in a team, alongside the roles of team members, the competencies of individuals in the team are equally important in order to address the issues and demands together. In Table 7.5 Engel (1994) has listed the competencies for collaboration in teams. Since the mid-1990s much has changed in the structure and outlook of the health and

Table 7.4 The roles of team players to create an effective team

Belbin (1981)	Parker (1990)
Leaders	*Collaborators* who focus on goals
Shapers	Flexible
Resource Investigators	Open to new ideas
Company workers	*Contributors* who focus on tasks; contribute good
Completer-finishers	information, hard work and are dependable
Chairs	*Communicators* who focus on the team process; resolve
Teamworkers	conflicts; are good listeners
Monitor-evaluators	*Challengers* who focus on questions and issues; evaluate
Plants	standards; push the team forward

Table 7.5 A model for some competencies for collaboration in teams

Abilities	
Superordinate	*Subordinate*
Adapting to change	Coping with ambiguity and uncertainty
	Critical reasoning
Participating in change	Continuing own education
Managing self and managing with others	Identifying and analysing problems; selecting appropriate means towards their resolution; monitoring progress; evaluating outcomes
Communication	Practising empathy

Source: Engel (1994: 69).

social care services, wherein an ever increasing emphasis has been placed on partnership and joint working but the competencies needed have changed little.

By the start of the twenty-first century, under 'subordinate' one might add being involved with interprofessional education. Under 'superordinate', a further item might be the capacity to work with ever limited funds for ever extending demands. However, the latter item could be nutshelled under 'managing'. Certainly the importance of adapting to and participating in change remains as key a feature as ever. In discussion with Professor Charles Engel in the autumn of 2001, as to whether any present item should now appear in the listings with regard to competencies for collaboration, an important development would suggest placing 'emotional intelligence' under 'superordinate'. Drawing on work by Goleman (1996), the issues refer to verbal and non-verbal appraisal and to the expression of emotion as well as the utilisation of emotional content in problem solving. Within an interprofessional context, for example, the personal relationships between people – the likes and dislikes across teams, the place of control – would be relevant to 'emotional intelligence' where the regulation of emotion in the self and with respect to others plays a part, among other needs, in balance and reconciliation.

The need to control expenditure on health and social care has led to an increasing requirement to establish team effectiveness that much depends on the criteria used. Although teamwork can be challenged by problems when different professional groups work together, conflict can also be used to creative benefit for collaboration.

AGENCIES, SECTORS AND ORGANISATIONS WORKING TOGETHER

One crucial factor in the provision of health and social care has been the need to bring various professional groups to work together across agencies and sectors. A selection of models now looks at this angle then considers wider possibilities for organisational joint working. The first model (Figure 7.3) shows an approach with regard to service provision for child health and social services for children in need.

Here is a model that accommodates specific professional input for certain aspects of the health and social services but is a clear arena for joint working. A neat division of responsibilities can be seen but, as the Audit Commission (1994a: 3) has pointed out, the overlap of responsibilities between social services and health authorities requires major adjustments to the way agencies work and relate to each other. However, change can soon shift the boundaries. In discussion with practitioner M.Sc. students, other good points have been raised such as that the centrepiece looks like a black hole for joint working; that boundaries are not static but tend to move to respond to needs and events; and that the division of activities between the NHS and social services is not necessarily equi-distant. The charm of models is to show ways forward and possibilities but also to enliven critical analysis.

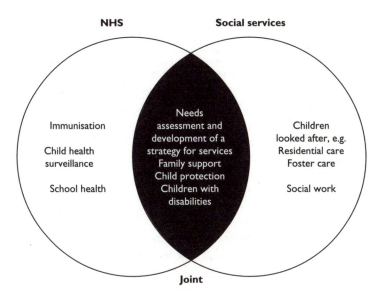

Figure 7.3 Services provided by the NHS and Social Services. Many activities fall within the remit of both NHS and Social Services.

Source: Audit Commission (1994a: 3). Exhibit 2, reproduced by kind permission of the Audit Commission.

PUBLIC/PRIVATE PARTNERSHIPS

A further analytical advantage of Figure 7.3 is the potential for application. As the public and private sector have been increasingly drawn together within specific contexts, one can reset the model (Table 7.6) for a different sphere of evaluation.

The interest for analysis can be to assess the customer and cost-effectiveness of ventures across the separate forms of provision in Table 7.6 in comparison with joint working and partnership outcomes as well as the potential for drawing up the advantages and disadvantages of each section. However, the problem in the application of the model in Table 7.6 is the sheer complexity of the issues whether in the public or private sector or with regard to working in partnership.

Table 7.6 Public/private partnerships in health and social care

Public sector Specific separate provision	Partnership/joint working	Private sector Specific separate provision

NHS health care provision
Local authority community
   care provision
	Private finance initiatives (PFI)[a]
	Public sector payments for private
	   health care provision
	Public/private partnerships
		Hospitals
		Dental care
		Osteopathy
		Physiotherapy
		Care homes

Note:
[a] PFI: A private sector consortium pays for a new hospital. The local NHS trust pays the consortium a regular fee for hospital use, which covers construction costs, the rent of the building, the cost of support services and the risks transferred to the private sector. See Chapter 2 for private concordats.

The next model concerns a review of mental health services for adults in which the Audit Commission (1994b) has acknowledged that a range of service provision is necessary to meet individual needs.

The interest in this field of work is, as Figure 7.4 displays, the wide range of different services involved that cut across the boundaries of social services, health care, social security and housing. Further, poverty and inadequate housing are high priorities for users but which are often overlooked by professionals who tend to focus on treatment and therapy (Audit Commission 1994b: 17). Therefore, one critique of the model is that the services tend to appear to be of an equal level of involvement and access to users, which is not necessarily the case. However, many people with mental health problems live in the community so mental health teams have a demanding role in seeking to coordinate the various services across different sectors to meet user needs. Again in discussion with practitioner M.Sc. students, looking at this model, two interesting points have been made. First, the family, friends and clients seem trapped within the circle with no way out. A second, very different issue raised, is that the encircled users sometimes simply do not wish to be helped

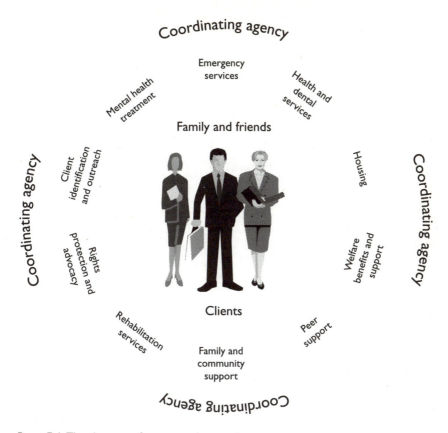

Figure 7.4 The elements of an appropriate service.

Source: Audit Commission (1994b: 17). Adapted from J. Carson and T. Sharma (1994) 'In-patient psychiatric care. What helps? Staff and patient perspectives', *Journal of Mental Health* 3, 99–104. Reproduced by kind permission of the *Journal of Mental Health* (http://www.tandf.co.uk).

nor receive care. The above model therefore presents an arena for consideration within a complex field of caring, but widely dispersed, services.

A model for carers and services

Seen from the angle of carers, a wide range of services can be of benefit, either directly or indirectly. However, the way agencies and professions have structured themselves, services are often separately organised and packaged in an array of different arenas, as illustrated by Powell and Kocher (1996: 15).

The model (Figure 7.5) reflects a basic problem in that the support and provision for carers' needs do not fit neatly into the way services are organised

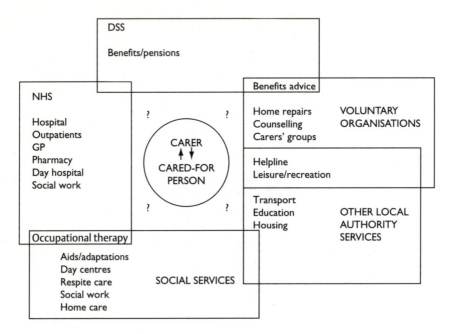

Figure 7.5 Carers and services.

Source: M. Powell and P. Kocher (1996: 15) *Strategies for Change: A Carers' Impact Resource Book*, London: King's Fund Publishing. Reproduced by kind permission of the King's Fund (www.kingsfund.org.uk).

and delivered. Unlike the field of mental health, no central team is necessarily available to coordinate the services. While the carer usually wants to be able to assemble a flexible package of care and support, a further issue is that needs are likely to change over time, both for the cared for and the carer. As Powell and Kocher (1996) contend, the key challenge for community care is the requisite to alter the system to become more responsive to the needs of service users and carers. By the twenty-first century, a further factor would be for interprofessional and interagency collaboration to play a lead part in this complex arena.

The jigsaw model

A rather different approach is to consider the purpose and outcome of working together. Drawing on the field of the mental health services, the Audit Commission (1994b: 55) has argued that the requirements for a comprehensive service must all be drawn together at a strategic level. In other words, strategic planning should determine the level and balance of resources, the priorities for the resources available and, importantly, the means of coordination and collaboration between them. Figure 7.6 shows how, starting with

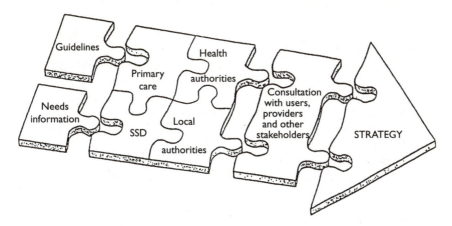

Figure 7.6 The jigsaw model: developing a strategy for mental health.
        SSD: Social Services Department.

Source: Audit Commission (1994b: 55). Adapted for the 2001 structure in Britain. Exhibit 26: Reproduced by kind permission of the Audit Commission.

guidelines and information on needs, the steps towards strategy can interlock across the services, the authorities and user consultation, towards a strategic goal.

In the field of mental health, the potential sources of information on needs cover a range of arenas from directors of public health, contract managers, general practitioners, mental health teams, local authority social services and housing, voluntary organisations, users and carers, as well as the criminal justice system. By the mid-1990s, the Audit Commission (1994b: 54) still found that individuals and groups often worked in isolation nor was information shared, thus effort was often duplicated. The 2002 development of care trusts, based on integrated provision, should be in a better position to address a collaborative strategy.

A model for mergers

Strongly influenced by the impact of the internal market from 1990–97 to curb costs, mergers increasingly took place among the purchasers of health care. Mergers developed between district health authorities, and between family health service authorities, both of which then merged into health authorities by 1996; GP fundholders started to work together, then more widely, with all the various purchasers to form total fundholding groups with health authorities.

Similarly, by the mid-1990s, hospital trusts also saw the potential for providers to merge. Following the proposals under *The NHS Plan* (Secretary of State for Health 2000), a rush towards mergers across primary care groups and trusts and between health authorities took place, which has led to the re-evaluation of health authority roles as much of their commissioning role is to be relinquished in favour of a strategic focus across greater geographical areas (McGauran 2001).

The pressure to merge organisations across health care provision can be set out under the following perceived advantages among others:

- Substantial savings especially cutting management costs
- The potential to act as a catalyst for change and improvement in services
- Measurable benefits for patients and users
- Demonstrating long-term benefits despite short-term disruption (Edwards and Passman 1997)

However, experience has shown that health service mergers can be problematical regarding the length of time for implementation; the predicted financial benefits – often somewhat disappointing (Audit Commission 1995); the likely tensions between professional groups; or a stronger and weaker organisation on merging, which may then be perceived as a take-over; mergers can also be a blunt instrument for improving management (Edwards and Passman 1997). The most certain result of a merger is, according to the Audit Commission (1995: 11), uncertainty. Figure 7.7 therefore sets out one useful model for the merger of two organisations.

Although the model depicts the merger of two former organisations (District Health Authorities), which could no longer be compared in scale or scope with present structures, the merger pattern is still of value as a way to overcome some of the inherent problems. Stages are agreed where the easier steps are undertaken first, to be followed by the more ambitious forms of working together, in order to establish an eventual merger. Each stage on the pathway also has a clear purpose to ensure a single entity for organisational permanence. The Audit Commission (1993: 11) acknowledged that many months may be needed for merged staff to work together effectively, particularly where partnership has come without the full commitment of all the participants. The run-up to the formation of a merger can also create uncertainty for staff that can itself become an obstacle to progress. Even when a merger has been carefully planned and handled with sensitivity, staff can still experience long-term upset and distress as in the case of the merger between Epsom Health Care and St. Helier trusts (Gillett 2000). Nevertheless, in principle, the model for working more closely together (Figure 7.7) provides one pathway to enable an effective merger.

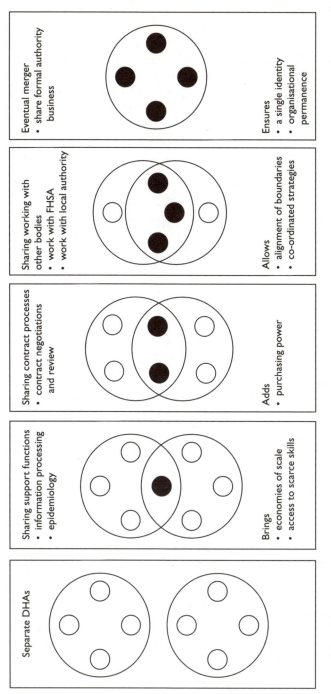

Figure 7.7 Working more closely together.

Source: Audit Commission (1993: 10) stated that 'many different models have evolved of joint working between the (former) DHAs (District Health Authorities) and the FHSA (Family Health Service Authority), under Exhibit 3'. Reproduced by kind permission of the Audit Commission.

MODELS FOR INTEGRATING HEALTH AND SOCIAL CARE PROVISION

The culmination of breaking down boundary divisions can be perceived as working towards achieving integration between health and social care services. The development of care trusts in England from 2002 is one way forward. Under *The NHS Plan* (Secretary of State for Health 2000), two types of care trust are envisaged: (1) a new level of primary care trusts that will provide for even closer integration of health and social services; and (2) the joining of secondary care NHS mental health trusts with social services. The two types are now considered under models for integration to indicate the potential for care trusts in the future.

Under the first type, the compilation in Table 7.7 is based on the work of the Joint Unit at the Department of Health, which spans social care and health services policy with lead responsibilities for partnerships, joint investment plans, continuing care policy, and, in particular, the development of care trusts. Within this context, the cultural, professional and constitutional differences and difficulties are acknowledged such as tribalism, territorialism and traditionalism.

Table 7.7 Integrating health and social care – emerging policies

Management	Finance; accountability	Innovative service models
Unified management for commissioning and integrated provision	Pooled funds/budgets not obligatory but with flexibilities	One-stop shops
		Integrated teams
		Resource centres
Whole systems approach to training, information and finance	Partners make proposals about governance with service level agreements and extent of delegation	Opportunities to include all health-related local authority functions including housing
Local flexibility tailored to local circumstances		
Single assessment	Targets with standards to be attained	
Single management structure	Trusts to be corporate bodies responsible both to NHS and LAs*	
Aims for care trusts	**Partnership schemes**	**Patients, users, customers**
Organisational stability to develop innovative approaches and integrated teams	Intermediate care	Patients' forum involvement
	Learning disabilities	Partnership integral to user focus and quality improvement
	Mental health	
	Joint equipment	
Coordinated services	Drug and alcohol services	
Enshrined in partnership – building on 1999 Health Act	Speech and language therapy	Patients make proposals about governance
		Customer-focused care

Source: Table adapted and modified from Bell (2001).

Note:
*NHS (National Health Service); LAs (local authorities).

Nevertheless, despite an overall vision of seeking to integrate services across the board, one element omitted is the charging for services that remains unquestioned, as a local authority responsibility based on means-tested needs assessment, while NHS services remain 'free' at the point of use.

A model for effective service integration

As the first integrated care trust in England, Somerset Partnership NHS and Social Care represents the second type of care trust. However, the local social care director has commented that, in deciding to integrate health and social care, the local area drew on a strong history of joint working (Okell 2001). However, as the Somerset Partnership went live in April 1999, the context does not entirely match the envisaged clinical governance or detailed arrangements for newly formed care trusts from 2002. Nevertheless, as new care trusts begin to take shape, the value of the developments in Somerset is to see how integration has been successfully achieved.

What had been integrated by 2001? Care trusts were confirmed under the Health and Social Care Act 2001. Statutory powers are thus available to permit the establishment of combined NHS mental health trusts with social services social care trusts. The emerging outcome has enabled four localities to become coterminous with primary care groups; each locality is managed by a manager and an assistant who come from opposite backgrounds (one from health and one from social care). Social care is represented at every level to include an executive director of social care; all managers are officers of the county council and the mental health trust who can thus spend against either budget; all staff are co-located in multidisciplinary teams while one integrated care process brings together the Care Programme Approach (health) with care management (social services) so that clients have one key-worker, care plan and review. How was integration then achieved successfully? (see Table 7.8)

From one model of successful integration, once again the different charging policies remain an unresolved issue wherein an integrated policy has certainly not taken place. Further, as elsewhere, approved social workers cannot be employed by care trusts in this capacity, so a mechanism has had to be found to employ approved social workers by social services although managed by the Somerset Partnership. Nevertheless, despite the challenges, integration has been achieved, above all, through effective communication (Okell 2001).

A model for needs assessment

Whether in care trusts or across the whole spectrum of health and social care, needs assessment plays a central part in securing cost-effectiveness, alongside strategic planning and service evaluation. One model (Figure 7.8) is now set

Table 7.8 Key contributing factors towards effective service integration

- A joint commissioning board (first, in shadow form then, to bcome fully operational) made up of officers from the social services and the health authority
- Integrated information technology systems
- Extensive consultation that led to a 'bottom-up' development and widespread commitment
- Commitment to the vision of integration throughout the organisations
- Notable 'champions'
- Political will
- Historical background of good multi-agency working
- Clear goals and objectives regarding the need for better services
- Trust and commitment
- Involvement of all the stakeholders in the review and implementation process

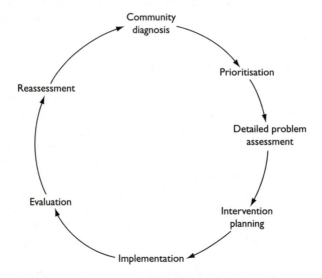

Figure 7.8 An assessment of the population's health needs.

Source: Gillam et al (1998: 54). Reproduced by kind permission of the *Journal of Interprofessional Care.*

out, drawn from the field of community-oriented primary care, to show a useful approach in the assessment of needs.

Although the model is related to health, the approach can equally well be linked to social care. The assessment of the population's needs can be carried out in seven stages. First for *community diagnosis*, a team of professionals define the health problems of the community on the basis of the available quantitative and qualitative data. The second stage is *prioritisation* where a simple grid is used to score each health problem in relation to specific criteria (the size and severity of the problem; the availability of effective intervention, the acceptability to the team and the consumer; feasibility, community involvement and cost-effectiveness). Having selected the issue for investigation, the team then assesses the extent of the priority problem in the total population (*detailed problem assessment*) that constitutes the base line for later evaluation. The *intervention planning* defines the relevant activities as to who is responsible for *implementation* in terms of the records and resources required, the training needs, the liaison across services and the deadlines involved. Under *evaluation*, the team then considers the methods to use in assessing how far the programme objectives have been met. Finally under *reassessment* in the light of the evaluation, a decision is made as to whether to continue with the particular intervention. Gillam et al's (1998) model helpfully provides a useful way to approach the assessment of the population's needs, which can be applied to an integrated health and social care approach, as the steps outlined have relevance to both forms of provision within a collaborative context.

Models for users

How far users have gained from interprofessional collaboration remains somewhat unclear but the first of two models show the potential. In Figure 7.9, Hornby and Atkins (2000) present a resource pool that represents the sum total of help to a particular individual or family living in a locality. From a user-centred and community-oriented perspective, rather than profession-centred and agency-oriented viewpoint, the resource pool takes on a different look.

Rather differently from most other interprofessional models, Figure 7.9 shows how the user can be placed at the centre as a potential self-helper but surrounded by faceworkers: the human face of help and provision. The approach suggests that four types of help can then be applied according to need: personal, community, general and special help. Within a community care approach, the importance of the ordinary life sector is emphasised, which extends the range of potential helpers (Hornby and Atkins 2000: 83–4).

Figure 7.10 shows, again, the user at the centre of the resource pool but surrounded by a complex arena of services and settings. Although guided by faceworkers at the ground (as distinct from the management) level, Hornby and Atkins (2000: 9) draw attention to the need for close collaboration, as an integrative approach does not necessarily weaken the boundaries between agencies or different types of helper. In order to maximise the full use of each potential source of help, there is a need to clarify the differences of input and the areas of overlap.

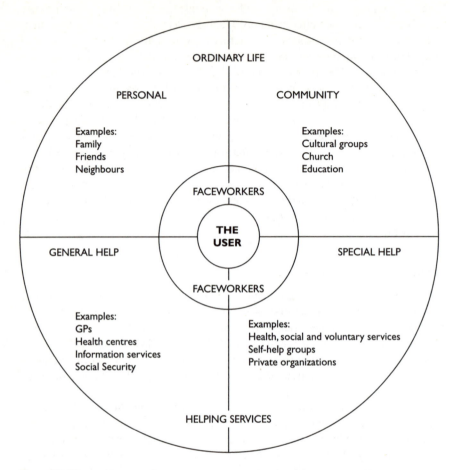

Figure 7.9 The resource pool.

Source: S. Hornby and J. Atkins (2000:84) *Collaborative Care: Interprofessional, Interagency and Interpersonal,* 2nd edn., Oxford: Blackwell Science. Reproduced by kind permission of Blackwell Science.

A model for user empowerment

The next step towards enabling patients and users to be at the central focus of provision is user empowerment. Figure 7.11 displays some key initiatives suggested by Braye and Preston-Shoot (1995) to further empowering practice in social care.

Figure 7.11 envisages an ascending pathway of possibilities from recognising the centrality of values towards appropriate empowering services. Forces resisting change are recognised in power or orthodoxy and convention; professional mistrust and fears (lack of status and expertise); user mistrust; fear of change and uncertainty; organisational constraints; and legislative

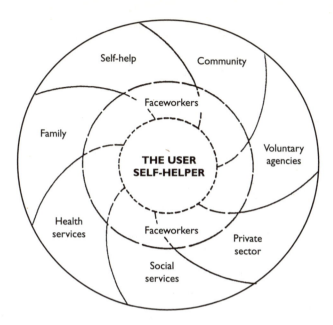

Figure 7.10 The user-centred model of help.

Source: S. Hornby and J. Atkins (2000: 9) *Collaborative Care: Interprofessional, Interagency and Interpersonal*, 2nd edn., Oxford: Blackwell Science. Reproduced by kind permission of Blackwell Science.

ambiguity. However, forces that can work positively for change include legal and policy mandates, professional mandates as well as user self-advocacy mandates. Overall, Braye and Preston-Shoot (1995) argue that much of what is labelled partnership practice is at best participation in worker and agency controlled agendas that represent a two-dimensional power relationship. Partnership practice does, however, have the potential to engage with power issues within a three-dimensional perspective, which thus involves also working together with service recipients, and thus contributes to user empowerment.

A model for change

The Sigmoid Curve sums up the pathway for change. As Handy (1994) describes, initiatives, organisations, even empires start slowly and experimentally, rise successfully, then wane. Applied to interprofessional ventures over the last decade, a similar start has been made. However, as Figure 7.12 shows, to sustain constant growth and development, a new Sigmoid Curve at point A is needed, otherwise the first curve peters out to B, as various corporations and companies have found to their cost.

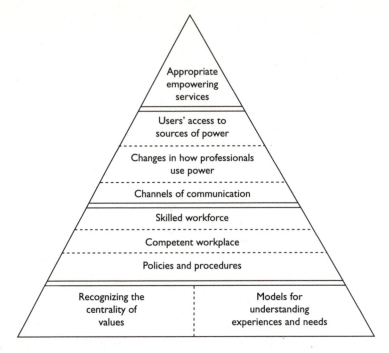

Figure 7.11 Key initiatives for empowerment.

Source: S. Braye and M. Preston-Shoot (1995: 113) *Empowering Practice in Social Care*, Buckingham: Open University Press. Reproduced by permission from the Open University Press.

Meanwhile, the shaded area in Figure 7.12 shows the turmoil, contentions and challenges involved with change, when time, resources, energy and vision are needed to enable a further curve upwards towards a renewed future. Working towards collaborative integration, health and social care may reflect

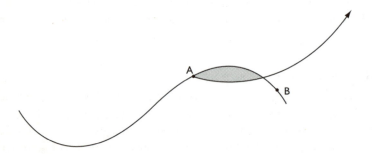

Figure 7.12 The Sigmoid Curve

Source: Handy (1994: 51); 'The Sigmoid Curve' from THE EMPTY RAINCOAT by Charles Handy published by Hutchinson. Used by permission of the Random House Group Limited.

an upward curve but, as Handy (1994: 50) warns, units of time are becoming smaller (once generations, then decades, then years and sometimes months) so the accelerating pace of change shrinks every Sigmoid Curve.

CONCLUSION

One present drawback with models for interprofessional collaboration is the limited evaluation in practice. As the Sigmoid Curve reflects, the quickening pace of change in the provision of health and social care tends to race past the opportunity for considered evaluation of inputs and outcomes to guide the future.

Interprofessional evaluation has therefore been limited with the exception of significant assessments from the field of interprofessional education (see Chapter 19) as well as from studies that focus on specific policy initiatives, for example, on health improvement programmes (Arora et al 2000) and Health Action Zones (Judge 1999). Meanwhile, research from the National Primary Care Research and Development Centre in Manchester has increasingly made an impact in the field of primary care where the work of Caroline Glendinning and Kirstein Rummery (see Chapter 13) has particular relevance for interprofessional and interagency issues with regard to older people. However, the more extensive research has been in the field of teamwork from McGrath's (1991) earlier work on community mental handicap teams in Clywd, Wales onwards. Nevertheless, on reviewing the studies undertaken, Rink et al (2000) have pointed out that the relationship between teamwork and patient outcome remains poorly understood as well as limited with regard to the enhancement of the quality of care, although some evidence does point to the beneficial effects of teamwork on the team members themselves.

This chapter therefore concludes with a compendium, from more recent research, on ways to achieve effective teamworking, first from Poulton and West (1999) whose work has extended across the last decade.

- *Individuals* should feel important to the team and to the team's success; should have an interactive and meaningful role; which should be identifiable and subject to evaluation
- *Teams* should have intrinsically and interesting tasks to undertake, with clear goals set, shared objectives and built-in performance feedback
- *Quality* emphasis and support for innovation are also important

The compendium could be usefully supplemented, by findings from Rummery and Glendinning's (2000) study on looking at *Developing New Partnerships for Older People*, in order to feature three further factors:

- *Commitment* from key managers and budget-holders
- *Acknowledging barriers* to collaboration
- *The need to involve patients/users* through, for example, surveys or direct participation on relevant boards

Overall, while change can soon shift boundaries and team structures, compendiums and models have their moments and assessment value. One positive feature is the gain to be derived from the application of models and subsequent modifications to improve services overall.

REFERENCES

Armitage, P. (1983) 'Joint working in primary health care' (Occasional Paper), *Nursing Times* 79, 75–8.

Arora, S., Davies, A. and Thompson, S. (2000) 'Developing health improvement programmes: challenges for a new millennium', *Journal of Interprofession Care* 14 (1) 9–18.

Audit Commission (1993) *Their Health, Your Business: The New Role of the District Health Authority*, London: HMSO.

Audit Commission (1994a) *Seen But Not Heard: Co-ordinating Community Child Health and Social Services for Children in Need*, London: HMSO.

Audit Commission (1994b) *Finding a Place: A Review of Mental Health Services for Adults*, London: HMSO.

Audit Commission (1995) *Less Dangerous Liaisons: Early Considerations for Making Mergers Work*, London: HMSO.

Belbin, R. (1981) *Management Teams: Why they Succeed or Fail*, London: Heinemann.

Bell, C. (2001) 'Integrating Health and Social Care – Emerging Policies', in *Integrating Health and Social Care*, Harrogate: Harrogate Management Centre. (No editor but a conference compilation.)

Braye, S. and Preston-Shoot, M. (1995) *Empowering Practice in Social Care*, Buckingham: Open University Press.

Carson, J. and Sharma, T. (1994) 'In-patient psychiatric care. What helps? Staff and patient perspectives, *Journal of Mental Health* 3, 99–104.

Edwards, N. and Passman, D. (1997) 'All mixed up', *Health Service Journal* 107 (5557) 30–31.

Engel, C. (1994) 'A functional anatomy of teamwork', in A. Leathard (ed.), *Going Inter-professional: Working Together for Health and Welfare*, London: Routledge.

Gillam, S., Joffe, M., Miller, R., Gray, A., Epstein, L. and Plamping, D. (1998) 'Community-oriented primary care – old wine in new bottles', *Journal of Interprofessional Care* 12 (1) 53–61.

Gillett, S. (2000) 'Turn of the Screw', *Health Service Journal* 111 (5699) 22–3.

Goleman, D. (1996) *Emotional Intelligence*, London: Bloomsbury Publishing.

Gregson, B., Cartlidge, A. and Bond, J. (1991) *Interprofessional Collaboration in Primary Health Care Organizations*, (Occasional Paper 52), London: Royal College of General Practitioners.

Gregson, B., Cartlidge, A. and Bond, J. (1992) 'Development of a measure of professional collaboration in primary health care', *Journal of Epidemiology and Community Health* 46, 48–53.

Handy, C. (1994) *The Empty Raincoat: Making Sense of the Future*, London: Hutchinson.

Hornby, S. and Atkins, J. (2000) *Collaborative Care: Interprofessional, Interagency and Interprofessional*, 2nd edn., Oxford: Blackwell Science.

Hudson, B. (1998) 'Prospects of Partnership', *Health Service Journal* 108 (5600) 26–7.

Judge, K. (1999) 'National Evaluation of Health Action Zones', in A. Bebbington and K. Judge (eds), *PSSRU Bulletin*, Canterbury: Personal Social Services Research Unit.

McGauran, A. (2001) 'Size isn't everything', *Health Service Journal* 11 (5746) 16–17.

McGrath, M. (1991) *Multi-disciplinary Teamwork*, Aldershot: Avebury.

Okell, S. (2001) 'The Care Trust – The Somerset Model', *Integrating Health and Social Care*, Harrogate: Harrogate Management Centre.

Parker, G. (1990) *Team Players and Teamwork: The New Competitive Business Strategy*, San Franciso: Jossey-Bass.

Payne, M. (2000) *Teamwork in Multiprofessional Care*, London: Macmillan.

Poulton, B. and West, M. (1999) 'The determinants of effectiveness in primary health care teams', *Journal of Interprofessional Care* 13 (1) 7–18.

Powell, M. and Kocher, P. (1996) *Strategies for Change: A Carers Impact Resource Book*, London: King's Fund Publishing.

Rawson, D. (1994) 'Models of Inter-professional work: likely theories and possibilities', in A. Leathard (ed.), *Going Inter-Professional: Working Together for Health and Welfare*, London: Routledge.

Rink, E., Ross, F. and Furne, A. (2000) *NT Monographs: Integrated Nursing Teams in Primary Care*, London: Emap HealthCare.

Rummery, K. and Glendinning, C. (2000) *Primary Care and Social Services: Developing New Partnerships for Older People*, Abingdon: Radcliffe Medical Press.

Secretary of State for Health (1997) *The new NHS: Modern – Dependable*, Cm. 3807, London: The Stationery Office.

Secretary of State for Health (2000) *The NHS Plan: A Plan for Investment; A Plan for Reform*, Cm. 4818-1, London: The Stationery Office.

Steinberg, D. (1989) *Interprofessional Consultation: Invitation and Imagination in Working Relationships*, Oxford: Blackwell Scientific Publications.

Part II

From policy to practice

Working together across
professions, sectors and
communities

Chapter 8

Clinical teamwork

The impact of policy on collaborative practice

Carolyn Miller and Marnie Freeman

SUMMARY

The study of how different health and social care professionals work together in the team caring for a patient reveals the value to patients of integrated teamworking. But research also shows how organisational policies can militate against effective interprofessional working. Two examples are discussed from a study by the authors: the impact of bed-filling policies in fragmenting teams and the exacerbation of divisions in teams produced by the Care Programme Approach. Clinical governance demands good communication between care professionals but this can be compromised by policies that inadvertently draw team members apart. Solutions require scrutiny and modification of policy, structure and process.

INTRODUCTION

The study of how members of clinical teams work together gives us important insights into what makes teams function well to the advantage of patients and clients. But can the findings say anything else about the broader factors that serve to foster or detract from collaboration between professionals? A great deal of what has been written about teams and teamwork, particularly in group and organisational psychology (e.g. Sundstrom et al 1990; West 1990; Belbin 1993), focuses on teams that have been set up to complete a specific task or solve a problem. Such research has analysed the personal attributes of team members and how they contribute to working together to complete the task. This research does not necessarily translate well into the workplace to illuminate behaviour in complex organisations, such as the National Health Service (NHS). In these situations it is the work context that can assume a dominant place in determining how individuals interact with others. In our research studies of multiprofessional teams[1] in various clinical settings, we have sought to understand teamwork as it takes place in busy clinical environments (see Miller et al 2001).

We found that individual beliefs about working with other professionals, and their combined consequences on the operation of the professionals as a group, were important in the success or otherwise of interprofessional working. However, the attributes of members of multiprofessional clinical teams and the identified qualities of 'good teamwork' could be undermined by the impact of the management policies operating in the day-to-day realities of the working environment. These organisational policies, themselves influenced by government directives, could substantially enhance or detract from the opportunities that clinicians had to work together for the patient or client in unexpected and unintended ways. The study of teamworking in practice throws light on the influence of management policies in a way that the study of the policies themselves, which are likely to be directed at different ends, may not evince. Examples that illustrate the interaction of team function and wider policy are discussed below and the broader implications for interprofessional collaboration are explored. The examples are taken from a three-year research study that included intensive research on how teams worked.

The research process

In this research, six multiprofessional clinical teams working in the UK were studied for three months each from the following specialisms: neuro-rehabilitation, medicine, child development assessment, diabetes, general practice and community mental health. These teams included nurses, doctors, physiotherapists, occupational therapists, speech and language therapists and social workers. Little was known about five of these teams before beginning the study except that they involved several health care clinicians from different professions. The sixth team (neuro-rehabilitation) was chosen for its national reputation for collaborative interprofessional working. The research methods used were non-participant observation of the team's activities, semi-structured interviews with clinical staff and managers and document analysis. Patterns of behaviour within the teams were observed, for example, in communication: what was being said, how was it said and to whom; and in awareness of role contribution: what team members did in certain situations; what their expectations of others' roles were; and what happened at the boundaries of those roles. These observations were followed up by interview questions to team members related to specific incidents and to their more general understandings of teamworking. Interviews with managers discussed their views of multiprofessional working, shared learning and trust initiatives that involved interprofessional collaboration, such as integrated patient care policies (for examples of this approach, see Garside 1993).

Collaborative working

The findings showed that among these teams, effective, collaborative team-working was only seen in one team as a whole team process. In two others, part of the defined team consistently worked collaboratively, while other members were observed to be peripheral to the collaborative core. The characteristics of collaborative working, which we observed, were as follows:

- A highly developed shared vision of teamworking and a shared philosophy of patient care
- All relevant team members were expected to contribute to the problem solving and decision-making processes about their particular patients
- Shared responsibility for team actions
- Communication was multi-layered: information and knowledge-sharing and the acknowledgement of professional concerns were all recognised as important for the development of effective teamwork
- Role understanding was also multi-layered: team members felt it was important that they knew what a role comprised, how it was performed and what were the underpinning rationales for action
- Role boundaries were flexible according to patient requirements, with team members learning skills and knowledge to ensure continuity of care
- A pool of team skills and knowledge had developed, enabled by joint practices, such as joint note-keeping, assessment, monitoring, evaluating and therapeutic intervention

Although we were not looking for advantages to patients and carers of different ways of working, these became clear from our observations. In our research, the greater the level of collaboration across the whole team, the greater the number of incidents observed that showed: continuity and consistency of care from one professional to another; a reduction of ambiguous messages between team members and between them and their patients/clients and carers; appropriate referral, both in terms of who was referred to and the timing of that referral; a wide range of knowledge being used on which to base team decisions; and a problem-solving approach across the team being used to determine care programmes.

The reasons why teams were unable to achieve effective teamworking with such clear benefits for patient/clients were multifaceted with both organisational and interpersonal factors involved. Fragmenting organisational structures were fuelled in part by traditional hierarchies and by responses to resource shortages but also, as we illustrate, by government policy. Conditions of fluidity and unpredictability in clinical environments led to fragmentation of specialist skills and inhibited communication and the development of role understanding between professionals. Interpersonal relationships were undermined by power structures and differences in beliefs about teamworking and were challenged further where professionals' roles needed to be reconstructed in the light of new policy.

POLICY IMPLEMENTATION AND INTERPROFESSIONAL COLLABORATION

To illustrate in particular the impact of government policy on interprofessional working, two situations seen in the clinical teams studied are discussed below. Both policies were introduced to improve the efficiency of care for patients. The first was bed-management policy in acute hospitals. The second was the introduction of key workers (now called care coordinators) into community mental health teams as a result of the Care Programme Approach (CPA). Each case shows how the policy changes affected clinicians' ability to achieve all the characteristics of collaborative working.

Bed-filling policy

The bed-filling policy was brought in by the previous (Conservative) government to maximise the number of patients being cared for in hospital at any one time. Previously, specialist care teams under a consultant had a ward(s) with a reserve of empty beds ready to take in patients to be treated within that specialist area. This practice was changed so that the pool of empty beds was made available for any patient who required admittance to hospital. It was intended that this would reduce waiting lists by streamlining the management of patient throughput. Disregarding whether the policy has indeed had the intended effect, a by-product of its implementation has been the fragmenting of supposed multiprofessional teamworking in the acute sector and the creation of an extremely unpredictable working environment. The alternative locating and rapid throughput of patients had a series of important consequences for the development and maintenance of multiprofessional teamwork. These effects were epitomised in one of our case studies – a 'respiratory' medical ward.

In order to fill as many available beds as possible at all times in the hospital within which the ward was located, it was often the case that patients were placed as outliers to specialist areas of care. This arrangement resulted in a wide variety of specialisms being managed within the wards; for example elderly, orthopaedic, gastro-intestinal problems and even surgical patients. The outcome of this configuration was that large numbers of relevant professionals (apart from ward-based nurses) were required to visit a large number of wards to see their patients; in some cases eight or ten instead of one or two as had traditionally been the case. One doctor made the point:

> most of the time I have been walking on my feet not seeing the patients,

just walking from ward to ward. My actual working time is four or five hours and walking time is three hours. (HO)

By the same token, the outcome for an individual ward, such as the respiratory medical ward, was that a large number of specialist doctors and other professionals such as physiotherapists, occupational therapists and specialist nurses would need to visit their own patients, in a constantly changing pattern. The latter was compounded by the fact that the acute sector was now only expected to house patients for as short a time as possible – with the emphasis having shifted to community care provision. The combination of these factors changed the nature of professionals' interaction with others within a central practice base of the ward. Despite the medical ward's designation, the large group of visiting professionals from the different specialisms were not a 'team' at all. In many cases they did not necessarily need to have contact with each other, their point of reference chiefly being the nurses.

Many people declared that, historically, a particular consultant's ward round and the pre-ward round visit by house officers and registrars would have taken an appreciable part of the day, since they would have been seeing many patients. This routine allowed multiple opportunities for communication and observation of professional practice. Now, a consultant and his 'firm' were seeing fewer patients in a particular ward over a shorter time. Because of the range of wards being attended by professionals, the possibility of being able to predict arrival at any one ward was limited, thereby creating further problems for the ward staff. The nurses would also need to manage several similar events throughout the day. In this situation, interactions between various professionals were perforce brief, if there was interaction at all. Ensuring that, in the flurry of activities, the appropriate nurse was available to talk to the relevant visiting professional was extremely difficult.

The impact of bed-filling policy on collaborative working

Not surprisingly, this situation greatly compromises communication, and understanding of what other 'team' members are doing, or why, becomes hard to determine. For example, nurses on the ward did not know when other professionals would arrive on the ward, nor who they would be. By the same token, despite a named nurse system, with the shift rotation of nurses and the use of 'bank' staff, visiting professionals did not know who to go to for advice and information. In the former case, lack of knowledge about when various professionals would be coming to the ward was compounded by the fact that visiting professionals did not demonstrate consistent patterns of communication with the nurses. Some professionals would wait until a nurse was available to inform them of what had occurred and any decisions made; others did not. The nurses, since they were often engaged in caring for patients with the bed curtains pulled, often did not realise that other professionals were in the ward. For many visiting professionals, it was simpler to write in the medical notes and assume that the nurses and other relevant professionals would read them. As attested by several of the nursing staff, this was by no means always the case and either information was not communicated at all, or it was miscommunicated. For example, one detrimental situation resulted where a patient was 'fasted' for several hours unnecessarily, and one where a patient missed a long-awaited appointment because the timing was misunderstood.

The missed opportunities for communication resulted in inconsistencies in patterns of care, some of which were vital for the patient's well-being. For example, one of the respiratory physiotherapists (PTs) expressed concern that lack of communication had led to disjunction in the care process. Because of the breadth of her patient care interventions across the hospital, the predictability of her visits to the 'respiratory medical' ward was limited. As a result, there was difficulty in linking her intervention with that of the nurses in order to maximise the effects for the patient. The PT came to the ward to perform chest exercises with particular patients that required the prior giving of drugs through a nebuliser, which was to have been organised by the nurses. The PT had indicated that the drugs needed to be given about an hour prior to treatment to maximise the effect of her therapy. However, the PT felt that the nurses were often late in doing their drug rounds, so that when the PT arrived not enough time had elapsed, or the patients had not had the drug at all. In either case, there was the possibility that the PT would be unable to do the treatment on that day. However, the PT was also observed to attend the ward in a random fashion, sometimes early in the morning, other times not until the afternoon.

Existing in an unstable and unpredictable environment severely limits the knowledge that individuals within a 'team' could develop about other professional's practice, that is their roles in action. For the greater part of the working day, these roles may be hidden from each other. A direct result of their not knowing the pattern of professional input and thereby missing communicating with other professionals was that the ward nurses contacted them at times when they may be busy in other areas. For example, nurses regularly contacted doctors using their 'bleep' system, which was a source of frustration for the nurses and resentment for the doctors. Some doctors were clearly stretched with work in other areas, and felt that the nurses did not understand how hard they *were* working and contacted them unnecessarily.

The brief and unexpected visits made by other professionals compromised nurses' availability to attend the patient, and so witness what the professional was doing, and how. This problem was seen even where roles were well established. How much more difficult then was the situation where new roles were introduced. This aspect was highlighted by the introduction of a discharge planning role to help support the bed-management policy. A specialist nurse had been employed to coordinate the discharge of elderly patients in particular. She was aware that, despite the fact that she reiterated her role on a regular basis, lack of ongoing visibility made it hard for her to build up the credibility of her contribution to the process of care. Attribution of a successful discharge may or may not come to her; people would simply observe that a discharge process had or had not been achieved smoothly.

Policies such as bed management have had far-reaching effects on the ability of professionals to form collaborative teams. Means of ameliorating some of the fall-out of the policy is a task that should be tackled by senior trust management and there was evidence of such developments within our study. The introduction in some trusts of, for example, medical admission wards, where professionals are attached to the ward rather than to a particular specialism, have provided better opportunities for the development of collaborative working.

The Care Programme Approach (CPA)

The CPA system was introduced as a framework for the community mental health teams (CMHT: including community psychiatric nurses (CPNs), social workers, occupational therapists (OTs) and psychiatrists) following an acknowledgement by government that the Community Care Programme was not offering sufficiently effective care for clients once they had been discharged into the community (DoH 1990a, 1990b). The programme resulted in a change of emphasis for the CMHTs towards the more severely mentally ill and meant that the roles of social worker and CPN, to a larger extent, overlapped; the boundaries between 'social' and 'health' input became more blurred. Because of the severity of mental illness, and the subsequent chaos that was often created in housing and employment, clear divisions in client care were now inappropriate. A fundamental role within the CPA was key-working (now called care coordination) with clients based on the development of a care plan. Within a team framework this approach was intended to ensure that such complex health and social issues would be dealt with comprehensively.

The introduction of the policy created two main problems for a CMHT in our study. The first related to cross-organisational incompatibilities and the second, to role boundary defensiveness (these issues have been identified in other recent work, e.g. Onyett et al 1996; Simpson 1999). The problems in our study arose largely because the policy was based on an *assumption* of close collaboration between team members which, as we demonstrate, was unlikely to be achieved. In this situation the policy was introduced without the guidelines and resources to ensure that the organisations involved were able to implement appropriate structures, processes and training, successfully. The health and social services had paid scant attention to infrastructure or cross-organisational cultural differences that might need to be addressed. As a result, differences in structure and process and differences in the interpretation of the key-worker role, created miscommunication, missed communication and professional defensiveness.

As suggested above, part of the CPA was the development of a care plan based on three levels of mental ill health suffered by the client. It was the intention that those clients with the greatest needs, or who were the most severely ill, received the fullest range of services and the most stringently monitored plan. Initially, at senior management level, the local trust, in consultation with social services, had developed joint documentation that included both psychological and social assessment for use with all potential clients. However, only health professionals used these documents. Supported by their own management, the social workers continued to use their own social assessment forms, which all the team agreed provided a much fuller social needs' assessment. The use of the two types of forms was a source of frustration for two reasons. First, and most unfortunately, the rating of the levels of mental health ran in opposite directions. Not surprisingly, this situation created confusion when clients were being discussed, with the potential for mistakes to be made in terms of attention to the severity of a client's illness. Second, because the social services' form was much more complex, the CPNs reasoned it should be completed by the social workers, despite the duplication of information that this entailed. In the process, this procedure reinforced existing dissent between the professional groups related to the keyworker role.

The key-worker role

The development of the care plan, prior to a patient's discharge from in-patient care, required the appointment of an appropriate key-worker. This professional would be responsible for coordinating the '*registration, assessment, planning and review*' of their client's care. Ideally, the key-worker should be a professional who already has knowledge of the client and has built a relationship with him or her, however, the choice of professional depends on the level of mental ill health to which a client has been allocated. The most seriously ill people would need full risk assessment and regular and frequent monitoring. For this reason such people may be deemed to require either CPNs or social workers as key-workers, as these professionals in the CMHT work most regularly and closely with clients.

The allocation of the key-worker role was a cause of much dissent and frustration and related in part to the nature of the role, which was contested between the health and social services. As far as the trust and many CPNs were concerned, understanding of this role was that the key-worker would need to be *aware* of all psychological, medical and social interventions in order to *coordinate* a client's care. However, they would not be responsible for *actioning* the interventions. In *this* sense, as a key-worker, the CPNs would still do their own assessments but leave the more complex social assessment to the social workers. The CPNs argued that this was important because of social workers' greater depth of understanding of social assessment. However, the social workers had a different understanding of the key-worker role that related to their service's previous practice. Social workers had for some time been involved in case management. For them, the key-worker role meant that an identified case manager would be responsible for not only coordinating aspects of a client's care plan, but also *executing* all aspects of that care plan. The social workers subscribed to this interpretation of key-working. With the introduction of the CPA keyworker role, the social workers felt that the CPNs in that role should include more social awareness in their thinking, and take on a social aspect to their work. However, this response did not readily occur. Key-working became: '*the ball that nobody wants to catch*'.

Protecting role boundaries

The CPNs argued that they had neither the time nor the skills to manage all aspects of client care. They protested that the social workers had smaller caseloads that allowed them to pursue housing or financial problems thoroughly. The social workers felt that the depth of work they were expected to do with each client made *their* caseloads comparable to the larger ones of the CPNs. This situation was further heightened by the fact that social worker numbers were reduced within the teams. As a result, social workers began to decline taking on, not only the key-worker role, but also housing and financial problems where CPNs were key-working. Both professional groups felt overburdened with the work, but the CPNs felt that they were unprepared for this new role and therefore unwilling to carry out the complex assessment and intervention required for the clients.

The CPNs' earlier role had been to engage in both therapeutic and health prevention work with less severely mentally ill clients. Now CPNs were being required to manage clients with chronic and severe mental illness and to look more broadly at the influence of social aspects of their clients' lives in order to offer the most appropriate care. Indeed, they may need to be involved in managing some of these aspects of care. For many in the team this would mean the loss of skills they had spent years acquiring; the CPNs valued the one-to-one therapeutic relationship with their clients, and viewed encroachment on this role with distaste.

The social workers felt that the CPNs were being professionally defensive in the face of the demand to work in new ways in the team. The social workers recognised that CPNs might need guidance and assistance in the more complex cases, but still they felt that this was appropriate for members of a CMHT. The difficulties were compounded by the fact that the two professions tended to hold very different beliefs about teamworking. A number of the CPNs operated from a standpoint where they emphasised the one-to-one relationship with their clients and were poorly motivated towards a team approach that required in-depth communication. The social workers, however, were largely great believers in the power of collaboration to manage the complexity of patients' lives. Given these differences, the potential for developing a systematic approach to the keyworker role was undermined. Unfortunately, there was little active support from either professional groups' management to resolve these issues and, as a result, people became evermore entrenched in unhelpful positions. Far from being a mechanism for including and coordinating team members' activities with a client as a 'team' process, the keyworker role was used to reinforce the professional role boundaries further (this problem is corroborated by Simpson 1999).

The impact for clients

Care for one client in this team was compromised as a result of the conflict between the two professional groups, and the lack of action by the management in both organisations. The staff nurse from the day hospital, which was attached to the team, had a particular problem with a client who was attending that facility. He had been evicted and now needed money and a place to live. The staff nurse had spent a great deal of time trying to find out who was the named person to investigate these issues and help the man, but had not received any response from either the CPNs or the social workers in the team. She raised the issue at a team meeting and was told by one of the CPNs that the day hospital staff should provide the key-worker; that neither the CPNs nor the social workers could take on the case. The staff nurse pointed out that this client was one of eight other people without key-workers, and that the CMHT needed to address this problem as clients were feeling unsupported, and potentially unable to maintain their place in the community. In an interview the staff nurse commented that she felt disturbed that those present in the meeting had not dealt with the client. In this situation professional role protection seemed to override patient focus.

Unlike the introduction of the bed-management policy, the CPA demanded effective collaboration among the various members of the CMHT. However, the way it was introduced, with the implications for practice apparently not thought through sufficiently, only served to further divide some professional groups. Cross-organisational working is fraught with problems of mismatching policies and mismatching cultures. Here, one policy was introduced for both, but each interpreted the working of the policy differently. This outcome highlights the importance of the need for ongoing discussion at all levels in order to identify and work through these differences in understanding. However, even given structural and process congruence between the organisations, differences in beliefs and attitudes between professionals about the very nature of their work in relation to others are potentially damaging to the development of collaborative practices. Introducing policies, which presume effective teamworking, seem naïve unless there is also the introduction of a systematic team development programme that addresses and ameliorates cultural and interpersonal differences.

CONCLUSIONS

This chapter has identified how the introduction of government policies can directly or indirectly inhibit interprofessional collaboration. The study emphasised that team development is not only an interprofessional issue in the setting of a particular ward or community patch, but also has to be addressed in terms of the impact of wider organisational policies, processes and cultures.

One of the most difficult issues that trusts struggle with is the conflicting nature of some policies. For example, in the search for maximum clinical efficiency, the bed-filling policy can substantially undermine the opportunities for professionals to communicate effectively with each other. By contrast, policies such as clinical governance (DoH 1997) are intended to address actively the concept of professional interaction in order to maximise clinical effectiveness. Juggling these conflicts may demand considerations such as which policy is paramount in terms of trusts' performance ratings and how that impacts on the interpretation of other policies. In terms of clinical governance, there is certainly an incentive at the higher levels of management to avoid negative incidents leading to litigation. In order to do this, there is a recognition of the need to improve the day-to-day communication and collaboration between professionals. However, whether this recognition is made explicit through the development of organisational structures and processes to achieve such collaboration may well be constrained by the need to provide maximum patient throughput.

Even where such structures and processes *are* implemented, then creating an environment where middle managers are motivated and able to support grass roots workers in developing collaborative practices may be undermined by the plethora of other legitimate priorities. For example, a further, recent outcome from our research was the development of a system of team training in trusts (Jefferies 1999). We found that, while trusts showed great initial interest in setting up these programmes for their teams, the uptake and consistent involvement by team members was often hampered because of workload commitments and shortages of staff. Despite middle managers being interested in the concept of team training, the reality of providing patient care in the often resource-poor acute wards resulted in limited success in the implementation of the team training programme.

Means of ameliorating these difficulties identified above must be tackled. Our research showed quite clearly that collaborative working had beneficial outcomes for patients and clients, and for the professionals themselves. Where such working was not seen, patient and client care was compromised.

Thus, senior managers face difficult challenges. They need to struggle with the implications of government policies demanding resources that may be unavailable. They also need to juggle the conflicts between policies that emphasise throughput of patients versus those that emphasise quality of care. These dilemmas are the context in which collaborative practices for the benefit of patients have to grow and survive. An increasing body of evidence, including our own, suggests that fostering the development of interprofessional collaboration is essential to enhance the quality of patient care.

NOTE

1 Multiprofessional and interprofessional definitions: a distinction has been made between 'multi' as being composed of many who may not interact, and 'inter', which implies an interaction between team members (e.g. Luszki 1958; Petrie, 1976). In our research we referred to 'multiprofessional' teams as being composed of members of different health and social care professions. The nature of their 'interaction' was for us to establish before we could describe them as 'interprofessional'.

REFERENCES

Belbin, R. (1993) *Team Roles at Work*, Oxford, Boston, Mass: Butterworth-Heinemann.

DoH (Department of Health) (1990a) *NHS and Community Care Act*, London: HMSO.

DoH (1990b) *The Care Programme Approach for People with Mental Illness*, London: HMSO.

DoH (1997) *The New NHS: Modern and Dependable*, London: HMSO.

Garside, P. (1993) *Patient-focussed Care: A Review of Seven Sites in England*, Leeds: NHS Management Executive.

Jefferies, N. (1999) *The Team Development Workbook Package*, Kent, East Surrey and Sussex Workforce Development Confederation, East Surrey Health Authority, Epsom, Surrey.

Luszki, M. (1958) *International Team Research Methods and Problems*, New York: National Training Laboratories.

Miller, C., Freeman, M. and Ross, N. (2001) *Interprofessional Practice in Health and Social Care: Challenging the Shared Learning Agenda*, London: Arnold.

Onyett, S., Pillinger, T. and Muijen, M. (1996) *Making Community Mental Health Teams Work*, London: Sainsbury Centre for Mental Health.

Petrie, H. (1976) 'Do you see what I see? The epistemology of interdisciplinary inquiry', *Journal of Aesthetic Education* 10 29–43.

Simpson, A. (1999) 'Focus on training', *Nursing Times* 95 (47) 66–68.

Sundstrom, E., DeMause, K. and Futrell, D. (1990) 'Work teams: application and effectiveness', *American Psychologist* 45, 120–33.

West, M. (1990) 'The social psychology of innovation in groups', in M. West and J. Farr (eds), *Innovation and Creativity at Work*, Chichester: John Wiley & Sons.

Chapter 9

New primary care policies

From professions to professionalism

Geoffrey Meads

SUMMARY

As part of the modernisation of primary care services in the UK, recent organisational developments have supplied new frameworks for interprofessional collaboration. These have gained momentum since 1997 through the political leadership of a government committed to cross-boundary programmes in its pursuit of a stronger corporate commitment to the 'new' National Health Service (NHS). As a result, the professionalism of function is replacing the traditional focus on person-specific individual professions. A case study from a central London district illustrates the growing effectiveness of this policy in local practice.

THE SIGNIFICANCE OF POLICY

The principal purpose of policy is to provide meaning. Progressive policies go with the grain and operate prospectively, shaping behavioural change in advance in accordance with politically legitimised values and criteria. Post-1997 'new NHS' policies in the UK have been of this kind. Indeed, as a systematic attempt to re-frame fundamentally the activities and attitudes of all the participants in a major public institution, they have been arguably without parallel in a modern democratic state. The conversion of the multi-tiered traditional NHS into one of just two organisational boundaries – central and local – and the translation of a closed managed market model into a politically led and administered open systems approach constitute a genuinely radical policy formulation. This has been accompanied inevitably by an unprecedented volume of government circulars and directives to the NHS in the country.

For the professional recipients of these communications, this has been a novel experience. Such new government policies as those on clinical governance, intermediate care and community health development are targeted directly at the professions. These policies possess the explicit aim of corporately re-engineering both the structures and processes through which individual members of professions undertake their professional roles. Indeed, on occasion, this plethora of central policy has actually brought into question the future viability of these roles themselves. For example, the position of the general medical practitioner as the sole gatekeeper to the wider NHS looks increasingly unsustainable in the context of multiple new access points for primary care referrals and services (e.g. walk-in centres, NHS Direct helplines and nurse practitioners). The pace and scale of the post-1997 policy onslaught has caught most professions on the back foot; a situation that has been compounded for those in London, Wales, Scotland and Northern Ireland by the arrival of another new source of political influence in the form of devolved assemblies and either regional mayors or ministers.

In contrast to this progressive approach, British professions in the past have generally approached the need for policy reluctantly as a reactive or retrospective requirement. Its purpose has usually been to give meaning to developments stimulated by self-determining professions, assured of their separate status, within a NHS that based and indeed titled its structures on their individual specialisms. For general practice-based primary care, this has meant the licence to develop through diversity with national policies emerging hurriedly as a means of rationalising disparate initiatives in such areas as health promotion, minor surgery and, most recently, health and social care commissioning. Suddenly, this individualism is no longer legitimate. By definition care programmes, integrated care pathways, resource centres, assessment wards, health action zones, healthy living centres and shared care protocols transcend and supersede conventional boundaries and disciplines. Working interprofessionally is becoming a prerequisite for each profession. Professionalism, with its focus on function, is a far more important concept in the contemporary health system than that of a person-based profession.

Accordingly, post-1997 policies are resolutely generic and 'profession-blind' in their approach to what is required of personnel to reform and revive the NHS. The following statement makes clear what is the bottom line.

> The effective engagement of *all* interests will be critical in rebuilding public confidence.
>
> (HSC 1998/167: S.10)

The two critical targets for this engagement are local 'staff' and 'communities' (of both public and patient groups). The two words litter the official literature, particularly in relation to the new primary care organisations. The latter are charged with the main responsibilities for 'giving front-line staff and patients the opportunity to think and work differently to solve old problems in new ways (as) the only way to deliver the improvements set out in the (July 2000) NHS Plan' (DoH 2001: S.56). For the 300 primary care trusts established in April 2002 'local staff involvement plans' and 'leadership' are mandatory requirements (DoH 2001: S.63). These are an integral part of their new organisational accountabilities for professional development, education and training (HSC 1998/228: 3).

In assuming these responsibilities, the management framework of primary care trusts (and groups) is that of the central Department of Health's guidance on non-profession specific *Human Resources* for *Working Together* (NHSE 1999). This guidance is not derived from the royal colleges and professional associations but rather from business school theories of 'collaborative advantage' and 'the learning organisation' (e.g. Senge 1990, Huxham and MacDonald 1992). Pointedly, the new primary care organisations have been reminded that 'the lead person for education and training, professional development and workforce planning', almost invariably a senior general medical practitioner in the past, 'need not necessarily be a doctor' (HSC 1998/228: S.23). The message in the government's guidance to the multiprofessional executive teams of primary care trusts on *Working Together* is similarly sharp edged. Neither the general practitioner (GP) nor any other primary care professional are mentioned by name for the first 12 pages or 26 paragraphs of a relatively brief (21 pages) document (NHSE 1999).

The future 'staff' position could scarcely be expressed more unequivocally than in the introductory exhortation to primary care trusts. They are informed that they

> have a unique opportunity to set high standards for all HR (human resources) from the beginning. All NHS employers are bound by requirements under employment law and NHS employment practice as set out in central guidance and are required to demonstrate a commitment to good equal opportunities practice. The HR framework for the NHS *Working Together* demonstrates the Ministerial commitment to valuing all staff employed in the NHS which includes primary care. PCT's (primary care trusts) will therefore be expected to follow the values, practices and targets for action identified in this document.
>
> (NHSE 1999: S.3)

Such an injunction is, of course, only possible because in the 'new NHS' the central and local organisational boundaries are in a relationship of direct encounter. A little more than a decade ago, general practices had six levels of NHS hierarchy between themselves and the central political administration, and minimal monetary responsibilities. Now the NHS primary care trusts have direct resource accountabilities for over 70 per cent of the whole NHS budget. This is currently in excess of £40 billion. In organisational terms, they *are* the central-local interface.

On the one hand, this new position has meant a transfer to primary care organisations of responsibilities for terms of service and employment previously the jealous central preserve of national professions and their negotiating representatives. On the other hand, it has signified a realignment of responsibilities at the local boundaries of the NHS. The uni-professional business partnership is no longer the sovereign organisational unit. The previous British government's genuinely groundbreaking White Paper on the future of primary care in August 1996 paved the way for the radical changes ahead. It established the strategic planning objective of a multidisciplinary workforce rooted in 'local flexibility enabling different approaches to be taken to meet different local needs and circumstances' (Secretary of State 1996a: v). This White Paper spawned the 1997 NHS (Primary Care) Act with its revolutionary provision for alternative (non-GP) providers subject to local contracts.

Since this time, as the local case study that follows illustrates, the development dynamic of British primary care has shifted rapidly away from its historically almost exclusively intra-practice orientation. Local service and subsequently organisational developments in primary care are now increasingly the property of the community network, the locality, the inter-practice and social care collaboratives, and even, occasionally, the whole area of health economy. Contemporary research, for example, details innovations in nurse-led personal medical services, combined mental health and primary health care teams and extended roles for community pharmacists and optometrists; as well, of course, as novel cooperative models generated by general medical practitioners themselves (e.g. Armstrong and Tylee 1999; Meads 1999; Heywood 2000: 26–42; Coleman 2001: 187–98; Lewis 2001: 29–47). These new enterprises are often characterised by different skills' mix and substitution.

It would, emphatically, be premature to write off the power of the individual GP principal, but the 'modernising' direction of travel seems clear. The last Conservative government's core values for primary care, and for the other public services and utilities as well, were often defined in terms of 'choice', 'competition' and chance (or 'opportunity') (e.g. Secretary of State for Health 1996b). The 'New' Labour government's stated principles seem softer, emphasising three alternative 'C's of 'cooperation', 'consensus' and, above all, 'collaboration' (e.g. Secretary of State for Health 1997: chapter 2). In practice, however, the two sets of political forces are neither so separate as they seem nor so sequential. In reality, they converge and powerfully coalesce. The effect is that the move towards the professionalism of role flexibilities, virtual organisations and intersectoral alliances in today's primary health care appears just as hard-headed and determined as the protectionism that previously surrounded the individual separate professions in yesterday's era monopolised by primary medical care.

A LOCAL CASE STUDY

Since 1997, a team of university-based facilitators[1] have worked with the changing primary care organisations of a central London health district on their implementation of 'new NHS' policies. In this district, of considerable economic and social deprivation, where efficient resource utilisation is a constant concern, the unifying theme has been that of interprofessional collaboration. Under the terms of several action research contracts, the facilitators have offered a series of developmental inputs as detailed in Table 9.1. Their twin aims have been to apply research to practice and to enable the evidence of developments in practice to inform and influence emerging policies. Accordingly, a variety of methods have been applied ranging from partnership profiling to frameworks for interactive or interprofessional learning and joint development (e.g. Barr 1994). These are exactly those now required by new NHS strategies for integrated workforce planning (DoH 2000: 4; 20).

Different partnership profiling techniques have been used both periodically to audit progress (or otherwise) on working together, and to prepare for the new collaborative organisational arrangements required by the government's 'modernising' strategies. Figure 9.1 is an illustration of the second of these functions. It draws on Schluter and Lees' analysis of the non-affective structural preconditions needed for successful relationships: directness of communication and contact; continuity, multiplexity in terms of breadth of understanding and awareness; parity of contributions and respect; and commonality through shared values and objectives (Schluter and Lee 1993: 68–92). Used in time-limited role play it has highlighted, especially for general medical practitioners, both the changing volume and the profile of their new relationships. Social services and non-statutory organisations have, for example, emerged as key future partners sometimes at the expense of past secondary care-oriented clinical relationships.

The group exercise described in Figure 9.1 was undertaken with local professionals on a 'Progress in Partnership' programme after earlier relational stocktakes had revealed a paucity of effective interprofessional collaboration. In March 1998, for example, a group session with 11 different primary care professional representatives was able to identify inter-GP combinations as the only currently effective peer relationships available to promote the improvements generally recognised as required in local primary care services. As a result, the achievement of the latter – from diabetic retinopathy screening to integrated nursing teams and oral health promotion – were seen to depend on the future relationships' management role of the overarching primary care group or trust. Moreover, the service improvement targets themselves were prioritised in strict accordance with the local NHS professional pecking order: from general medical practitioners and senior specialist community nurses at the top to community pharmacists and optometrists on the bottom two rungs. It seemed very unlikely that this list of relative status really

Table 9.1 Interprofessional collaboration programme: developing new primary care organisations in a central London district, 1997–2002

Timescale	IP project
1 January 1997–July 1998	Ocular primary health care services project with health authority-nominated optometrists (6), GPs (2) and social services and ophthalmology department 'links'
2 April–October 1998	Monthly management development day workshops for 15 senior GPs and practice managers including 'partnership' and 'policy' sessions
3 January–July 1999	Monthly half-day workshops for formal representatives of local primary professional associations on 'partnership' working
4 October 1998–August 2000	Individual PCG board team development half-day sessions
5 August 1999–March 2000	Monthly half-day workshops for 10 new team managers (health) appointed by local authority to outposted NHS settings: on interagency collaboration and organisational change issues
6 September 1999–February 2000	Three half-day conferences on interprofessional practice implications of new primary care policies for 120 front-line older people's services staff
7 July 2000–February 2001	Four half-day seminars for six senior social work practitioners on partnership policy and skills development
8 January–March 2002	Monthly half-day 'integrated care management' workshops for over 40 senior community and practice nurses, PCG managers, voluntary organisation members and social services practitioners and team leaders
9 October 2001	Site-specific workshop with SWOT analysis of four combined professional roles in developing unified local health centre information system
10 April 2001–March 2002	Pan-London five site shared learning project on interprofessional collaboration involving local GP, district nurse and senior social work practitioner representatives

reflected the comparative strengths of their potential contributions to health and health care.

Three years later, despite several changes in individual personnel, the relational profile looked very different. Over 40 participants from the family

You are a newly formed PCG Board. Bearing in mind both your immediate and long-term responsibilities, identify and agree the five relationships that are most important to maintain or develop (these may be either within the PCG or with other organisations, groups or individuals). For each of these relationships rate their relative strengths and weaknesses for each relational precondition on a 1–5 scale (5 = high). Discuss the reasons for any notable areas of strength or weakness. Suggest one or two actions for strengthening the weakest aspects of each of these relationships.

Relationship (e.g. between member practices)	Relational preconditions				
	Directness 4	Continuity 3	Multiplexity 3	Parity 2 (Identify areas for increased participation by 'fringe' practices)	Commonality 2
1					
2					
3					
4					
5					

Figure 9.1 Relational mapping.

health, community and social services in March 2001 were able to agree on a series of strategic and corporate objectives. These were not simply confined to such pressing operational issues as 'being responsive to all emergencies' and 'ensuring safe levels of clinical and care provision'. They also included such informal aims as seeking to establish 'a common culture of corridor conversations', and the following areas for joint development:

- a shared framework for Quality
- combinations of community services, including GPs in cross-boundary teams
- common assessment approaches
- unified information systems
- integrated training and skills development. ('Integrated Care Management' Workshop, Camden, March 2001.)

In terms of interactive learning theory, such joint developments represent the final stage in a linear progression that witnesses behaviour being modified, and common ground established, once mutual understanding has been achieved and dysfunctional bias or stereotypes have been addressed (Barr 2002). Our experience is that this sequence is rarely so linear in practice. Realising reciprocal understanding is a constant challenge and interprofessional prejudices are remarkably deep-rooted. Figure 9.2 sets out a pro forma for an introductory exercise employed at one of the local multiprofessional workshops that actually became the basis for two sessions each of three hours' duration, such were the severe knowledge deficits of the participants about each other.

These sessions also revealed the importance of addressing the partnership agenda required by modernisation policy imperatives across a broad range of learning fronts. Rather than being linear, interactive learning is complex, iterative and multifaceted. These epithets may apply even when a single professional group is the specific educational focus. Table 9.2, for example, is the actual learning audit prepared by six senior social work practitioners, following their relocation in NHS premises, in readiness for their contribution to the forthcoming primary care trust and the combined older people's assessment programmes it will promote.

Personal, professional, interprofessional and organisational learning and development priorities have proved distinct and equally important. They are also interdependent. Restructuring organisational units to incorporate small general practices, for example, will not be productive unless personal valuations of different employment status are reappraised. Similarly, interprofessional 'unfreezing' could not begin in the particular context of our local case study, until the social work practitioners recognised that local district nurses' aspirations to care management roles represented not so much rivalry as a legitimate professional development path actually required and approved by

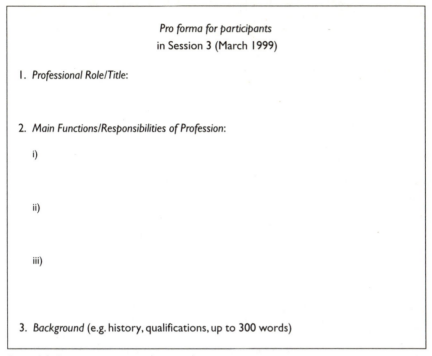

Pro forma for participants
in Session 3 (March 1999)

1. *Professional Role/Title:*

2. *Main Functions/Responsibilities of Profession:*

   i)

   ii)

   iii)

3. *Background* (e.g. history, qualifications, up to 300 words)

Figure 9.2 Progress in partnership – with new primary care groups.

the relevant royal college and national nursing accreditation agencies. Accepting as authentic each of these dimensions of learning and development can be difficult and challenging. But they can also be remarkably productive, generating genuinely dramatic advances in collaborative working and for interprofessional approaches as normative practice.

Accordingly, the title for the latest interprofessional learning programme in this London locality includes the words 'working together as if we are one organisation'. Joint micro- and macro-level initiatives now extend from shop-based provision of low-vision aids to multidisciplinary rapid response and refugees' services. There is a broad consensus in favour of an early application to become fully integrated borough-wide care trusts in 2002/3. One of the existing primary care trusts has sought national 'education provider' recognition. The other leads on research. An April 2001 internal report to the health authority included the following paragraph (Meads 2001).

> Modern service organisations are unlike traditional bureaucracies or professions. Given the changing environment they need to learn to be more flexible and adaptive. People in them need to learn together. Recognising this (local) health and social care staff are looking to move incrementally

Table 9.2 Social work service senior practitioners' learning needs audit in the changing world of primary care

	Attitude	Action
Level 1: Personal	• Overcoming prejudices and stereotypes • Maintaining motivation to lead self and others • Sustaining convictions about import of individuals self-determination and relationships • Valuing own status	• Identifying and addressing knowledge shortfalls • Mapping future flexible career paths
Level 2: Professional	• Adopting cross-boundary mindsets • Clarifying new boundaries • Thinking 'quality' systems • Promoting prevention • Valuing own status	• Converting SW values into joint performance measures • Spreading practice and philosophy of care management • Making quality tangible • Representing 'client' versus professions • Honing therapeutic roles
Level 3: Interprofessional	• 'Unfreezing' so that working together can get started • Strengthening mutual awareness • Seeing service gaps as joint opportunities • Supporting each other on shifting primary/secondary care interface	• Sharing skills in practice and learning together • Collaborating to prevent client breakdowns/critical incidents • Arranging information exchange on relevant roles and responsibilities • Profiling and aligning different accountability, funding, regulatory structures and processes
Level 4: Organisational	• Inclusion of small/shorthand practices • Interactive learning mindsets • Respect reciprocal values • Learn together about good practice models elsewhere	• More joint policy development forums • Further combined referral and assessment arrangements • Jointly commissioned local, practice-based research and evaluation • Joint long-term staff education strategies and sponsorship • Pooled budgets and unified resources

through practical steps, from a virtual team to a system of unified management in a care trust. This will require strength of vision and leadership to move people forward together along the journey, with the primary care group phase of development used to resolve conflict and heal residual wounds. There is a willingness to take the trip rooted in convictions that local participants do share a common purpose, and would like to reach a single ethos which embraces not only those in the local authority but all those committed to their services.

The report goes on to employ a model of collaborative advantage to specify no fewer than 13 operational functions where 'omissions' or 'duplications' apply (Huxham and MacDonald 1992). In every instance an interprofessional response is recommended. This case study is indicative of a wider trend across the country as policies for professionalism begin to bed down. In primary care these policies are clearly making their mark.

CONCLUSION

This chapter started by noting that successful policies are usually those that go with the grain. If such a statement can now be applied to new primary care policies in the UK – as well as countries as distant as Colombia, Chile and Cuba – why is this, given that the professions of primary care have been characterised by reactive or even reactionary approaches to policy in the past? The emerging practice of interprofessional learning and development, as illustrated in the local case study above, appears at least part of the answer. It is the bridge between policy and professionalism.

Following the 1999 staff conferences detailed in Table 9.1, a classroom exercise witnessed several groups of general medical and care management practitioners separately listing their individual and then their institutional professional values. The convergence between the former was a revelation to the participants. Some words were actually identical: 'holistic', 'confidentiality' and 'self-determination'. Others were clearly complimentary or compatible: 'acceptance', 'longitudinal', 'personal' and 'continuity'. The popular notion that doctors and social workers belong to rival camps was instantly dismissed.

All the actual areas of divergence and dispute were at the level of their separate cultures and organisations. 'Expert' versus 'semi-professional', 'individualistic' versus 'community', 'non-cash limited' versus 'budgets', 'traditional' versus 'new sciences' were some examples. But when placed in the context of interprofessional goals for the newly formed corporate primary care organisations, none of these any longer represented insuperable barriers. Local needs and functions were perceived as not only transcending individual professions' interests but also, significantly, as better able to draw on the converging personal professional values quoted in the previous paragraph. The impact was motivational.

In the UK, it has become clear that new primary care policies do offer a realistic prospect of shifting the balance towards interprofessional learning, development and collaboration. The new organisational structures and the processes they create are forcing a fundamental review of the role of separate professions. With those geographic areas containing the most acute health and social care needs for once in a position to take a lead in shaping the mainstream of primary care practice, it may well be that the old adage of 'form following function' could yet apply. In this context, and adhering to this principle, the move from professions to professionalism can confidently be asserted as a hallmark of 'modernising' policies.

NOTE

1 In addition to the author: Nancy Craven, Lecturer in Health Management, City University; Yvonne Cornish, Lecturer in Public Health, University of Kent; Derek Cramp, Visiting Professor of Medical Systems, City University, and Mark Exworthy, Research Fellow, University College London.

REFERENCES

Armstrong, E. and Tylee, A. (1999) 'Primary mental healthcare', in J. Sims (ed.), *Primary Health Care Sciences*, London: Whurr.

Barr, H. (1994) *Perspectives on Shared Learning*, London: Centre for the Advancement of Interprofessional Education.

Barr, H. (2002) *Interprofessional Education: Today, Yesterday and Tomorrow*, London: The Learning and Teaching Support Network.

Coleman, D. (2001) 'Prescribing: remedy for chronic inflation', in G. Meads and P. Meads (eds), *Trust in Experience: Transferable Learning for Primary Care Trusts*, Oxford: Radcliffe Medical Press.

DoH (Department of Health) (2000) *A Health Service of all the Talents: Developing the NHS Workforce*, London: Department of Health.

DoH (2001) *Shifting the Balance of Power within the NHS: Securing Delivery*, London: Department of Health.

HSC (Health Service Circular) (1998/167) *Health Improvement Programmes: Planning for Better Health and Better Health Care*, Leeds: NHS Executive.

HSC (Health Service Circular) (1998/228) *The new NHS Modern and Dependable. Primary Care Groups: Delivering the Agenda*, Leeds: NHS Executive.

Heywood, P. (2000) 'The changing character of service provision', in P. Tovey (ed.), *The Challenges of Change*, Buckingham: Open University Press.

Huxham, C. and MacDonald, D. (1992) 'Introducing collaborative advantage: achieving inter-organisational effectiveness through Meta-strategy', *Management Decision* 30 (3) 50–56.

Lewis, R. (2001) 'Nurse-led PMS pilots', in R. Lewis, S. Gillam and C. Jenkins (eds), *Personal Medical Services Pilots: Modernising Primary Care*, London: King's Fund Publishing.

Meads, G. (1999) 'Streaming into the river', *Journal of Interprofessional Care* 13 (3) 271–6.

Meads, G. (2001) Personal communication.

NHS Executive (1999) *Working Together: Human Resources Guidance and Requirements for Primary Care Trusts*, Leeds: NHS Executive.

Schluter, M. and Lee, D. (1993) *The R Factor*, London: Hodder and Stoughton.

Secretary of State for Health (1996a) *Primary Care: The Future*, Leeds: NHS Executive.

Secretary of State for Health (1996b) *Primary Care: The Future – Choice and Opportunity*, London: HMSO.

Secretary of State for Health (1997) *The new NHS: Modern, Dependable*, Cm. 3807, London: The Stationery Office.

Senge, P. (1990) *The Fifth Discipline: The Art and Science of a Learning Organisation*, London: Century.

Chapter 10

Journeys into thirdspace?

Health alliances and the challenge of border crossing

Alan Beattie

SUMMARY

There has been in the UK in the past few years a remarkable surge of investment in the development of 'health alliances' (interagency and intersectoral
partnerships for health) – and to a lesser extent in their evaluation. As yet this
has not been accompanied by a marked improvement in understanding what
makes for success or failure in such initiatives. Two new perspectives are
offered as ways of encouraging dialogue and informing critical and creative
practice in this field of work. Both are illustrations of the broadly socio-
cultural approach that seems essential in a situation where contested and
competing frames of thought are prominent.

First, the idea of 'multiple metaphors' in reading and designing organisations is used to draw attention to the 'trap' that linear, mechanistic, additive ('hard systems') thinking still poses in work on health alliances, and to
highlight the range of non-linear models now emerging that offer promise for
future development and evaluation work. Second, the concept of 'thirdspace'
– borrowed from cultural and urban studies – is adapted to suggest an agenda
for working directly 'at the edge' where multiple viewpoints, difference and
discordance are juxtaposed; an agenda that requires negotiating across such
barriers and borderlines in order to create new, 'hybrid' entities and new
shared meanings at several levels. By working across the 'bar of difference',
the much talked about benefits of health alliances may be achieved, but – this
'interstitial perspective' insists – only so long as nobody (and nothing) stays
the same.

It is suggested that the future of alliances for health at local level will hinge
on the readiness of agencies to learn to change their root metaphors, to
abandon stereotypic thinking, to move towards new, more flexible and open
deployments of power and to renegotiate continuously their own boundaries
and their various institutional identities. The agenda is challenging; but if it is
not taken forward, the radical promise offered by new partnerships for health
at local level will not be fulfilled.

HEALTH ALLIANCES AS A TEST BED FOR INNOVATION, EXPERIMENT AND THEORY-BUILDING

By the early 1990s, 'health alliances' had emerged as a major vehicle for conjoint action bringing together at local level the diverse services (health, social services, environment, education, voluntary organisations etc.) essential to deliver health promotion and the 'new public health'. It was clear that health alliance projects provided 'a vital test-bed for innovation and experiment in multidisciplinary collaboration' – as in the World Health Organization's Health for All 2000 and Healthy Cities projects and the UK Government's Health of the Nation programmes (Beattie 1994: 110). But it was also clear at that time that this was a field that had been seriously under-researched; there was an 'embarrassing poverty' of systematic and theoretically informed analysis of the health alliances newly emerging at many different levels. Through the mid-1990s, research and development on 'partnership working' in the field of public health and health promotion (PHHP) did gather momentum (Leathard 1997).

Then from 1997 onwards in the UK, an unprecedented volume of public money was invested in health alliances (Scriven 1998), following the arrival of a new Labour government with an explicit commitment to using local area-based health initiatives as a vehicle for tackling issues of health inequalities and social exclusion. The evaluation of these initiatives (notably Health Action Zones, Sure Start and New Deal for Communities), as well as the considerable range of related projects with a remit of 'social regeneration' that also explore partnership working at local level (e.g. City Challenge and Safer Cities) has now begun to create an extensive body of documentation on health alliances (Stewart 2000; Russell 2001) which is attracting considerable attention from policy analysts (Clarence and Painter 1998; Hudson et al 1999; Powell and Moon 2001).

One clear focus of interest has been whether the recent round of area-based health alliances can serve as a test case regarding what New Labour's 'third way' political philosophy might mean in practice (Blair 1998; Powell 1999). A second focus of interest is whether the hopes attached to the post-1997 waves of interagency action for health were perhaps premature, naïve and doomed to be disappointed – because such new initiatives went ahead with little appreciation of how poorly developed our understanding is of the complexity of such partnership work in multiagency contexts (Medd 2001).

In this chapter, I would like to examine an issue that is closely related to these first two issues, namely the multiple and competing frames of thought that are in play in recent reports on the development and evaluation of health alliances. I will do so by taking further the type of socio-cultural analysis of health alliances that I have employed in previous publications (Beattie 1993, 1994, 1995); and I will draw attention to a new direction for theory-building that may help to achieve a better understanding of these complex initiatives and may offer particular promise for future development work.

MULTIPLE FRAMES OF THOUGHT IN THE DEVELOPMENT AND EVALUATION OF HEALTH ALLIANCES

There has been a vast proliferation of health alliances since 1997 at many different levels (Markwell and Speller 2001). Much of this has been accompanied by an unexamined recycling and amplification of the rhetoric of 'synergy through partnership'. As Medd (2001) observes, this is often backed up by a literature that consists of 'how-to-do-it' tips and hints, lists of prerequisites for 'success' in health alliances, of a normative and prescriptive kind, insufficiently informed by systematic evidence or by critical, theory-based argument. At the same time, a conspicuous feature of the recent development and evaluation of health alliances is that the theoretical underpinnings of projects often turn out to be marginal or shadowy, sometimes entirely undeclared. For example, one strand of the government-commissioned large-scale evaluation of Health Action Zones in England (Judge et al 1999) (see also Chapter 2, Table 2.5 for the background) has been concerned with investigating the processes of 'building capacity for collaboration', which has taken the form of five in-depth case studies. It is reported that all five cases lack an explicit 'theory of change' as regards local partnership strategies (Barnes et al 2000).

An earlier national study of intersectoral collaboration for health arrived at the view that to find just one single theory for understanding health alliances may remain an elusive goal (Delaney and Moran 1991; Delaney 1994a, 1994b, 1996). But it is striking that, in fact, authors writing about health alliances from different theoretical viewpoints rarely refer to one another's work. Thus, when crucial insights and urgent matters for debate do emerge from such work, the variety of different approaches to analysis (Davies et al 1993) means that different lines of argument are not brought together in ways that can help to fuel critical reflection and dialogue between protagonists. This feature of the academic investigation of health alliances mirrors the larger problem in the practice domain, of fragmented 'separate spheres' of organisational and professional work – that such alliances are set up to deal with in the first place. So there has not yet emerged a constructive 'paradigm dialogue' (Guba 1990) around health alliances of the kind that has helped to encourage the growth of reflective and critical practice within many of the separate disciplines of professional work in public services (e.g. nursing; social and community work; health promotion; and teaching).

To guide an analysis of this multiplicity of theories in health alliances, I will draw on the work of Morgan (1986) who has argued that one way of avoiding cognitive traps or straitjackets in organisational development is to pay close attention to the metaphors that are embedded – often buried – in the models and frameworks that are in play within organisations. Morgan (1986) enumerates 'seven types of metaphor' that are widely taken for granted by managers and professionals in the ways that they 'read' and 'design' organisations. Table 10.1 sets out a slightly modified and extended version of the seven core or root metaphors identified by Morgan (1986); listed alongside them are the clusters of key concepts that are closely linked to each particular metaphor.

This scheme can immediately serve to highlight a feature of recent developments in theory-building related to health alliances. In other words, too often both in government policy documents and among practitioners and researchers, the conceptualisation of health alliances still appears straitjacketed by a mechanistic and 'additive' way of thinking – the first metaphor of Table 10.1 – that emphasises the outputs and/or benefits that are directly 'caused' by putting agencies together into partnerships. One of the sources of the argument in official policy documents for new interdisciplinary and multiagency public health initiatives appears to be the 'structures and systems' approach (Beattie 2001); yet the design and evaluation of new health alliances seems only rarely to deploy even the most modest shifts from linear thinking, for example the organismic or cybernetic metaphors (numbers 2 and 3 in Table 10.1) that were prominent in the early phases of whole systems work. But some new and promising attempts to understand or develop health alliances are beginning to emerge from conceptualisations that are informed by the metaphors beyond number 1 on the list above – all of which represent a break with linear 'hard systems' thinking. What follows is an attempt to map some of the ways in which these six 'non-linear, non-deterministic' metaphors may come into use in the development and evaluation of health alliances.

Table 10.1 Seven types of metaphor used in reading and designing organisations (modified after Morgan 1986)

Core metaphor	Illustrative concepts and models
1 Mechanistic	e.g. cause-and-effect pathways; direct 1:1 determinations
2 Organismic	e.g. growth and development; adaptation; fitness to environment
3 Cybernetic	e.g. feedback loops; double-loop learning; triple-loop learning
4 Holographic	e.g. information spaces; codifications; translations
5 Cultural	e.g. stories, sayings; testimonies; legends; myths; rituals; ceremonies
6 Political	e.g. schismatics; constructive conflict; loosely-coupled systems
7 Dialectical	e.g. interplay; framing/reframing; self-organising; autopoietic

Six non-linear metaphors in the development and evaluation of health alliances

1   An organismic metaphor would suggest viewing health alliances as entities that move through what developmental and evolutionary biologists call 'epigenetic landscapes', unfolding and adapting in response to their diverse and changing ecologies (Ho and Saunders 1979; Goodwin and Saunders 1989). This way of seeing health alliances is illustrated in Douglas (1998), who refers to it as a shift from Newtonian to Darwinian views of organisational life; and also in Backet-Milburn and MacHardy (1998), who identify developmental groupwork as a useful approach to the nurturing of alliances through interpersonal relationships.

2   A cybernetic metaphor would suggest the view that health alliances require not merely classical 'feedback on performance' ('single-loop' learning) but that – crucially – they entail shared action/reflection cycles of the sort described in whole systems theory and in the concept of the 'learning organisation' (Senge 1990, 1994, 1999) as 'double-loop' and 'triple-loop' learning. This way of seeing health alliances is exemplified in Springett's (1998) monitoring and evaluation of the Liverpool healthy city project.

3   A holographic metaphor would suggest looking at health alliances as a system of information exchange made up of an array of different 'information spaces', the flow between which is structured through a set of different encodings and decodings (Boisot 1994, 1995). One glimpse of the usefulness of this way of seeing health alliances is provided in earlier work by Springett (1995) that used network exchange theory to analyse alliance work across a range of healthy city projects.

4   A cultural metaphor would suggest viewing health alliances in terms of the way in which they give scope for dialogue, 'story exchange' and the exercise of the 'narrative imagination' as a basis for the building of shared understandings and shared visions (Winter et al 1999). This way of seeing health alliances is illustrated by Elliott and Jackson (1998: 67) who reported that their approach to building an alliance was to structure 'arenas to facilitate and promote collaborative exchange' and to set up a 'strategic framework that would provide a sense of direction and a value base to work within'.

5   A political metaphor would suggest looking at health alliances as inescapably 'arenas of conflict' where diverse partners emerge from their previously well-defended boundaries, encounter one another and begin to recognise they are dealing with 'essentially contested concepts' (of which 'health' itself is one of the most obvious examples: Beattie 1991). This way of viewing health alliances is seen in Dalley (1993) and in Beattie (1995), both of whom apply the metaphor of 'tribal warfare' to interprofessional work; also in Markwell (1998) who recommends

conflict theory as an approach to alliance work, drawing on Handy's (1995) argument that organisations are made up of distinct tribes each worshipping their own separate, different 'gods of management'; and also in Wall (1998) who suggests that conflicting values across the 'different worlds' brought together in health alliances may best be analysed and dealt with in terms of ethical theory.

6   A dialectical metaphor would suggest viewing health alliances as a zone in which the interplay of competing ideas and visions can create self-sustaining spirals of dialogue and mutually agreed change – sometimes displaying 'runaway' behaviour, setting up their own spirals of self-renewal at different levels, on occasions evading complete analysis and understanding, perhaps best seen as 'a continuation of chaos by other means' (Stacey 1996, 2000). A start on viewing health alliances in this way is apparent in the King's Fund 'working whole systems' project on partnerships for health in London and elsewhere (Harries et al 1999; Pratt et al 2000).

An important result of the analysis of health alliances in terms of 'multiple metaphors' – as set out here – is that the analysis supports the argument that no one single theory could or should ever come into the ascendancy. It is not merely that any theoretical framework proposed for or used within the development of health alliances would do well to be tentative; rather – like Routledge (1997) in a different context – we should anticipate that no single over-arching theory will 'hold true' for all health alliances, in all their diversity and local particularity, in all times and places. So, if health alliances have since the early 1990s offered a test bed for innovation and experiment in social policy and social action, health alliances can now also be seen to offer fertile grounds for the critical and creative interrogation of contemporary social theories – theories that are at the forefront of policy debates: theories of local change, theories of organisational governance, theories of equity and social inclusion in welfare delivery.

BEYOND THE BOUNDARIES: AN INTERSTITIAL PERSPECTIVE ON HEALTH ALLIANCES

I would like now to explore the so-called 'interstitial perspective', drawn from recent work not in the fields of organisation studies or health studies but in cultural studies. This perspective has the particular attraction of representing not merely a decisive shift away from mechanistic and linear modes of thought, but also of spanning in an intriguing way the whole range of 'non-linear' models (as set out above).

A key concept in the interstitial perspective is that of 'thirdspace', an idea originally devised as a way of trying to define some of the distinctive features of 'postmodern' architecture, where 'thirdspace' refers to unexpected juxta-positions, discordances that generate newness, interstitial structures that are de-centred and create ambivalence – perhaps make you (as an inhabitant or visitor) temporarily 'lose your bearings' (Jameson 1991). Another cultural studies commentator has seized on this concept and elaborated it as a tool of thought for exploring the dynamics of encounters between people of dif-ferent cultural backgrounds (as in race relations); with the suggestion that thirdspace opens up 'where the negotiation of incommensurable differences creates a tension peculiar to borderline existences' (Bhabha 1994: 218). Such a space is 'neither One nor the Other, but something else besides, in-between ... continually opening out, remaking the boundaries ...' (Bhabha 1994: 219). It is a space of 'hybridity', a space of discursive contestation, at the borderlines and crossing borders; and the inhabitants of thirdspace depend for their survival on discovering 'how newness enters the world', by making links through newly created, still unstable interventions, rather than by employing the ready-made, the already-named and the pre-set (Bhabha 1994: 227). Setting up thirdspace permits 'the creation of agency through incom-mensurable (not simply multiple) positions' (Bhabha 1994: 231).

The cluster of concepts around thirdspace is a striking instance of the challenge and potential of postmodern and 'postcolonial' thinking, and is proving to be of enormous interest in the field of human and social geog-raphy. Rose (1994) used thirdspace to give an account of the production and reception of two 'protest' films made by local community groups in east London, in particular to articulate the 'cultural hybridity' of the film forms; and also in a study of a range of community arts projects in Edinburgh (Rose 1997). Law (1997) used the concept to illuminate how 'encounters with otherness' are negotiated and new meanings are defined, in a tourist bar in the Philippines. Soja (1996, 2000) has devoted two linked book-length studies to 'exploring the spaces that difference makes' in historical and contempor-ary city life, using thirdspace as the key concept to articulate how ethnic and social diversity and inequality (the Other, multiple Others) create 'borderline' existences. Soja (1996) argues that the new margin, the edge, is always a stimulus to 'move on', to open up paradoxical 'thirdspace'; and continuously to increase the openness of this new domain through dialectical processes; or what Soja (1996: 7, 53): calls 'trialectics' that is, a triple dialectic of interplay between 'the real' + 'the imagined' + 'what is simultaneously real-and-imagined'.

Thirdspace as a guiding metaphor for health alliances?

The new 'geometry of knowledge' defined as thirdspace offers an immediate yield of tools of thought that can be useful in the development and evalu-ation of health alliances. From the lines of research using the interstitial perspective outlined in the previous section, several key ideas can be drawn together into an agenda for that needs to be addressed by all those embarking on interprofessional and/or interagency collaboration for health (see Table 10.2).

The concept of thirdspace offers a way of engaging in the 'uneasy politics of instability', where the risk is taken of leaving things under-defined, of destabilising the previous certainties of power/knowledge, of celebrating definitional uncertainty. The concept of thirdspace addresses situations that are multiple, composite, heterogeneous, plural and indeterminate (Rose 1997). I find this an exciting way of looking at situations – as in health alliances – where protagonists are often not 'natural bedfellows' (Smith 2001), yet where people must work together in new ways, across complex lines of protection or resistance, outside the boundaries of their own agencies or institutions (Barnes et al 2000) – must engage in 'border crossings'. The concept of thirdspace in this context helps to articulate more precisely what challenges can be anticipated, and what principles are at stake, in moving towards the 'new republic of health' that has been argued for elsewhere (Beattie 1995: 20).

In a paper written – trenchantly and cogently – from the standpoint of a practitioner, Ewles (1998: 195) comments that working together across agency boundaries is 'fundamental to health promotion practice, and rightly so'; yet, insiders, like Ewles (1998), often end up 'wondering whether alliance work can ever be worth it', when the rhetoric surrounding health alliances so spectacularly outstrips the actuality, and when the costs of joint work

---

Table 10.2 'Thirdspace principles' as a basis for the theory-and-practice of health alliances

---

1   Start from a recognition of 'difference'; focus on 'otherness' and on how it can be negotiated

2   Address issues simultaneously at three distinct levels: the level of the protagonists who encounter one another; the level of the real practice contexts (e.g. organisational arrangements) that shape the encounter; and the level of the preconceived ideas (e.g. stereotypes) that shape both the protagonists and the contexts

3   Deal with *multiple* viewpoints and *multiple* levels *at the same time*

4   Recognise that protagonists can speak – can learn to speak, can be encouraged to speak – from positions beyond their conventional (stereotypical) location, beyond their assigned or preconstituted identities

5   Envisage and try out new deployments of power – ambivalent, or subversive of existing familiar arrangements

6   Negotiate and elaborate new spaces; seek or devise or develop new sites of collaboration

7   Construct new shared meanings together 'across the bar of difference'

8   Explore together and elaborate the grounds of difference and dissimilarity in new directions – beyond mere 'dualisms'

9   Acknowledge that new spaces are themselves continually fragmented and fractured, and treat them as always incomplete and uncertain

10 Subject all newly created identities to processes of continuous negotiation

sometimes clearly exceed the gains. Ewles (1998) notes that there is a whole spectrum of forms (and degrees) of joint work, and that it is important to 'think through' where any alliance is, or may need to be – at different points in time – on 'the spectrum'. Ewles (1998: 202) concludes 'we should all aim for an approach to alliance working based on an open, honest, critical appraisal, not hype'. I would want to add that in order to conduct 'open, honest critical appraisal' of health alliances – when multiple and competing frames of thought are in play – it is essential to try to construct and/or use powerful theoretical models, so as to clarify and challenge and perhaps turn upside-down or inside-out the terms of reference that are taken for granted, in fact to 'renew the discourse' – by 'changing our metaphors' (Table 10.1), and/or by adopting the interstitial perspective and 'journeying into thirdspace' (Table 10.2).

The magnitude of the challenge must not be underestimated; it is a challenge that professional practitioners will feel at the personal and interpersonal as well as at the organisational level; and that must make an impact at the national level as well as locally. But if these kinds of challenges are not acknowledged and addressed and the shifts towards greater openness and flexibility are not made – by individuals and by institutions – systems for promoting more equitable health are unlikely to be brought into being.

REFERENCES

Barnes, M., Sullivan, H. and Matka, E. (2000) *Context, Strategy and Capacity: Initial Findings from the Strategic Level Analysis*, Report of National Evaluation Team for Health Action Zones, Birmingham: University of Birmingham (http://www.haznet.org.uk).
Backet-Milburn K. and MacHardy, L. (1998) 'Healthy alliances depend on healthy social processes', in A. Scriven (ed.), *Alliances in Health Promotion: Theory and Practice*, London: Macmillan.
Beattie, A. (1991) 'Knowledge and control in health promotion: a test-case in social theory and social policy', in M. Calnan, J. Gabe and M. Bury (eds), *The Sociology of the Health Service*, London: Routledge.
Beattie, A. (1993) 'The changing boundaries of health', in A. Beattie, M. Gott, L. Jones and M. Sidell (eds), *Health and Wellbeing: A Reader*, London: Macmillan.
Beattie, A. (1994) 'Healthy alliances or dangerous liaisons? The challenge of working together in health promotion', in A. Leathard (ed.), *Going Inter-Professional: Working Together for Health and Welfare*, London: Routledge.
Beattie, A. (1995) 'War and peace among the health tribes', in K. Soothill, L. MacKay and C. Webb (eds), *Interprofessional Relations in Health Care*, London: Arnold.
Beattie, A. (2001) 'Health promotion', in C. Dowrick (ed.), *Medicine in Society*, London: Arnold.
Bhabha, H. (1994) 'How newness enters the world: postmodern space, postcolonial times and the trials of cultural translation', in H. Bhabba (ed.), *The Location of Culture*, London: Routledge.

Blair, T. (1998) *The Third Way*, London: Fabian Society.

Boisot, M. (1994) *Information and Organization: The Manager as Anthropologist*, London: Harper & Collins.

Boisot, M. (1995) *Information Space: A Framework for Learning in Organizations, Institutions and Culture*, London: Routledge.

Clarence, E. and Painter, C. (1998) 'Public services under New Labour: collaborative discourses and local networking', *Public Policy and Administration* 13 (3) 8–22.

Dalley, G. (1993) 'Professional ideology or organisational tribalism: the health service-social work divide', in J. Walmsley, J. Reynolds, P. Shakespeare and R. Woolfe (eds), *Health, Welfare and Practice: Reflecting on Roles and Relationships*, London: Sage.

Davies, J., Dooris, M., Russell, J. and Petterson, G. (1993) *Healthy Alliances: A Study of Inter-agency Collaboration in Health Promotion*, London: South West Thames Regional Health Authority.

Delaney, F. and Moran, G. (1991) 'Collaboration for health: in theory and practice', *Health Education Journal* 50, 97–9.

Delaney, F. (1994a) 'Making connections: research into intersectoral collaboration', *Health Education Journal* 53, 474–85.

Delaney, F. (1994b) 'Muddling through the middle ground: theoretical concerns in inter-sectoral collaboration and health promotion', *Health Promotion International* 9, 217–25.

Delaney, F. (1996) 'Theoretical issues in intersectoral collaboration', in A. Scriven and J. Orme (eds), *Health Promotion: Professional Perspectives*, 1st edn., Basingstoke: Macmillan.

Douglas, R. (1998) 'A framework for healthy alliances', in A. Scriven (ed.), *Alliances in Health Promotion: Theory and Practice*, London: Macmillan.

Elliott, M. and Jackson, D. (1998) 'Developing a strategic alliance using a soft systems approach', in A. Scriven (ed.), *Alliances in Health Promotion: Theory and Practice*, London: Macmillan.

Ewles, L. (1998) 'Working in alliances: an inside story', in A. Scriven (ed.), *Alliances in Health Promotion: Theory and Practice*, London: Macmillan.

Goodwin, B. and Saunders, P. (eds) (1989) *Theoretical Biology: Epigenetic and Evolutionary Order from Complex Systems*, Edinburgh: Edinburgh University Press.

Guba, E. (ed) (1990) *The Paradigm Dialog*, London: Sage.

Handy, C. (1995) *The Gods of Management: The Changing Work of Organisations*, London: Arrow.

Harries, J., Gordon, P., Plamping, P. and Fischer, M. (1999) *Elephant Problems and Fixes that Fail: The Story of a Search for New Approaches to Inter-agency Working*, London: King's Fund.

Ho, M. and Saunders, P. (1979) 'Beyond neo-Darwinism: an epigenetic approach to evolution', *Journal of Theoretical Biology* 78, 573–91.

Hudson, B., Hardy, B., Henwood, M. and Wistow, G. (1999) 'In pursuit of inter-agency collaboration in the public sector: what is the contribution of theory and research?' *Public Management: An International Journal of Research and Theory* 1 (2) 235–60.

Jameson, F. (1991) *Postmodernism Or, the Cultural Logic of Late Capitalism*, Durham: Duke University Press.

Judge, K., Barnes, M. and Bauld, L. (1999) *Health Action Zones: Learning to Make a*

Difference, Report of National Evaluation Team for Health Action Zones, Canterbury: University of Kent (http://www.ukc.ac.uk/pssru).

Law, L. (1997) 'Dancing on the bar: sex, money, and the uneasy politics of third-space', in S. Pile and M. Keith (eds), *Geographies of Resistance*, London: Routledge.

Leathard, A. (1997) 'Collaboration: united we stand, divided we fall?' in L. Jones and M. Sidell (eds), *The Challenge of Promoting Health: Exploration and Action*, London: Macmillan.

Markwell, S. (1998) 'Exploration of conflict theory as it relates to healthy alliances', in Scriven (ed.), *Alliances in Health Promotion: Theory and Practice*, London: Macmillan.

Markwell, S. and Speller, V. (2001) 'Partnership working and interprofessional collaboration: policy and practice', in A. Scriven and J. Orme (eds), *Health Promotion: Professional Perspective* 2nd edn., Basingstoke: Palgrave.

Medd, W. (2001) 'Complexity and partnership', in D. Taylor (ed.), *Breaking Down Barriers: Reviewing Partnership Practice*, Brighton: University of Brighton.

Morgan, G. (1986) *Images of Organisation*, London: Sage.

Powell, M. (1999) 'New Labour and the third way in the British NHS', *International Journal of Health Services* 29 (2) 353–70.

Powell, M. and Moon, G. (2001) 'Health Action Zones: the "third way" of a new area-based policy?', *Health and Social Care in the Community* 9 (1) 43–50.

Pratt, J., Plamping, D. and Gordon, P. (2000) *Working Whole Systems: Practice and Theory in Network Organisations*, London: King's Fund.

Rose, G. (1994) 'The cultural politics of place: local representation and oppositional discourse in two films', *Transactions of the Institute of British Geographers*. NS 19, 46–60.

Rose, G. (1997) 'Performing inoperative community: the space and the resistance of some community arts projects', in S. Pile and M. Keith (eds), *Geographies of Resistance*, London: Routledge.

Routledge, P. (1997) 'A spatiality of resistances', in S. Pile and M. Keith (eds), *Geographies of Resistance*, London: Routledge.

Russell, H. (2001) *Local Strategic Partnerships: Lessons from New Commitment to Regeneration*, Bristol: The Policy Press.

Scriven, A. (ed) (1998) *Alliances in Health Promotion: Theory and Practice*, London: Macmillan.

Senge, P. (1990) *The Fifth Discipline: The Art and Practice of Organisational Learning*, New York: Doubleday.

Senge, P. (1994) *The Fifth Discipline Fieldbook: Strategies and Tools for Building a Learning Organization*, London: Brealey.

Senge, P. (1999) *The Dance of Change: The Challenges of Sustaining Momentum in Learning Organisations*, London: Brealey.

Smith, T. (2001) *Common Knowledge: The Tyne and Wear Health Action Zone's Arts and Health Project*, Report, Centre for Arts and Humanities in Health and Medicine, Durham: University of Durham.

Soja, E. (1996) *Thirdspace: Journeys to Los Angeles and other Real-and-Imagined Place*, Oxford: Blackwell.

Soja, E. (2000) *Postmetropolis: Critical Studies of Cities and Regions*, Oxford: Blackwell.

Springett, J. (1995) *Intersectoral Collaboration Theory and Practice: Lessons for the WHO Healthy Cities Project*, Institute for Health, Occasional Paper Series, Liverpool: Liverpool JM University.

Springett, J. (1998) 'Quality measures and evaluation of Healthy City policy initiatives: the Liverpool experience', in J. Davies and G. Macdonald (eds), *Quality, Evidence and Effectiveness in Health Promotion*, London: Routledge.

Stacey, R. (1996) *Complexity and Creativity in Organisations*, San Francisco: Berret-Koehler.

Stacey, R. (2000) *Strategic Management and Organisational Dynamics: The Challenge of Complexity*, Harlow: Pearson.

Stewart, M. (2000) *Collaboration and Co-ordination in Area-based Regeneration Initiatives*, Regeneration Research Summary Number 35, London: Department of Environment, Transport and the Regions (http://www.regeneration.detr.gov.uk/rs).

Wall, A. (1998) 'The ethics of getting on with others', in A. Scriven (ed.), *Alliances in Health Promotion: Theory and Practice*, London: Macmillan.

Winter, R., Buck, A. and Sobiechowska, P. (1999) *Professional Experience and the Investigative Imagination*, London: Routledge.

Chapter 11

Supporting families

An interprofessional approach?

Lonica Vanclay

SUMMARY

The experience of a UK voluntary organisation, Family Welfare Association (FWA) is used to show that different forms of collaboration between many people and agencies are required for high quality, effective family support services. Although the practical difficulties of collaborative work have long been experienced and are well documented, they are deep-seated and continue to occur. FWA has found that leadership; communication, trust and mutual respect between those involved; and having clear, shared, service focused goals and objectives helps to deal with the difficulties. However, successful collaboration in family support will only be achieved with the development of a culture of collaboration in all organisations, a process that will take time, sustained effort and commitment and coordinated policy support.

THE NATURE OF FAMILY SUPPORT

Types of family support

Family support services promote and support the welfare and upbringing of children by their families. Services are targeted in different ways, with different levels of intervention (Hardiker 1988). Universal services include playgroups, toy libraries, pre- and postnatal care and some parenting education activities.

Second-level services provide community-based early intervention and support to exclude families in disadvantaged localities to prevent problems arising. Their aim is to promote integration, enhance coping and parenting, develop skills, strengthen networks, develop new services and change the environment. Family, neighbourhood and community centres, self-help groups and community development activities are examples (Gibbons 1990; Canaan and Warren 1997).

More specialised services target referred vulnerable families experiencing early stress and provide help to prevent problems escalating. Family centres, intensive home support, counselling and multidisciplinary child and adolescent mental health teams are examples. The most targeted services work with families defined as having a child in need of protection or at risk of neglect or abuse, and aim to avoid the need for involvement of statutory child protection services and children being looked after by the state.

Different forms of family support are appropriate at different times for different families and different organisations adopt different approaches according to their own aims, experience, interests and resources.

A holistic approach to family support

The family is central to the personal experience of each individual whether this is the family of origin, the co-residential group or whether an individual is living alone, separated through choice, accident or circumstance, from other family members. Adults and children are supported by grandparents, relatives and significant others as well as by their immediate family. Services should promote and assist the development of supportive relationships between a wide network of family members. To support the family as a whole, services will need to support individual family members at all stages of the life cycle with their own problems.

Family life and individual and family well-being also encompass many relationships with the wider environment. Problems result from the complex interaction of individual, familial, community, societal, environmental, economic, biological, educational, emotional, legal and social factors. Individuals and families will need and want contact with different agencies to help them resolve difficulties. Family support, therefore, requires collaboration with a wide range of partners including community groups, voluntary agencies and statutory organisations in the housing, economic, welfare, education, police, justice, leisure and transport sectors in addition to health and social care. Policies and services in all these sectors have a major impact on family well-being and coordination between them is essential for family support.

This chapter focuses on front-line social support services that provide a wide range of individual, family, group and community activities to help individuals and families deal with issues of concern to them; services that aim to empower people, help them build on their strengths, increase self-esteem, strengthen social networks, improve functioning, promote health and well-being and reach their full potential.

Key features of family support services

User consultations and evaluations of UK family support services show services are valued by users, have significant benefits and require collaboration to be effective (Macdonald and Roberts 1995; Utting 1995; Robbins 1998; Buchanan 1999; Little 1999; Mental Health Foundation 1999; Aldgate and Statham 2001; Henricson et al 2001). Important points highlighted by the research follow.

- Providing a continuum of early intervention support services can prevent problems escalating, reduce family breakdown, prevent social exclusion and enhance a sense of community
- Families want, need and use such services, especially when they are non-stigmatising and accessible
- Services that work with the whole family and provide a combination of practical and emotional help have a greater impact
- Much of the expertise for the solution of problems rests with people themselves. Effective prevention and intervention requires that professionals build on people's own strengths, experience and skills
- Effective services should be welcoming, flexible and reliable, with staff who users can trust, who respect users and listen carefully to them
- Providers must ensure services reach and are appropriate for groups, such as men, minority ethnic families and teenagers, who are often marginalised and do not access family support services.

The research concludes that a range of services are needed to meet different needs at different stages, that no one off the shelf model of family support works for all. Services need to be responsive to local needs and linked in to other local services. The studies also show that people do not want to be asked the same questions over and over, to be given conflicting advice, to receive fragmented or separate, parallel services or to be sent from one agency to another. They want, need and deserve coordinated support and integrated services. Effective family support requires interagency working and partnerships across many sectors.

POLICY INFLUENCES ON COLLABORATIVE WORK IN FAMILY SUPPORT

Collaboration and coordination is also required and encouraged by government. The unification into generic social services departments in 1968 of the children's, health and welfare services, which had been spread across several departments, signalled the beginning of a coordinated approach to family support in England. These new departments were to provide community-based social care and support services for the family as a whole (Seebohm 1989).

Cooperation and joint working between health and social services developed during the 1970s. Teamwork in the health service and a community focus in social work were encouraged and recognition of the importance of social factors in health increased. Several successful but short lived projects began, with social workers attached to general practitioner (GP) practices to support children in need and their families or to improve older people's services (Huntingdon 1981; Clare and Corney 1982).

During the 1980s, the government promoted greater separation between services, distinguished provider and purchaser roles and emphasised competition. With the added impact of rapid organisational changes, increased social pressures and inequalities and the squeeze on resources, professionals and organisations became more concerned with internal developments. The little interest there had been in coordinating family support services across health, education and social care decreased.

Several enquiries in the late 1980s concluded that poor interprofessional communication and interagency collaboration were important causes of child protection and community care service failures. Calls for greater coordination, improved interprofessional working and joint planning and commissioning made throughout the 1990s in community care, mental health and primary health care policies affected family support services (Department of Health 1990a, 1990b, 1994, 1996; Loxley 1997).

In children and family services, the need for a team approach, partnership with parents, provision of a range of services appropriate to children's needs and coordination between health and social services were also emphasised (Department of Health 1989; Home Office et al 1991; Department of Health et al 1999). Interagency planning was introduced (Department of Health et al 1996). Subsequent guidelines (Department of Health et al 2000) require interagency collaboration in assessment to ensure full understanding of children's needs and families' circumstances and an effective service response.

In addition to targeted help for families with particular problems, family support in the UK includes government help for all families through fiscal and benefit policies. Concerns emerged in the 1990s that family breakdown and social disadvantage and exclusion were increasing. Questions about the effectiveness of the considerable public resources spent were raised. The government acknowledged that intervention was provided too late, that services needed to pre-empt problems and tackle them earlier, using cross-sectoral approaches (Department of Health 1992; Acheson 1998; Gordon 2000).

The government set out an early intervention strategy for supporting vulnerable families with children (Home Office 1999). This included five strands:

- Improving parenting through ensuring parents have access to advice and information on how to bring up children (coordinated by the National Family and Parenting Institute)
- Amending aspects of the tax and benefits system to increase the income of low income families

- Helping families balance work and home by promoting family-friendly employment practices and employee rights
- Improving support for adult relationships
- Improving services for families with acute problems with children's learning, youth offending, teenage pregnancy and domestic violence

The Social Exclusion Unit was established in 1997 with cross-departmental membership to look at reducing the social exclusion of disadvantaged families and to promote the regeneration of deprived neighbourhoods. A plethora of initiatives with family support components and designated funding to reduce exclusion and inequality and improve health and well-being were introduced (Table 11.1). All these initiatives require team, interagency and partnership working. Although there is some overlap between them and they are not always coordinated locally or integrated nationally, the number and variety signifies considerable policy support for collaborative working in family support.

Many initiatives require the establishment of partnerships with representatives from different statutory, business and voluntary organisations (Table 11.2). All specify the need to consult, actively involve and listen to users and

Table 11.1. Interagency initiatives with a family support element

Education/employment	*Social care and housing*
Early excellence centres	Youth offending teams
Education action zones	On track
Pastoral and behavioural support programmes	Quality Protects
Sure start	Supporting people
Children and young people's fund	
Connexions	
Employment action zones	
Neighbourhood nurseries	
Health/public health	*Regeneration*
Health action zones	Single regeneration budget
Healthy living centres	New deal for communities
Modernisation plans	Rural development areas
Improved access to services	Neighbourhood renewal
	New deal for lone parents
	New opportunities fund

Table 11.2 Partnerships relevant to family support

- Early years' development and childcare partnerships
- Education action zone partnerships
- Children and young people's partnerships
- Sure start partnerships
- Regeneration partnerships (SRB and New Deal)

local residents. The partnership is responsible for planning programmes of activities, for funding received and for ensuring activities are provided, usually by a number of different organisations. The roles of lead agency and accountable body may be taken by one or two organisations for the partnership.

The government requires that partnerships compile different strategic plans (Table 11.3). Central government has also introduced national strategies, implementation plans that are to be developed locally, including the National Childcare Strategy and the Teenage Pregnancy Coordination Strategy.

The need for coordination between these many initiatives (often with overlapping geographical boundaries) and partnerships (many with overlapping membership) has been acknowledged by the requirement that local areas set up Local Strategic Partnerships (LSPs) involving the public, private, business, voluntary and community sectors (Social Exclusion Unit 2000). The role of LSPs is to prepare and implement a community strategy that promotes the well-being of the area, bring together local plans, partnerships and initiatives and develop and deliver a neighbourhood renewal strategy. It is increasingly recognised that having coterminous boundaries makes integrated work easier.

Responsibility for aspects of family support is spread across many government departments, as this section shows. In 1998 the Family Policy Unit was formed in the Home Office, which has the responsibility for coordinating family policy across government. Largely, this coordination takes the form of the Ministerial Sub-committees on Active Communities and Family Issues, chaired by the Home Secretary. This committee makes decisions on major areas of family policy.

The Family Policy Unit also runs a Family Support Grant programme that provides funding to voluntary organisations to address the gaps in the support currently available to parents. The focus of the Unit's work is to support all those in a parenting role, promoting the ethos that asking for help is a sign of responsible parenting and not an admission of failure and aiming to reach those needing particular support through providing universal support.

The government is becoming increasingly coordinated with growing interdepartmental liaison. Planning guidance for the Children's Services Plans, for example, was issued in England jointly by the Departments of Health,

Table 11.3 Plans relevant to family support

- Health improvement plans
- Early years and child care partnership plans
- Education development plans
- Children's services plans
- Children and young people's strategic plans
- Youth justice plans

Education and Employment, Environment, Transport and Regions, Culture, Media and Sport and the Home Office, Treasury and Cabinet Office. Establishing one continuing body to lead and coordinate a holistic approach to family support policy at national government level would be a major step forward.

PRACTICE ISSUES

Providing family support services requires collaboration with others, as the previous sections show. However, implementing this approach in practice is not easy. The experience of the FWA, a British voluntary organisation registered as a charity, is used as a case example to consider ways of dealing with the difficulties encountered in providing front-line family support services in collaboration with others. FWA has a long history of coordinating services (it was established in 1869 as the Charity Organisation Society to coordinate charitable giving), of pioneering innovative services (it set up one of the first Citizens' Advice Bureaux) and of working across health and social care (it seconded a social worker to be the first hospital social worker). It runs services and distributes grants, so provides both practical and emotional support.

FWA provides a range of holistic family support services including child and family services and mental health day care and residential services, funded from different sources, across the south-east of England. Involvement in different types of collaborative working is an integral component of its family support service provision.

FWA employs staff from different backgrounds in its services who work as a team; its staff work with other professionals from other agencies in different ways and it participates in many partnerships to plan, develop and provide new services and to better coordinate the planning and provision of existing services. Family support requires more than interprofessional collaboration. Intra-agency teamwork, interagency working and participation in partnerships are essential.

Teamwork within the agency

In its home-based family support services, family centres, mental health day care and residential services, FWA employs staff with different professional backgrounds, including community and nursery nursing, social work, therapy, youth and community work, education and psychology. Services also have staff with no formal professional qualifications, including people who have undertaken counselling courses, playgroup workers, support workers, administrative and reception staff, cooks, cleaners, peer mentors and volunteers. Some are full time, some part time and others sessional (e.g. group tutors). All work together to provide high quality, responsive and coordinated services.

The difficulties of teamwork summarised in the literature (Miller et al 2001), continue to be experienced by FWA staff, who have found two factors to be particularly important in facilitating and sustaining teamwork – leadership and clear objectives.

Senior staff encourage services to value and prioritise teamwork. Project managers have designated responsibility for developing a mutually supportive, positive team culture among staff and a way of working that values collaboration and information-sharing. Through facilitating discussions, workshops, regular staff meetings and case reviews, the managers help staff members recognise, value and understand the particular approach, role and contribution of each colleague. Project managers help sustain the commitment and enthusiasm of staff through team reviews, individual supervision and developmental activities. Attention is given to ensuring part-time and new staff are integrated into the team. While some staff are usually more involved with certain users or situations, managers value all staff equally and let them know they are equally important to the overall success of the service.

Facilitating a shared vision with clear objectives that all staff own and helped to develop is another important task for managers. All staff are expected to uphold the core shared values that FWA consulted on and set out. Managers oversee the allocation of roles and responsibilities and regular reviews of plans, progress, priorities and difficulties. Constant communication is necessary. Managers support each team member in carrying out tasks, ensure all work together harmoniously to deliver the service and mediate discussions between staff when differences or conflicts arise.

Interagency working

Definitions of collaboration highlight that shared purpose and agreed goals are equally important when different agencies work together. Mutual respect and willingness to negotiate and share information, responsibility, skills, decision-making and accountability are also necessary (Pugh and De'Ath 1989; Beresford and Trevillion 1995).

FWA's family support staff have found that providing appropriate integrated services for users requires that they regularly work collaboratively in different ways with staff from different agencies. Sometimes, occasional liaison and information-sharing is required; for example staff in a mental health day centre obtain information about a referral from the community mental health team and liaise with the GP. At other times, frequent cross-referral and regular joint working are necessary. Staff in a family centre work jointly with the local authority social worker and a health visitor to support a young parent. They visit together, exchange information and meet with the family and all agencies involved to ensure that everyone understands each other's roles and plans and reviews progress together.

FWA has developed two models of service to work explicitly across agency and client group divisions: Building Bridges and WellFamily services. In both, staff take a holistic approach and work in collaboration with other professionals and agencies to foster a coordinated approach. In adult mental health services, the focus is on the adult's mental ill health, the adult's parenting responsibilities are overlooked and any children in the family are not supported. Children's services lack the skill and remit to support the adult with their mental illness. In contrast, the FWA's Building Bridges and Well-Family services take an integrated approach and work with the whole family.

Building Bridges services provide information, counselling support, practical help and group activities for parents and children together and separately, helping adults with their parenting role, helping children understand parental mental illness and supporting children with their caring role. Well-Family services provide individuals of all ages and families as a whole who self-refer or are referred with information, advice and counselling support on a range of social and emotional problems affecting their health and well-being. The worker is based in primary health care settings and sees users in their own homes or in GP practices. The non-stigmatising primary care base and flexible, holistic, collaborative and responsive approach facilitate access to and usage of the service by a very wide range of people, including those who often fall through the service nets (Clarke et al 2001). A practice guide (Vanclay 2001) further describes the model.

These services require constant interagency working, hence difficulties are brought into sharper focus. At first, staff did not always understand or value the role of others. Sometimes other professionals were concerned that their role was being taken over by FWA staff. Differences in educational experience, knowledge, status and styles of intervention between different staff complicated collaboration. These problems of staff defensiveness, tribalism and territoriality also occur within an agency. However, when staff are from different agencies, difficulties increase as there are fewer opportunities to meet and develop good working relationships. There is more potential for miscommunication and role conflict and confusion.

FWA staff work hard at developing good relationships of trust and understanding with colleagues. They are flexible, responsive and enthusiastic about collaboration. They persistently take the initiative in creating and using opportunities for contact. Being in the same building helps but does not guarantee good interagency working. Interagency working was effective when staff gave time to building relationships and developed good networks and formal and informal links. Practice experience of working together with particular families also helped the growth of mutual respect between staff and a better understanding of their respective roles.

FWA's WellFamily and Building Bridges staff found that clarifying and agreeing the tasks needed to achieve the common shared goals was very important, just as it is with intra-agency teamwork. It was necessary to identify which staff in which agencies could best undertake those tasks and to foster an attitude where all are equally valued. Staff had to learn to understand the role and culture of other staff and other agencies and to understand and respect differences and boundaries. Staff also had to be confident about their own identity and agency's role so they could describe and contribute their particular strengths and skills to the overall task. Regular review and evaluation of progress towards agreed goals by staff from different agencies and the opportunity to learn together from this process helped interagency work grow.

The process of developing and sustaining coordination between agencies working with families needs facilitation. In early intervention family support services there is seldom a designated keyworker. The job description of FWA's Building Bridges and WellFamily staff included responsibility for ensuring coordination. This included bringing professionals together to plan, monitor completion of allocated tasks and review progress and link with family members to ensure that they understood the respective roles of different agencies. As voluntary organisation employees, FWA staff found that their authority and competence was sometimes first questioned by statutory agencies who assumed voluntary organisation staff were volunteers and amateurs. They also found that over time, their independence, flexibility, holistic approach and user focus enabled them to work effectively across and between organisational boundaries. Agencies and families valued this greatly and having someone with this role was very important in ensuring coordination was achieved.

Interagency work is further complicated by differences between agencies in management, organisational structure, operational focus, priorities, style, eligibility criteria, resources, influence, boundaries, constitutional arrangements, funding sources and budgetary procedures. With constant structural changes in services and workload and resource pressures, staff inevitably prioritise their own work and the concerns of their own agency and give interagency work less time and priority than it needs. FWA's services have found that collaboration is easier when all staff and each agency understand why it is necessary, support it, prioritise it and put resources, time and effort into making it work. Taking a collaborative rather than a competitive approach and being willing to negotiate, concede autonomy and share power is not easy. Senior management support for collaboration and effective communication at senior management level between agencies will help. Having established interagency structures and relationships at strategic levels, which value interagency working, highlight it as a criteria for success and build it into local service plans will help facilitate collaboration between front-line staff.

FWA's conclusions from its service experience about what helps interagency work reflect the lessons from another recent interagency family support initiative, which highlights the importance of support at all levels, clear roles, formal and informal contact, shared activities and having someone with clear responsibility for coordination in facilitating collaborative work (Wigfall and Moss 2001).

Participating in partnerships

FWA is a member of many local partnerships (see Table 11.2) and provides family support services on their behalf in several areas. It also participates in and contributes practice experience and views on needs and gaps to locality Health and Social Care Boards that plan and coordinate new and existing services and allocate resources.

Unlike interagency working where different professionals from different agencies collaborate at times to help plan and deliver services, partnership staff (whether employed by the partnership, one lead agency and/or several different agencies) work towards the common partnership goal all their time while delivering separate components of the agreed overall programme.

Although there is a common management framework, a specified form and structure for coordination, common goals, shared tasks and many opportunities for joint working and communication in partnerships, staff still experience difficulties.

Workers can feel they have split allegiances between their employer and the partnership as a whole, especially if the employer's knowledge of or support for the overall partnership goal and activities is limited or if views differ. Because staff in partnership programmes constantly work together, they are very aware of the different approaches, status, expectations, salary, levels of funding, management styles and cultures of different professionals and agencies. This can create tension and mistrust between staff. The greater power, resources and influence that large statutory organisations have over small community groups and voluntary organisations contributes further to unequal and uneasy relationships between partners. Local residents and representatives from community groups often feel especially marginalised.

FWA has found that effective leadership, facilitation of a teamwork approach and commitment from all partners are needed to develop the trust, openness and mutual respect and understanding necessary for all partnership members to agree a shared vision with achievable goals and to allocate tasks and funds. It takes time for partners to establish ways of effectively involving users, sharing responsibility, information and decisions and developing simple and transparent processes for accessing and accounting for funds.

CONCLUSION

The difficulties of intra-agency team, interagency and partnership working have long been experienced and are well documented in the literature (Huntingdon 1981; Ovretveit 1993; Audit Commission 1994; Owens et al 1995; Vanclay 1996; Atkinson et al 2001; Hornby and Atkins 2001; Scriven and Orme 2001). That FWA staff still experience these difficulties despite the considerable current policy support for collaborative work at all levels highlights how challenging and complex it is to develop and maintain collaborative working.

Despite being difficult to achieve, collaborative work is necessary. Government policy requires it. Most importantly, users need, want and deserve access to a wide range of skills and flexible, seamless, high quality, holistic family support services that respond to their needs as a whole person. Team, interagency and partnership working are essential for the planning and provision of high quality holistic family support services.

There are no quick or easy solutions for overcoming the difficulties. There are, however, as FWA staff have found, common themes for success, whether the collaboration is with users, staff, agencies or partnerships. Leadership, mutual respect, communication, trust and shared, clear goals and objectives are fundamental. Most importantly, considerable continuous effort and commitment is needed from all staff at all levels in all organisations to work together, reflect together on that work and learn together from that process. It will take time and sustained commitment to develop this new culture of learning and partnership.

The skills needed for collaboration have been identified (Vanclay 1996; Whittington and Bell 2001). Greater emphasis must be given to incorporating the development of such skills into all stages of the training and development of all staff. The process will need prioritising and resourcing and will be achieved not through short-term projects but by ensuring team, interagency and partnership working are integral components of each individual's and organisation's family support work.

REFERENCES

Acheson, D. (1998) *Independent Inquiry into Inequalities in Health Report*, London: The Stationery Office.

Aldgate, J. and Statham, J. (2001) *The Children Act Now: Messages from Research*, London: The Stationery Office.

Atkinson, M., Wilkin, A., Stott, A. and Kinder, K. (2001) *Multi-agency Working: An Audit of Activity*, Slough: National Foundation for Educational Research.

Audit Commission (1994) *Seen But Not Heard – Coordinating Community Child Health and Social Services for Children*, London: HMSO.

Beresford, P. and Trevillion, S. (1995) *Developing Skills for Community Care: A Collaborative Approach*, Aldershot: Arena.

Buchanan, A. (1999) *What Works in Family Support?*, Essex: Barnardos.

Canaan, C. and Warren, C. (eds) (1997) *Social Action with Children and Families: A Community Development Approach to Child and Family Welfare*, London: Routledge.

Clare, A. and Corney, R. (ed.) (1982) *Social Work and Primary Health Care*, London: Academic Press.

Clarke, K., Sarre, S., Glendinning, C. and Datta, J. (2001) *FWA's WellFamily Service: Evaluation Report*, London: Family Welfare Association.

Department of Health (1989) *An Introduction to the Children Act 1989*, London: HMSO.

Department of Health (1990a) *The NHS and Community Care Act*, London: HMSO.

Department of Health (1990b) *The Care Programme Approach*, London: HMSO.

Department of Health (1992) *Report of the Inquiry into London's Health Service, Medical Education and Research (The Tomlinson Report)*, London: HMSO.

Department of Health (1994) *Implementing Caring for People: The Role of the GP and Primary Healthcare Team*, London: Health Publications Unit, Department of Health.

Department of Health (1996) *Building Bridges: A Guide to Arrangements for the Care and Protection of Severely Mentally Ill People*, London: HMSO.

Department of Health and Department for Education and Employment (1996) *Children's Services Planning Guidance*, London: The Stationery Office.

Department of Health, Home Office and Department for Education and Employment (1999) *Working Together to Safeguard Children*, London: The Stationery Office.

Department of Health, Department for Education and Employment and Home Office (2000) *Framework for the Assessment of Children in Need and their Families*, London: The Stationery Office.

Gibbons, J. (1990) *Family Support and Prevention*, London: HMSO.

Gordon, D. (2000) *Poverty and Social Exclusion in Britain*, York: Joseph Rowntree Foundation.

Hardiker, P. (1988) 'Children still in need indeed: prevention across five decades', in O. Stevenson (ed.) *Child Welfare in the UK*, Oxford: Blackwell Scientific.

Henricson, C., Katz, I., Mesie, J., Sandison, M. and Tunstill, J. (2001) *National Mapping of Family Services in England and Wales – A Consultation Document*, London: National Family and Parenting Institute.

Home Office (1999) *Supporting Families*, London: The Stationery Office.

Home Office, Department of Health, Department of Education and Science and Welsh Office (1991) *Working Together Under the Children Act 1989*, London: HMSO.

Hornby, S. and Atkins, J. (2001) *Collaborative Care: Interprofessional, Interagency and Interpersonal*, Oxford: Blackwell.

Huntingdon, J. (1981) *Social Work and General Medical Practice*, London: Allen & and Unwin.

Little, M. (1999) 'Prevention and early intervention with children in need: definitions, principles and examples of good practice', *Children and Society* 13, 304–16.

Loxley, A. (1997) *Collaboration in Health and Welfare: Working with Difference*, London: Jessica Kingsley.

Macdonald, G. and Roberts, H. (1995) *What Works in the Early Years*, Essex: Barnardos.

Mental Health Foundation (1999) *Bright Futures: Promoting Children and Young People's Mental Health*, London: Mental Health Foundation.

Miller, C., Freeman, M. and Ross, N. (2001) *Interprofessional Practice in Health and Social Care*, London: Arnold.

Ovretveit, J. (1993) *Coordinating Community Care*, Milton Keynes: Open University Press.

Owens, P., Carrier, J. and Horder, J. (1995) *Interprofessional Issues in Community and Primary Health Care*, London: Macmillan.

Pugh, G. and De'Ath, E. (1989) *Working Towards Partnership in the Early Years*, London: National Children's Bureau.

Robbins, D. (1998) *Families in Focus*, London: The Stationery Office.

Scriven, A. and Orme, J. (2001) *Health Promotion: Professional Perspectives*, Milton Keynes: Palgrave/The Open University.

Seebohm, F. (1989) *Seebohm: Twenty Years On*, London: Policy Studies Institute.

Social Exclusion Unit (2000) *A New Commitment to Neighbourhood Renewal: National Strategic Action Plan*, London: The Stationery Office.

Utting, D. (1995) *Family and Parenthood: Supporting Families, Preventing Breakdown*, York: Joseph Rowntree Foundation.

Vanclay, L. (1996) *Sustaining Collaboration between General Practitioners and Social Workers*, London: CAIPE.

Vanclay, L. (2001) *The WellFamily Service Model: A Practice Guide*, London: FWA.

Whittington, C. and Bell, L. (2001) 'Learning for interprofessional and interagency practice', *Journal of Interprofessional Care* 15 (2) 53–169.

Wigfall, V. and Moss, P. (2001) *More than the Sum of its Parts: A Study of a Multi-agency Child Care Network*, London: National Children's Bureau.

Chapter 12

Safeguarding children together
Addressing the interprofessional agenda

Sara Glennie

SUMMARY

Research has substantially influenced the current policy agenda for interprofessional work in child protection and has driven the need for fundamental changes in practice at individual, organisational and interorganisational level. The intended changes in interagency practice have been promoted through the implementation of two important policy documents; *Working Together to Safeguard Children* (Department of Health et al 1999) and *The Framework for the Assessment of Children in Need and their Families* (Department of Health et al 2000). Nationally, strategies employed to ensure their implementation have differed from one area to another. Area Child Protection Committees (ACPCs) and interagency child protection training have been only moderately successful in supporting developments given the current interprofessional context.

INTRODUCTION

Predictably, discussions about child protection practice in the UK begin with a well-established mantra; effective protection for children is contingent on interprofessional and interagency commitment and collaboration at all levels. An early statement in the most recent, relevant government guidance is characteristic of the tone; 'promoting children's well-being and safeguarding them from significant harm depends crucially upon effective information sharing, collaboration and understanding between agencies and professionals' (Department of Health et al 1999: 2). Similarly, Stevenson (1994: 121) reminds us of the 'now widely accepted view that effective work in child protection requires interprofessional co-operation', as do recommendations from successive inquiries into child deaths (Reder and Duncan 1999). The message is clear and unequivocal. However, the translation of an agreed rhetoric, no matter how well formulated through policy, into recognisable interprofessional practice reality, remains both intellectually perplexing and practically challenging. This situation has been most acutely felt during the latter part of the 1990s, a time of rapid policy development in child welfare and complicated by simultaneous disturbance in the interprofessional environment due to structural change and chronic problems of staff recruitment, retention and morale within public sector organisations.

This chapter briefly outlines the key influences from research on the development of the current policy agenda for interprofessional work in child protection. Discussion focuses on the strategies that have been employed to ensure the achievement of the intended changes at individual, organisational and interorganisational levels through the implementation of two important policy documents; *Working Together to Safeguard Children* (Department of Health et al 1999) and *The Framework for the Assessment of Children in Need and their Families* (Department of Health et al 2000). (*Note*: Both documents are referred to in the subsequent text as *Working Together* and *The Assessment Framework*.) Tensions and difficulties experienced in the current context are highlighted. The role that ACPCs and interagency training play as key mechanisms for shaping interprofessional practice change is discussed.

RECEIVING THE MESSAGE

The year 1995 can be seen as a particularly significant watershed in the development of child protection policy and practice in the UK. During that year, the Department of Health published *Child Protection, Messages from Research* (DoH 1995). The publication summarised 20 research studies, also published in detail, commissioned in response to problems raised by a number of high profile inquiries into child protection practice during the 1980s. The studies are rich in data and enable a wide range of questions to be asked about particular aspects of the child protection system; for example, what outcomes for children and families can be expected? How are child protection conferences working? A number of the studies also posed the question; 'what about the focus of interagency work?' The answer to this latter question revealed one of the clearest messages arising from the research initiative:

> far too many cases are at present being dealt with under child protection procedures and . . . these should be dealt with under family support provisions. It is suggested that resources are being wasted by unnecessary investigations – or inquiries – under Section 47 of the Act (*The Children Act* 1989). The primary policy change should be to prioritise Section 17 and Part 3 of the Act in terms of helping and supporting families with children in need, thereby keeping notions of policing, surveillance and coercive interventions to a minimum.
>
> (Parton et al 1997: 216)

'Messages', as the research summary document became known, subsequently acted as a primary driver (Morrison 2000: 366) in shifting the direction of national policy and therefore the preoccupations of interprofessional practice as the government initiated the 'refocusing' of child protection.

> Research tells us that children are generally well protected when there are serious child abuse concerns. The challenge for us all now is to extend that successful collaboration to wider work in support of children and their families in need. Refocusing Children's Services is about avoiding too narrow a focus on alleged incidents of abuse or neglect. Instead it promotes the development of comprehensive children's services that incorporate the wide range of family and community support networks available.
>
> (Burns 1996)

The refocusing initiative, or debate, was well aired in interprofessional fora in an effort to appreciate the day-to-day implications of the proposed changes for the practice relationships between professionals on the ground.

What needs to change?

At that time, it can be argued that the great success of the previous decade, largely attributable to the efforts of ACPCs, had been the socialisation of large numbers of professionals working in the community into ways of working within an interagency child protection system that were systematic and, more or less, predictable, particularly in the early stages of the child protection process.

In part, this was due to the constant refinement of interagency child protection procedures and practice guidance, integrated into practice through interagency training and then reinforced by the supervision and management processes within individual agencies. In most areas, these efforts were effective in clarifying the multiple roles and tasks associated with the protection of children. Overall, the interagency system operated smoothly; Hallett (1995) refers to highly routinised collaboration, embedded in practice and procedures, which is most effective when individuals knew and trusted one another. Hallett (1995) also notes that social workers and police officers acted powerfully at the interface between other professional groups in the community and the child protection system. In the early stages of intervention, these two groups were considered by others as experts in the confirmation of cases needing to be managed within the child protection system while other professional roles could best be described as potential referrers and information sources.

Predictable as it was, the interagency system was not without difficulties (Farmer and Owen 1995). For example, initial child protection conferences provided a potential opportunity for professional groups other than social workers to exert influence and participate more widely in decision-making, but influence was dependent on attendance, and confidence in role. Furthermore, there were indications of superficially consensual behaviour among professionals at key decision points, attributable in part to be to the reluctance of other agencies to challenge the perceived wisdom of social services departments (SSD). As Corby (1987) had suggested earlier, 'A crucial influence in maintaining the no-conflict norm was the lead role of the SSD' (Corby 1987: 99). Farmer and Owen (1995) observed that new or unexpected information was not always welcome in conferences, pulling as it did against the need for certainty and consensus and potentially threatening to the foundations of the social network in which interagency work is grounded.

However, despite the difficulties, it can be argued that in 1995 the child protection system in the UK was characterised by an agreed set of codified interprofessional behaviours held together by a common language and conceptual templates, which were largely evidential and forensic in nature. A snapshot of communication between a voluntary sector family centre and a social services team about a severely neglected child clearly illustrates the forensic quality of interprofessional communication that was being highlighted:

> the primary medium of communication and exchange related to the evidence, or not, of physical signs on the child's body. So there were faxes about faeces in skin folds, bruises and nappy rash. All of these facts are important, however, the weight they were given appeared to define the relationship as one in which the family centre focuses on the search for evidence rather than full participation in the identification, promotion and evaluation of developmental goals for X.
>
> (taken from research notes by Sara Glennie in 1997)

This practice detail gives some indication of the challenges facing interprofessional work between individuals as efforts to 'refocus' began to be addressed. Horwath and Morrison (2000: 245) considered the task to be one of changing 'emphasis, from an investigative approach ... to a more balanced approach between preventive and tertiary interventions'. However, the 'change in attitude towards safeguarding and promoting the welfare of children requires an evaluation of agency values, core business, priorities and organisational structures . . .'. The change that was needed gradually became evident to individual agencies who make up ACPCs through the extended consultation process that was employed to inform the publication of *Working Together*. The document, the first revision of interagency guidance in relation to child protection since 1991, fully embodied 'Messages' and set clear developmental objectives for interagency work into the new millennium. Prepared and issued jointly by the Department of Health, Home Office and

Department for Education and Employment, *Working Together*, with an accompanying document, *The Assessment Framework*, was issued under Section 7 of the Local Authority Social Services Act 1970. This means that the guidance must be followed unless there are exceptional circumstances that justify a variation.

Although explicitly linked in their final publication, the above two documents differed in quality, had different developmental histories and carried dissimilar implementation directives from central government. These differences were to have a significant impact on the way in which implementation was approached and experienced.

The developmental history of new guidance

Essentially, *Working Together* was the product of an extended interagency consultation process and built on messages from research that had already been widely disseminated (if not acted upon) by other means. The document was a revision of guidance designed to inform interagency working and, although containing many new and challenging demands, there was a sense, across agencies, that the document was both familiar and provided them with 'a national framework within which agencies and professionals at local level – individually and jointly – draw up and agree upon their own more detailed ways of working together' (Department of Health et al 1999: vii). No explicit implementation timetable accompanied the publication.

On the other hand, *The Assessment Framework* was identified during its developmental stages almost exclusively with meeting the need to improve social work assessment activity. The document therefore appeared, to many ACPC partner agencies, to be a SSD responsibility. The publication was designed as a practice tool characterised by a holistic, needs-led and child-focused approach and was piloted extensively within SSDs. Only late in the day were training materials, designed to support its introduction, adapted for use with interagency audiences. On publication, in April 2000, it became clear that *The Assessment Framework* was 'intended to provide a valuable foundation for policy and practice for *all* professionals and agencies who manage and provide services to children in need and their families' (ministerial letter dated 4 April 2000 accompanying *The Assessment Framework*). The document carried an explicit expectation of implementation by 1st April 2001 and therefore formed a central part of the interprofessional child welfare agenda.

DESTABILISING THE INTERPROFESSIONAL PRACTICE SYSTEM

Changing policy is one thing; changing the behaviours of individuals within a complex system to conform to policy intention is another. Looking at the fine grain of interprofessional practice behaviour, the nature of change required by the refocusing initiative and subsequent new guidance looked like this: first, practitioners needed to reconceptualise the way in which they look at the population of children in the community and use a different language to name those revised concepts. Second, the roles and relationships of existing partners in interprofessional networks need to be renegotiated and new partners need to be integrated into practice environments. Furthermore, a rapidly expanding knowledge base needed to be understood and shared interprofessionally, along with the integration of a common assessment tool that enables a sharper interagency focus on outcomes for children. Finally, new protocols needed to be agreed across agencies; then developed and communicated at a local level in order to clarify and support all of the above. As Adams (2002: 1) graphically suggests, 'some of the messages which those of us helping schools to fulfil their child protection responsibilities had found especially pertinent are now becoming redundant as a sea-change washes over the whole field'.

The impact of change

Moving from the individual to the system level, the analysis developed by Benson (1975) in the USA and applied recently in the UK by Lupton et al (2001) is helpful in understanding the consequences for interprofessional work indicated by *Working Together* and *The Assessment Framework*. Benson's (1975) analysis employs two sets of concepts that are crucial to understanding interorganisational change. First, it is important to recognise that:

> patterns of interaction that derive from organisations' collaboration in the performance of their core functions . . . this interaction can be theorised in terms of the achievement of equilibrium across four key dimensions: *domain consensus* (agreement regarding the role and scope of each agency); *ideological consensus* (agreement about the nature of the tasks faced and the most appropriate way of approaching these tasks); *positive evaluation* (by workers in one organisation of the work of those in others); *work co-ordination* (patterns of collaboration and co-operation). Those networks in strong equilibrium are characterised by highly co-ordinated, co-operative interactions, based on consensus and mutual respect.
>
> (Lupton et al 2001: 15–16)

But in order to understand why a complex system, such as an interprofessional network, has particular characteristics, it is also necessary to 'examine a second set of concepts' (Lupton et al 2001: 16). These concepts relate to the deeper processes that influence individual organisational behaviour. Thus:

the dynamics of an interorganisational network should be viewed as a mini political economy in which the behaviour of each participant is determined in large part by its need to *secure its own objectives* (authors' emphasis). Achievement of domain or ideological consensus within the network, effective work cooperation or positive mutual evaluation will be possible only to the extent that it does not involve actions that undermine the . . . position of the collaborating agency.

(Lupton et al 2001: 16–17)

In order to implement *Working Together* and *The Assessment Framework* across agencies concerned with child protection, the system would necessarily be destabilised. As discussed by Lupton et al (2001), Benson's (1975) analysis suggests that implementation would require first of all, a realignment of *ideological and domain consensus*. In the process of realignment, *positive evaluation*, fragile at the best of times in anxious working contexts (Woodhouse and Pengelly 1991), would inevitably be jeopardised while *work coordination* was renegotiated and appropriately adjusted.

IMPLEMENTING NEW GUIDANCE

Morrison (2000: 368) reminds us that *Working Together* is but 'one of a raft of important inter-agency policy initiatives to address the needs of the most vulnerable groups in the population', which have flowed and continue to flow from the current Labour administration. The implementation challenge facing interorganisational partnerships, such as that which supports child protection, cannot be underestimated. Morrison (2000: 371) views it starkly, 'shifting the balance towards a more needs-led and preventive approach to child protection, in the context of continuous change, increasing public and political expectations about the management of risks, and centrally imposed outcome targets is a highly complex and possibly impossible task'. In attempting the impossible task, interagency child protection training plays a key role.

The developing role of interagency child protection training

Since the mid-1980s, interagency training has been identified as one of the primary mechanisms for delivering change in the interprofessional child protection system. With no common management or supervision structures, training is one of the few processes that successfully operates in the 'spaces between organisations' (Horwath and Glennie 1999: 203). Consequently, interagency child protection training has developed and matured significantly, usually under the umbrella of ACPCs, across the full range of training and development functions; from the establishment of need, to the development of method and delivery and the evaluation of impact on practice (Charles and Hendry 2000).

Promoting Interagency Training (PIAT)

While given scant attention in guidance at the time (Department of Health and Social Security 1988; DoH 1991) the important role of interagency child protection training was formally recognised in the late 1980s when the Department of Health commissioned work to explore its potential and complexity and to produce relevant training materials (Charles with Stevenson 1990). Further work has continued during the 1990s, particularly under the auspices of PIAT, a self-funding collaborative partnership between the NSPCC (National Society for the Prevention of Cruelty to Children), Sheffield University and the Professional Development Group at the University of Nottingham.

In advancing its aims, PIAT convenes a national conference annually, and provides a mechanism through which the collective 'voice' of interagency training can be heard at government level (PIAT 1998). Through publication and the facilitation of development groups, PIAT seeks to work actively with current preoccupations and concerns of those directly involved in interagency child protection training.

In anticipation of the likely central role that interagency training would play in delivering the changes in practice required by new guidance, PIAT, with supporting funding from the Department of Health, initiated an action research project in 1999. The research aimed to identify the different approaches to implementation of both *Working Together* and *The Assessment Framework* adopted across local authorities in England, to describe the approaches and the use of interagency training to generate change. A small group of health, education and social services representatives, drawn from a wide geographical distribution of unitary, shire county authorities and metropolitan boroughs in England were invited to work together as an action research group during the first year of implementation. Issues identified by the research group were further explored through the use of questionnaires and telephone interviews with an additional sample of 31 local authorities. The following discussion draws directly on their experience and findings.

Implementation: challenges and fertile conditions

The study (Charles and Glennie 2001) revealed some key issues in the translation of policy into interprofessional child protection practice. One was the identification of a set of 'fertile conditions' for implementation. The conditions read like a common-sense set of directions and confirm the 'key implementation factors' identified earlier by others (Morrison 2000: 372).

However, in the climate described above, the conditions identified proved extraordinarily difficult to achieve.

Ideological and domain consensus

Prior to initiating implementation, the study highlighted the need for extensive interagency planning based on accurate knowledge. It is crucial that the interagency practice context into which change is to be introduced is known and appreciated by all parties. Only then is it possible to move to the establishment of a shared vision across agencies about the nature of change required at policy, procedural and practice level. Horwath and Morrison (2000: 248) refer to this work as the 'contemplation stage' of organisational change during which it is important to acknowledge the need for alteration, establish ownership, as well as audit current strengths and weaknesses in order to identify what changes are needed. The establishment of these agreements proved to be a slow and imperfect process and implementation activity in the early stages was therefore severely hindered. One characteristic shared by all authorities represented was the absence of an explicit or agreed model of interagency change to inform action. Furthermore, there was little or no clarity about the desired outcomes. Implementation, it seems, had quickly become a word in common usage that carried no specific, actionable or agreed meaning within or across the agencies concerned. Several months into the centrally driven implementation timetable for *The Assessment Framework*:

> twenty three per cent of respondents to the questionnaire stated their authorities had no clear strategy for implementation, with a further 15 per cent being unaware of any implementation plan and process. Some planning approaches were described as 'piecemeal'. Whilst some authorities demonstrated evidence of a planned approach, many were less effective when they lacked inter-agency focus.
>
> (Charles and Glennie 2001: 6)

There were, at the same time, some areas reporting that the 'messages' contained in *Working Together* were not new. The guidance simply confirmed the incremental changes that had been made in local policy, procedure and practice during the late 1990s, particularly where there had been a proactive approach to the refocusing initiative. In those areas, the guidance was seen to be following and confirming developments in practice that had already been secured. This situation was more likely in unitary authorities, many of whom had used the opportunity that the structural and personnel changes, which local government reorganisation had brought to renegotiate and recast their child protection procedures and practice in line with contemporary research findings.

The Assessment Framework presented a different challenge. In the interprofessional environment, it was entirely new and, unlike *Working Together*, was not following, but was seen as *leading* practice. Implementation required that practitioners and managers in all agencies needed to be taken through a series of conceptually discreet steps, which began with helping them to answer the following questions; 'what is it?' and 'what has it got to do with me?' Having answered those questions, practitioners and managers could move on, individually and collectively, to think about how *The Assessment Framework* could be applied effectively to interprofessional practice.

Driving implementation

The responsibility for the implementation of *Working Together* was uncontroversial; it was clearly ACPC business. However, responsibility for *The Assessment Framework* was managed very differently across local authorities. The PIAT research showed two clear patterns; implementation activity was either led through the ACPC, or explicitly driven by SSDs, sometimes assisted by a perceived external 'expert'. A number of exogenous factors (Lupton et al 2001) appeared to predispose the adoption of one or other model. Predisposing factors predictably included the prevailing interagency culture of collaboration or otherwise, the presence or absence of leaders and their location, and pragmatic factors such as the size, flexibility and location of budgets (Charles and Glennie 2001: 3). While both approaches are legitimate, they generated different outcomes, particularly in relation to the sense of ownership and accountability that agencies demonstrate in relation to *The Assessment Framework*.

The identification of an interagency steering mechanism, whether or not it was the ACPC, was considered an essential prerequisite to commitment and agreed priorities (Morrison 2000; Charles and Glennie 2001). Referring to Benson (1975), Lupton et al (2001: 17) cautions, 'the behaviour of each participant is determined in large part by its need to secure its own objectives'. Therefore, by casting implementation as an interagency objective at the earliest opportunity, the risk of pulling in different directions is reduced. In fact, SSDs were identified as the driving force in the implementation of *The Assessment Framework* in a large majority of authorities. Only a small number implemented *The Assessment Framework* through the ACPC. Consequently,

> commitment levels varied within different parts of different agencies as
> well as between them. Where connections were easily established as to
> how implementation linked with individual agencies' core business,
> commitment was more likely. Competing priorities made an important
> difference in the capacity to give implementation a high priority . . . a
> significant number of authorities reported problems with commitment at

senior levels, with ... actions not matching words, and difficulties in engaging counterparts in partner agencies.

(Charles and Glennie 2001: 5)

Implementation progress

Implementation activity in relation to both *Working Together* and *The Assessment Framework* continues and while not the 'impossible task' that Morrison (2000: 368) prophesied, change is slow. A recently published summary of Children Act (1989) studies (DoH 2001a) confirms that it has been difficult for 'authorities to shift their views' and fully embrace the intention of *Working Together* guidance as child protection concerns continue to be 'the gateway to support services in many areas' (DoH 2001a: 44). In terms of the concepts and language that drive interprofessional decision-making, there is evidence that the continuing focus on incidents of abuse makes it difficult for workers to set children's need for protection into the wider context of their developmental needs and social context. For example, 'whilst domestic violence was present in nearly half of the cases in the safeguarding study ... it was rarely mentioned in child protection plans' (DoH 2001a: 45) suggesting that the holistic assessment of children's needs, including their need for protection, is not yet a reliable characteristic of interagency practice.

There are, of course, many reasons for this slow rate of change and it is still early days. However, there are encouraging signs, albeit anecdotal, for the faint hearted or discouraged. At a recent national seminar of those directly involved in the implementation of *The Assessment Framework*, it was reported that implementation activity had:

> provided some excellent opportunities for building and developing local networks and practice ... a multi-agency steering group illustrated how ownership of the Framework could be generated across all agencies. It became 'ours' not just Social Services ... an approach that required a mind shift on the part of social workers. They had to move from the position of having to 'do it all ourselves' as they recognised the possibility and desirability of collaborative work.

(Firth 2001: 3)

OVERSEEING THE INTERPROFESSIONAL AGENDA

During the last 15 years, ACPCs have been given an increasingly detailed remit to set the local conditions that enable 'agencies and professionals (to) work together to promote children's welfare and protect them from abuse and neglect' (Department of Health 1999 et al: vii). Although there are some common features, the structures and processes through which this is managed vary considerably from one authority to another. For example, ACPCs vary in their funding agreements, arrangements for chairing, the focus of sub-committee activity, and the range and robustness of interagency training activity. To some extent this is to be expected and many would argue that it is positively helpful, ensuring responsiveness to local conditions. However, this freedom may be challenged by two developments that have begun to jostle with implementation for priority on the interprofessional agenda in child protection. The first development concerns inspection. The second is the Laming Inquiry (2001).

A new agenda?

In 1998, it was proposed that all chief inspectors of services that are substantially involved with children should publish a joint report on child protection. Standards and criteria for joint inspection have recently been developed and in the current year, eight ACPCs will be inspected for the first time by teams led by the Social Services Inspectorate and including representatives from OFSTED (Office for Standards in Education), Commission for Health Improvement, HMI Probation, HMI Constabulary, HMI Prisons, HM Magistrates Courts Inspectorate and HM Crown Prosecution Service Inspectorate (DoH 2001b: 2). The inspection findings are likely to contribute to the debate that has been raised by the public inquiry into the shocking death of Victoria Climbie (Laming Inquiry 2001). Among other matters, the inquiry has focused attention on old questions about responsibility for the interagency agenda that need to be readdressed. To what extent can a non-statutory body, such as an ACPC, ensure effective interagency work when the forces that are pulling agencies apart are so unremitting? Should ACPCs be given a strengthened mandate? To what extent can practitioners be expected to effectively manage the differences among them when, as Lupton et al (2001) suggest when discussing Benson (1975), there is no secure overarching ideological or domain consensus? To what extent are we, as a society, prepared to tolerate difficulties, and sometimes disasters, in order to preserve the culture of 'voluntariness' that has characterised interprofessional work in this field for so long?

The implementation of *Working Together* and *The Assessment Framework* has provided an opportunity to critically evaluate the change processes currently adopted when attempts are made to develop the 'spaces between' professionals and the organisations they represent. Although a rather ragged picture has emerged, working through implementation has provided helpful understandings. The experience has highlighted again the difficulties of achieving joint vision, priority and ownership across organisations. Furthermore, questions have been raised about the mechanisms that are considered most appropriate and effective for overseeing change. These are not new concerns. However, they will need to be addressed with renewed urgency as the Laming Inquiry (2001) and the inspection of ACPCs shape a new agenda for the complex, and often chaotic, system that struggles to find the best way of promoting the life chances of vulnerable children.

REFERENCES

Adams, S. (2002) 'New guidance documents in child protection: New messages for schools', *Pastoral Care in Education* 20(2) 3–6.

Benson, J. (1975) 'The interorganisational network as a political economy', *Administrative Science Quarterly* 20, 229–49.

Burns, S. (1996) *Extract from Ministerial Press Release*, Association of Directors of Social Services Conference: London.

Charles, M. with Stevenson, O. (1990) *Multidisciplinary is Different!* Nottingham: University of Nottingham.

Charles, M. and Glennie, S. (2001) *The Implementation of Working Together to Safeguard Children and The Framework for the Assessment of Children in Need and Their Families*, Report to the Department of Health, PIAT.

Charles, M. and Hendry, E. (eds) (2000) *Training Together to Safeguard Children, Guidance on Inter-agency Training*, London: NSPCC.

Corby, B. (1987) *Working with Child Abuse*, Milton Keynes: Open University Press.

DoH (Department of Health) (1991) *Working Together under the Children Act 1989: A Guide to Arrangements for Inter-agency Cooperation for the Protection of Children from Abuse*, London: HMSO.

DoH (1995) *Child Protection Messages from Research: Studies in Child Protection*, London: HMSO.

DoH (2001a) *The Children Act Now, Messages from Research*, London: The Stationery Office.

DoH (2001b) *Inter-agency Inspection of Safeguards for Children, 2001/2002, Standards and Criteria*, Department of Health web site (www.doh.gov.uk).

Department of Health and Social Security (1988) *Working Together: A Guide to Interagency Cooperation for the Protection of Children from Abuse*, London: HMSO.

Department of Health; Department of Education and Employment; Home Office (2000) *The Framework for the Assessment of Children in Need and their Families*, London: The Stationery Office.

Department of Health; Home Office; Department for Education and Employment and the National Assembly for Wales (1999) *Working Together to Safeguard Children*, London: The Stationery Office.

Farmer, E. and Owen, M. (1995) *Child Protection Practice: Private Risks and Public Remedies*, Studies in Child Protection, London: HMSO.

Firth, B. (2001) *Report of a Professional Development Group Seminar on The Assessment Framework*, Nottingham: University of Nottingham.

Hallett, C. (1995) *Inter-agency Coordination in Child Protection*, Studies in Child Protection, London: HMSO.

Horwath, J. and Glennie, S. (1999) 'Inter-agency Child Protection Training: Gathering Impressions', *Child Abuse Review* 8 (3) 200–206.

Horwath, J. and Morrison, T. (2000) 'Identifying and implementing pathways for organisational change: using the Framework for the Assessment of Children in Need and their Families as an example', *Child and Family Social Work* 5 (3) 245–54.

Laming Inquiry (2001) *Victoria Climbie Inquiry* (www.victoria-climbie-inquiry.org.uk).

Lupton, C., North, N. and Khan, P. (2001) *Working Together or Pulling Apart? The National Health Service and Child Protection Networks*, Bristol: The Policy Press.

Morrison, T. (2000) 'Working together to safeguard children: challenges and changes for inter-agency co-ordination in child protection', *Journal of Interprofessional Care* 14 (4) 363–73.

Parton, N., Thorpe, D. and Wattam, C. (1997) *Child Protection, Risk and the Moral Order*, Basingstoke: Macmillan.

PIAT (Promoting Interagency Training) (1998) Submission to consultation process in relation to *Working Together to Safeguard Children*, Leicester: PIAT.

Reder, P. and Duncan, S. (1999) *Lost Innocents: A Follow-up Study of Fatal Child Abuse*, London: Routledge.

Stevenson, O. (1994) 'Child protection, where now for inter-professional work?' in A. Leathard (ed.), *Going Inter-professional, Working Together for Health and Social Welfare*, London: Routledge.

Woodhouse, D. and Pengelly, P. (1991) *Anxiety and the Dynamics of Collaboration*, Aberdeen: Aberdeen University Press.

Chapter 13

Collaboration between primary health and social care

From policy to practice in developing services for older people

Caroline Glendinning and Kirstein Rummery

SUMMARY

The history of collaboration between primary health and social services is neither extensive nor particularly rosy. This chapter first of all describes this history and outlines the new policy imperatives facing primary health and social services. It will then draw on the findings of an ongoing study to examine how primary care groups and trusts (PCG/Ts) are tackling the new collaborative agenda with social services. The chapter concludes with a discussion of the likely impact and effectiveness of these new measures on the lives of frail, older service users. The focus of the chapter will be on collaboration between primary health and social services in England; following devolution, differences between the four countries of the UK are increasingly apparent, both in the organisation of health services and the implications for collaboration (Rummery 1998).

INTRODUCTION

The boundaries between health and social care services for older people have long been regarded as major barriers to the delivery of integrated services for older people. Moreover, these boundaries have acquired a high political salience, as the two sectors have become increasingly interdependent. For example, the active involvement of local authority home care and other social services can be crucially important in preventing the admission of frail, older people to hospital or long-term care and in facilitating their prompt discharge from hospital once treatment is completed.

However, unlike previous efforts to promote intersectoral collaboration, an entirely new set of organisations – PCG/Ts – are now located at the heart of the current drive to demolish the 'Berlin Wall' between health and social care. PCG/Ts replace the adversarial, fragmented and inequitable system of fund-holding by general practitioners (GPs). PCGs were established in April 1999. Significantly, from the point of view of this chapter, GPs are the dominant professional group on PCG/T boards. PCG/Ts have extensive responsibilities, including improving the health of their local population; working in partnership to integrate primary and community health services; and leading the implementation of new service developments across the health–social care interface. By 2002, when all PCGs became freestanding PCTs, they were responsible for three-quarters of the total National Health Service (NHS) budget. This chapter discusses the impact these changes have had on collaborative working.

'Building on sand' – the history of primary health–social services collaboration

Prior to 1997, collaboration between primary health and social services took place primarily within the context of GP practices; it was therefore both fragmented and far from widespread. It is important to bear in mind the autonomy and independence of GPs, which has persisted since the inception of the NHS (Pater 1981). General practice is traditionally based on 'individualistic, small shopkeeper principles', in which 'the principles of free choice of doctors by patients and complete medical autonomy . . . remain sacrosanct' (Klein 1983: 14). Until very recently, GP practices remained fragmented both from each other and from the wider range of community health services (Glendinning 1998).

Nevertheless, many GPs and other primary health care team members found the need for closer collaboration with their local social services departments, particularly after the 1993 community care changes, when social services care managers took on a new 'gatekeeping' role in assessing older people's needs for residential and domiciliary care services. A common strategy among GPs to improve collaboration with social services was to attach or locate a social services care manager in a GP practice, alongside other members of the primary health care team. A review of published and 'grey' literature on such initiatives (Glendinning et al 1998; Rummery and Glendinning, 2000) showed that such 'outposted' social workers take referrals directly from practice staff; conduct standard social services assessments; and arrange appropriate local authority services.

Process evaluations of these initiatives have found improvements in information-sharing and better mutual understanding of the different professional roles, responsibilities and organisational frameworks within which social and primary health services are delivered. These benefits could be further enhanced by investments in joint training or team-building exercises. Communication and collaboration between social services staff and community nurses (district nurses and health visitors) in particular were enhanced, possibly more so than between social workers and GPs. In turn, closer relationships led to quicker and more appropriate referrals and better feedback on the outcomes of referrals. However, outposted social services staff could feel isolated from their colleagues and concerned about the creation of inequities *vis-à-vis* GP practices without 'outposted' social services staff. Additionally, although older people may have been able to obtain social services more quickly, there is no evidence that they obtained more services or that these were better coordinated. Finally, commentators have noted the tendency for 'relationships between doctors and social workers to develop in a dominant/dependent pattern, deriving from their unequal professional status' (Lymbery 1998: 203), and the consequent difficulties for interprofessional collaboration.

In contrast, GPs were rarely involved in the joint planning and service commissioning processes that developed between health and local authorities from the early 1980s onwards – despite the potential for collaboration in these broader, interorganisational activities to lead to strategic shifts in services and new investments (Rummery and Glendinning 1997). An evaluation of different joint commissioning initiatives found an 'apparent lack of interest on the part of GPs for engaging in joint commissioning with local SSDs' (social services departments) (Hudson 1999: 365). The Total Purchasing Pilot projects, where (groups of) fundholding GPs were given devolved budgets to purchase a very extensive range of services (including those on the boundaries of social and community care), were similarly preoccupied with improving practice-level interprofessional communication, or with purchasing additional social work services to relieve pressure on GP practice staff, rather than addressing the wider health and social care service needs of older people across the locality as a whole (Wyke et al 1999). This narrow, partisan approach inevitably created inequities between different groups of patients, which were of particular concern to local authority social services partners (Bosanquet et al 1998).

In summary, GPs have been described as the 'weak professional link in the collaborative chain' (Hudson et al 1998: 15). Moreover, interprofessional relationships between GPs and social workers have long been regarded by both academics and professionals as lacking in trust and mutual understanding, and therefore constituting an unhelpful basis for collaboration (Lymbery 1998).

Primary care, PCG/Ts and the new partnership agenda

With a political commitment to end the divisiveness of GP fundholding, the first Labour administration introduced PCG/Ts, to which *all* the GPs in a locality belong. Behind this lay the aim of building 'on the experience of previous initiatives that had involved primary care professionals in the process of shaping and negotiating local patterns of service provision' (Goodwin 2001: 4), by pushing decision-making 'down to the front-line worker, here the doctor, who is conceived to be closer to the needs and wishes of the consumer' (Walby and Greenwell 1994: 60). PCGs were governed by 12-member Boards, of whom seven are GPs, two are nurses and one a representative from the local social services department; other health professionals (physiotherapists, dentists etc.) have no right of representation at all (North and Peckham 2001; Sheaff et al 2002). The same pattern of professional representation is now replicated on the Professional Executive Boards of PCTs. GPs therefore now have a leading role in strategic service planning, through the new Health Improvement Plans (HImPs); in commissioning health services for older people through PCG/Ts, together with social services and other local authority colleagues; and in managing the delivery of these services, through close interprofessional working at the front line.

This collaborative imperative is built into the heart of PCG/Ts' obligations; 'exhortations to be decent about joint working have been replaced by [a] panoply of sanctions, incentives and threats' (Hudson 1999: 199). Like other NHS organisations, PCG/Ts have a statutory obligation to work in partnership with other services. Substantial financial resources have been 'ring-fenced' to support new health and social services collaborations. New 'flexibilities' removing structural barriers to collaboration have been introduced. These allow budgets for specified services to be pooled; commissioning responsibilities to be delegated to a single 'lead' organisation; and health *and* social care services integrated within one 'provider' organisation (DoH 1998; Hudson et al 2001). Impatient with the pace of change, the NHS Plan (DoH 2000) subsequently announced further investments in combined health and social 'intermediate care' services to avert hospital admissions and support early discharge; the location of social workers in primary care settings; integrated assessments of older people's health and social care needs; and the eventual merger of local health and social services commissioning, governance and service provision functions into a single organisation, a 'care trust'. Moreover, the 2001 Health and Social Care Act allows the Secretary of State to compel local health and social services organisations to use the new partnership flexibilities, where collaboration is judged inadequate.

Evaluating the new interprofessional collaboration

Despite their unpromising history, the challenges now facing primary health and social care collaboration are complex and tough. How they are responding is the focus of a study with two interlinking, longitudinal components. One is a survey of a representative sample of 15 per cent of English PCG/Ts; two 'waves' of fieldwork, on which this chapter draws, took place in autumn 1999 and autumn 2000 (Wilkin et al 2000; Wilkin et al 2001). The second study involves in-depth case studies of four of these PCG/Ts, also so far conducted on two occasions (Rummery et al 2001). Informants in both studies include PCG/T officers, GP and social services board members, and community health and social services staff at senior and middle management levels.

Interprofessional collaboration on the PCG/T board

The statutory obligation to have a social services representative on each PCG/T board represents a shift in the level of collaboration, from simply improving communication at the level of GP practices, to fostering collaboration that is both strategic (planning and developing services) and operational (improving front-line service coordination).

Despite the unpromising history and their minority status on the board, social services representatives report improvements in the attitudes of other board members towards them. In 2000, 77 per cent of social services representatives judged these attitudes to be friendly and constructive, compared with 58 per cent in 1999. Moreover, their influence over board decisions appeared to have increased, although still outweighed by the influence of GPs. In 1999, 54 per cent of PCG chief officers rated social services representatives as having little or no influence, compared to only 5 per cent who rated GP board members as having little influence; a year later, 44 per cent of social services representatives were rated as having little or no influence (Wilkin et al 2000, 2001).

Underlying this continuing gap in attitudes and influence are some major differences in professional values and orientation. Social services representatives (as well as health authority and nursing representatives) on PCG/T boards pointed out how GPs had difficulty in thinking beyond the medical needs of their individual patients:

> What the GPs on the board are concerned about is what happens to their individual patients. I don't think they're quite evolved to the stage where they are thinking strategically yet; they're still focused, quite rightly in a lot of respects, on what this is going to mean for GPs in their practice and for their patients.
> (Social services representative, PCG board, site C, year 1)

This perceived constraint reflected differences in the familiarity of the two professions with the task of planning services to meet the needs of a whole area, or population, rather than just the patients in their practice. In contrast, social services representatives were senior managers with strategic planning and service commissioning responsibilities and, frequently, extensive operational responsibilities as well (Glendinning et al 2001):

> That's been quite a different lesson for me in terms of being used to talking to the health authority on the same level in terms of let's talk strategic . . . high level plans. At the PCG board you have to come right in on the ground about the patient and the impact on the GP if you want the GP to engage . . . I have been the one that's banging on the table saying, 'It is your responsibility. When you're at the board you're still a

GP but you're taking the wider management role and accountability for the practice.'

(Social services representative, PCG board, site C, year 1)

Not only were GPs unused to thinking strategically about the needs of a population rather than their own patients; they and other health professionals on the board also often failed to understand how social services departments operated, what services they offered, who was eligible for services and how their accountability mechanisms were determined by the wider context of local government. One nursing manager explained:

> The one thing I can't get my head around with social services is their bureaucracy and the way in which they have to go through the committee structure and their elected members in order to do anything. It's really quite frustrating.

(Community nursing manager, site C, year 1)

Conversely, very few social services representatives had prior knowledge of the pressures and working methods of primary care in general, or GPs in particular:

> It's a whole different constituency, primary care; and understanding where primary care's coming from and the needs and demands and pressures that are on primary care to deliver their services and their focus has been for me one of the most important aspects of [working on the board].

(Social services representative, PCG board, site B, year 1)

> I was starting from a very low knowledge base of GPs and how they worked and what drove them. It took me a while to understand them and understand what drove them in terms of how they function.

(Social services representative, PCG board, site A, year 1)

These differences could lead to misunderstandings. For example, respondents in the case study sites referred to the fact that 'emergencies' to health professionals needed a response within an hour, while social services staff interpreted 'emergency' as a situation needing attention within a few days.

However, the actual experience of working together at the PCG/T board did go some way towards overcoming some of these interprofessional problems; a trend that was clearly apparent in the survey findings reported above:

> What has improved has been the understanding. What's developed is an understanding of what the social services agenda is and some of the social services issues.

(Social services representative, PCG board, site A, year 1)

Interprofessional difficulties also accounted in some ways towards the relatively slow pace of progress that PCG/T boards made towards commissioning services jointly with social services for older people. GP's lack of experience of strategic service commissioning meant that tasks such as improving primary and community health services were much easier to tackle than more difficult joint commissioning activities with social services. By autumn 2000, only 11 per cent of PCG/Ts had taken over from their local health authority all responsibility for the commissioning of older people's services jointly with the social services department and in 17 per cent of PCG/Ts, joint commissioning remained entirely with the health authority (in the majority of PCG/Ts, responsibility for joint commissioning with social services was shared between the PCG/T and the health authority).

Interprofessional collaboration between health and social care in the community

As suggested above, although much of the focus of evaluative research has been on GP practice-level collaboration between GPs and social services care managers, the roles of district nurses and health visitors are likely to bring them into much more direct contact with care managers, home help staff and other social services staff, in the course of day-to-day collaboration over the needs of individual older people. Indeed, in the course of implementing the 1990 NHS and Community Care Act, a few, highly innovative projects were developed, in which community nurses have worked alongside social services staff, providing integrated assessment and care management for older people whose needs cross the health and social care boundary (Tucker and Brown 1997).

GPs' and community nurses' different histories of interprofessional collaboration were apparent in the survey, which revealed much better relationships between social services and community health professionals than between social services staff and GPs in the early days of PCG/Ts (Figure 13.1).

One of the case study sites illustrated the history of close collaboration between social work and community nursing staff on which the PCG was able to build:

> I would say our links with social services have always been good, and prior to the PCG we were working jointly anyway. We've been operating joint care management since it started in 1994. So we did joint training – social worker, district nurses – and we've developed that. Those links were well-established and we've built on them.
>
> (Nursing manager, site B, year 1)

Even without joint care management, most case study respondents agreed

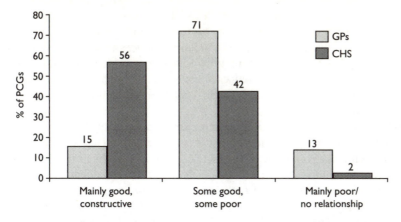

Figure 13.1 Relationships between social services, GPs and community health staff (autumn 1999).

that community nurses and social workers had a much stronger history of collaborative working than GPs and social workers:

> I think that the link with GPs has perhaps been more tenuous, certainly the link between the community nursing service and social services has again been quite active. There have been a number of initiatives even before [PCGs] when we were working with them ... like hospital at home, some of the discharge planning and fast response has always been quite a productive relationship between the community trust and ourselves.
>
> (Social services representative, PCG board, site C, year 1)

However, changes in the dynamics of interprofessional relationships resulting from the dominant position of GPs in the governance of PCG/Ts meant that these good relationships had not always been sustained. For example, in one of the case study sites, community nurses now felt sidelined by a focus on service developments that they felt reflected the interests and needs of GPs and social services rather than their own perspectives. In another case study site, respondents initially spoke enthusiastically about plans to realign services and integrate care management across nursing and social work boundaries, but a year later were expressing doubts about nurses' ability and willingness to take on such a role. Community nurses and social services managers in all four case study PCG/Ts expressed concern that difficulties in obtaining GPs' commitment to collaboration work might derail previous good relationships between community nurses and social workers. Indeed, the plans within many PCGs for becoming trusts, in which they would be able to take over and integrate community health with GP practice-based services, does indeed confirm the reality of this threat.

Figure 13.1 indicates that collaborative relationships between social services and GP practice-based staff may have been less developed prior to the formation of PCG/Ts. Indeed, in 1999 only 10 per cent of PCGs had social workers attached to all the practices in the PCG (albeit usually on a shared or sessional basis); and a further 20 per cent had social workers attached to some of the PCG's practices.

The qualitative case study interviews revealed some of the problems that PCG/Ts could experience in trying to improve this relatively low level of collaboration between GPs, their practice-based staff and social services. One PCG had tried to realign all their social work teams to cover primary care localities, based around GP practice clusters, but had run into problems implementing this because of lack of agreement by the local GPs on the board. Another PCG had failed in its initial bid to become a trust at least partly because of opposition from local GPs to plans that the trust would develop closer collaboration with social services. Here a respondent responsible for linking social workers to GP practices had hoped that this project would be rolled out across the PCG but was disappointed:

> We've got some very good links, but we've not had the kind of support I've wanted. The kind of support I wanted was for them to kind of spread the work, because there is only so far as frontline workers you can go. You can't get the hierarchy of health on board at this level, so you need someone quite high up in the PCG to get them on board, and we haven't really had that, we've had to slog away ourselves.
> (Social services manager, site A, year 2)

Despite these problems, within six months of PCGs being established, 85 per cent of social services representatives said relationships between their staff and local GPs had improved and 44 per cent said relationships between social services and community health had also improved (albeit from a better starting point).

DOES COLLABORATION BETWEEN PRIMARY HEALTH AND SOCIAL CARE DELIVER WHAT OLDER PEOPLE WANT?

PCG/Ts' priorities in developing services for older people were heavily influenced by national policy agendas. These factors include improvements in hospital discharge and admission arrangements and the development of intermediate care facilities. However, these priorities were not always those of either social services partners or of older people themselves:

Their [GPs'] focus is on reducing bed delays, reducing the amount of time people are in hospital for certain events like a broken neck of femur or a stroke. They're quite determined to reduce that at almost any cost to us.

(Social services manager, area A, year 1)

Such differences in priorities were often underpinned by differences between professional groups in the processes of identifying needs and developing new services to meet those needs; in particular, GPs and PCG/Ts tended to rely on professional assessments of needs, whereas social services partners preferred to involve users and their representative organisations. By the end of 2000, only 51 per cent of PCG/Ts had conducted comprehensive assessments of the needs of their older people; those which had been carried out had relied on information from health authorities (91 per cent of PCG/Ts that had assessed older people's needs), GP practices (89 per cent of PCG/Ts) or had consulted local health professionals (74 per cent of PCG/Ts). Only 66 per cent of PCG/Ts conducting assessments of older people's needs and services had consulted with voluntary organisations or patient groups. Similarly, few PCG/Ts consulted either patient or carer organisations in commissioning hospital or community health services (Figure 13.2)

In contrast, social services managers were keen to involve service users in planning services and had several mechanisms for doing so, including consulting with voluntary organisations over community care plans and broader community involvement in 'Best Value' reviews. Moreover, the outcomes of such consultation could reflect users' priorities more than those of professionals or their employing organisations:

One area that we consulted with the public in community care was bathing . . . we together sorted out a system that isn't wonderfully popular with professionals but is very popular with clients and patients.

(Social services commissioning manager, site B, year 1)

One of the case study PCGs held an annual open conference to consult widely with local voluntary organisations, but generally the approach to older people's involvement used by PCGs could be summed up thus:

I don't think at this moment in time we are in a position to consult on the [service development] changes because we haven't decided what they might be.

(PCG chief officer, site D, year 1)

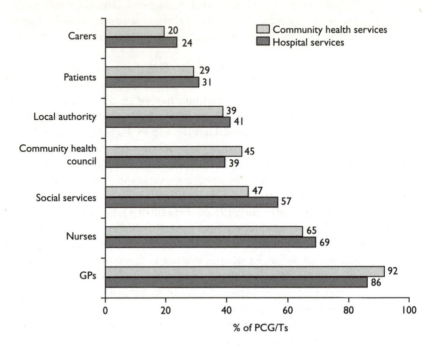

Figure 13.2 Percentages of PCG/Ts consulting different groups to inform service commissioning.

DISCUSSION AND CONCLUSIONS

In the first two years after PCG/Ts were established, some improvements in interprofessional collaboration between social services and primary health services are clearly apparent. Although greatly outnumbered by GPs, the inclusion of a social services representative on PCG/T boards has undoubtedly helped mutual understanding, not just of each other's roles but also of the organisational, financial and accountability frameworks within which the different professional groups operate. However, progress has been slow, partly because of the traditional focus of general practice on optimising arrangements for the practice and its patients; social services representatives, on the other hand, are much more familiar with the locality-wide and population-level strategic planning activities. Consequently, PCG/Ts have been slow to take over the strategic joint commissioning activities hitherto conducted by health authorities in partnership with social services.

Similarly, there is evidence that interprofessional barriers between primary health and social services are beginning to break down within the community, although progress is again slow. Relationships between social services and community health staff had a more positive history on which to build; but relationships between social services and GP practice-based professionals also showed improvements. However, the dominant voice of GPs on PCG/T boards may pose some threats by sidelining interprofessional collaboration between social services and community health staff.

Although these are promising signs, some considerable risks remain. Some of these risks reflect the continuing profound differences in the perspectives and values of social services professionals and GPs. Indeed, 38 per cent of social services representatives in 2000 identified an overconcern with clinical issues and the dominance of medical culture as major barriers to closer collaboration. One area in which differences in professional cultures are apparent is in the willingness to listen to older people and involve them in planning, developing, monitoring and reviewing new service developments, rather than relying on the views of other health professionals. Perhaps partly reflecting their position in the pre-1997 NHS internal market, as 'proxy' purchasers of secondary and community health services on behalf of their patients, the GPs who now dominate PCG/T boards appear still to prefer to consult their professional colleagues, rather than older people themselves. It is difficult to anticipate how this differential willingness to seek out and act on users' voices may affect the development of interprofessional relationships between primary health and social services in the future.

However, one major threat to improved collaboration was clearly apparent. This is the very considerable organisational turbulence that has affected both local authority and primary care organisations. Many local authorities have reorganised their structures – in particular the responsibilities of their elected members – into separate cabinet and scrutiny functions. PCGs have also undergone major evolution and development, as they moved towards trust status by 2002. In the process, many PCGs have merged with each other, in order to increase their administrative capacity and purchasing leverage. Within two years of their establishment, two-thirds of PCGs were actually involved, or are planning such mergers (Wilkin et al 2001). Whether these objectives are achieved, such mergers are likely to have significant costs (Bojke et al 2001).

One cost of both mergers and transition to trust status was the disruption of existing relationships, both at board and operational levels. Indeed, interprofessional collaboration appeared a common and early casualty of this organisational turbulence. When asked why they were seeking trust status, only a fifth of PCG chief executives placed the integration of health and social services among their three most important reasons. Similarly, a third of social services representatives in 2000 identified the pace of change as a barrier to closer collaboration. This organisational turbulence will also affect the creation of the new, integrated care trusts. It may take some considerable time for these changes to settle down; in the meantime, it will be difficult to build interprofessional relationships that are characterised by mutual understanding, trust and respect for the different contributions of primary care and social services partners.

REFERENCES

Bojke, C., Gravell, H. and Wilkin, D. (2001) 'Is bigger better for primary care groups and trusts?' *British Medical Journal* 322, 599–602.

Bosanquet, N., Jarman, B., Dolan, S., Watson, L. and Bruster, S. (1998) *The Bromsgrove Total Purchasing Project 1994–1996*, London: Department of Primary Health and General Practice, Imperial College School of Medicine at St. Mary's.

DoH (Department of Health) (1998) *Partnership in Action. New Opportunities for Joint Working between Health and Social Services*, London: Department of Health.

DoH (Department of Health) (2000) *The NHS Plan for England*, London: Department of Health.

Glendinning, C. (1998) 'From general practice to primary care', in E. Brunsdon, H. Dean and R. Woods (eds), *Social Policy Review* 10, London: Social Policy Association.

Glendinning, C., Abbott, S. and Coleman, A. (2001) 'Bridging the gap: new relationships between primary care groups and local authorities', *Social Policy and Administration* 35 (4) 411–25.

Glendinning, C., Rummery, K. and Clarke, R. (1998) 'From collaboration to commissioning; developing relationships between primary health and social services', *British Medical Journal* 7151, 122–4.

Goodwin, N. (2001) 'The long-term importance of English primary care groups for integration in primary health care and de-institutionalisation of hospital care', *International Journal of Integrated Care* 1 (2) 1–13.

Hudson, B. (1999) 'Joint commissioning across the primary health care–social care boundary: can it work?' *Health and Social Care in the Community*, 7 (5) 358–66.

Hudson, B., Lewis, H., Waddington, E. and Wistow, G. (1998) *The Interface between Social Care and Primary Care: National Mapping Exercise*, Leeds: Nuffield Institute for Health.

Hudson, B., Young, R., Hardy, B. and Glendinning, C. (2001) *National Evaluation of Notifications for Use of the Section 31 Partnership Flexibilities of the Health Act 1999*, Manchester: National Primary Care Research and Development Centre, Leeds: Nuffield Institute for Health.

Klein, R. (1983) *The Politics of the National Health Service*, London: Longmans.

Lymbery, M. (1998) 'Social work in general practice: dilemmas and solutions', *Journal of Interprofessional Care* 12 (2) 199–210.

North, N. and Peckham, S. (2001) 'Analysing structural interests in primary care groups', *Social Policy and Administration*, 35 (4) 426–40.

Pater, J. (1981) *The Making of the National Health Service*, London: King Edward's Hospital Fund for London.

Rummery, K. (1998) 'Changes in primary health care policy: the implications for joint commissioning with social services', *Health and Social Care in the Community*, 6 (6) 429–38.

Rummery, K., Coleman, A. and Jacobs, S. (2001) 'Uneasy bedfellows? The development of partnerships between primary care groups and local authorities concerning services for older people', in D. Taylor (ed.), *Breaking Down Barriers: Reviewing partnership in practice*, University of Brighton Press: Brighton.

Rummery, K. and Glendinning, C. (1997) *Working Together: Primary Care Involvement in Commissioning Social Care Services*, Debates in Primary Care 2, Manchester: National Primary Care Research and Development Centre.

Rummery, K. and Glendinning, C. (2000) *Primary Care and Social Services: Developing New Partnerships for Older People*, Oxford: Radcliffe Medical Press.

Sheaff, R., Dickson, M. and Smith, K. (2002) Is GP restratification beginning in England? *Social Policy and Administration* 36 (7) 765–79.

Tucker, L. and Brown, L. (1997) *Evaluating Different Models for Jointly Commissioning Community Care*, Report 4, Bath: The Wiltshire Social Services and University of Bath Research and Development Partnership.

Walby, S. and Greenwell, J. (1994) 'Managing the National Health Service', in J. Clarke, A. Cochrane and E. McLaughlin (eds), *Managing Social Policy*, London: Sage.

Wilkin, D., Gillam, S. and Leese, B. (2000) *The National Tracker Survey of Primary Care Groups and Trusts: Progress and Challenges 1999/2000*, Manchester: National Primary Care Research and Development Centre.

Wilkin, D., Gillam, S. and Coleman, A. (2001) *The National Tracker Survey of Primary Care Groups and Trusts 2000/2001: Modernising the NHS?* Manchester: National Primary Care Research and Development Centre.

Wyke, S., Myles, S., Popay, J., Scott, J., Campbell, A. and Girling, H. (1999) 'Total purchasing, community and continuing care: lessons for future policy developments in the NHS', *Health and Social Care in the Community*, 7 (6) 395–408.

Chapter 14

Disability, user-controlled services – partnership or conflict?

Colin Barnes

SUMMARY

Historically, the international disabled people's movement has been critical of both professionally and interprofessionally led services for their failure to enable disabled people to live 'independently' within the community. In response, groups of disabled people developed their own. Generally referred to as Centres for Independent Living (CILs), these organisations appeared, first, in the USA, Canada and 'developing' countries like Nicaragua and Costa Rica and, later, in European states such as the UK and Sweden. There are now at least 80 user-controlled service providers operating in various parts of the UK (Barnes et al 2000). However, there is a symbiotic but often uneasy relationship between the 'old' and the 'new'. This chapter charts that relationship and highlights some of the key issues that will inevitably confront all those involved in services for disabled people.

WHY USER-CONTROLLED SERVICES?

Quite simply, user-controlled services emerged in response to the perceived failure of traditional professionally led systems to enable disabled people to adopt a lifestyle of their own choosing within a mainstream environment. To varying degrees this perception, whether justified or not, is evident among both policy-makers and disabled people.

Due mainly to a combination of seemingly ever escalating costs and the heightened expectations of an increasingly cynical electorate, politicians and policy-makers became evermore critical of state and state-sponsored provision in the closing decades of the twentieth century. This resulted in a gradual but intensifying emphasis on market forces within health and social services at both the national and local levels couched within the rhetoric of consumer sovereignty and interests. The outcome has been a much greater involvement by non-statutory agencies from the private and voluntary sectors in service provision and delivery (Drake 1999).

One of the most significant developments over recent years has been the introduction of the Community Care (Direct Payments) Act 1996. Its aim is to enable local authorities to provide disabled people with appropriate funding to employ their own helpers or personal assistants (PAs), thus empowering them to eliminate their dependence on others such as professionals, relatives and friends. In so doing, disabled people are able to achieve a degree of autonomy and independence hitherto unprecedented within the British context. Subsequent legislation, namely, the Carers and Disabled Children Act 2000, has extended this provision to include other user groups such as 'carers', people with parental responsibility for disabled children and young disabled people aged 16–17. Furthermore, under Section 57 of the Health and Social Care Act 2001, it is possible that regulations will be introduced to ensure that direct payments are available to all those who are eligible and want them (DoH 2001).

The shift towards greater user control has received a further boost from the Scottish Executive who recently announced a £530,000 two year development project led by a consortium of voluntary and user-controlled agencies to set up and develop further locally based user-controlled support networks. The initiative aims to increase awareness of direct payments at local and national levels, establish appropriate mechanisms for information-sharing, provide training and guidance and build confidence among potential users, and coordinate and provide feedback to the Scottish Executive (SE 2001). All this suggests that there is a growing commitment on the part of government bodies to increase the number of people receiving direct payments and a move from a discretionary to a mandatory system. Direct payments therefore have: 'the potential for the most fundamental reorganisation of welfare for half a century' (Oliver and Sapey 1999: 175).

A major factor in these developments is the long standing pressure from groups of disabled people for greater control over the services on which they are forced to depend. The creation of the modern welfare state in the 1940s and the shift from institutional to community-based provision precipitated an unprecedented growth in the disability industry and the numbers of professional helpers working within it. But, rather than eliminate disabled people's perceived dependence on others, this simply served to perpetuate it. Professionally led provision is viewed as part of the problem rather than the solution.

Whatever the priorities of policy-makers, there is a wealth of evidence to suggest that professionals substantially influence the ways in which services are actually delivered. In many ways, disciplinary practices and procedures, professional vested interests and interprofessional rivalries coupled with the control of resources results in the deployment of services for professional convenience rather than user need (Wilding 1982; Patten 1990). It is also the case that from disabled people's perspectives, the emergence of interdisciplinary approaches to service delivery has made little difference to the problem and may even have made the situation far worse (Oliver 1991; Barnes 1994).

Moreover, there is substantive evidence from a variety of sources that rather than empower disabled people, conventionally led provision achieves the reverse (Barnes 1991; Morris 1993; Zarb and Nadash 1995; Barton 2001; Morgan et al 2001). For instance, in 1994 the British Council of Disabled People (BCODP) published the results of research based on interviews with 70 people from four case study local authority areas in the Midlands, the south of England and inner and outer London. This research highlighted several major disadvantages with statutory provision that included a lack of control over the type of support available; and who, how and when that support was delivered. In short, service users had little or no control over who came into their home and what they actually did once they were inside. Provision was also found to be both unreliable and inflexible. This resulted in a heightened sense of vulnerability and stress among users and caused very real concerns and fears about the future (Zarb and Nadash 1995).

Similar findings have been reported in a more recent national study – the 'Creating Independent Futures' project. Again, initiated by the BCODP and carried out by the Centre for Disability Studies at the University of Leeds the project involved a national survey of known user-controlled services and in-depth interviews with users and staff from user-controlled services in nine local authority areas in England, Scotland and Wales (Barnes et al 2000).

The sample of 76 users included almost equal numbers of men and women. The majority was in the middle-age ranges. Most participants described themselves as having one or more physical impairment/s but also included people who had been labelled 'with learning difficulties' and others who were 'mental health system' users or survivors. All participants had experience of a wide range of services provided by various statutory and voluntary agencies. Yet, although there was considerable variation in people's levels of satisfaction with the services received from non-user-controlled statutory and voluntary provision, general concerns were raised about assessment procedures, lack of control, reliability, flexibility and helper/helped relations (Morgan et al 2001).

Direct payments are seen by many as a user-friendly way of resolving these problems. It is also important to note at this juncture that it is widely recognised that many disabled people welcome the control of their support workers but, mainly because of the bureaucracy involved, are unhappy and/or unsure about becoming employers. This hesitancy should not be surprising given that like the population generally, the overwhelming majority of disabled people have neither the skills nor the experience for the role of employer. Consequently, the need for a well-developed infrastructure of user-controlled peer support services is a constant theme running throughout the literature on direct payments (Zarb and Nadash 1995; Hasler et al 1999; Witcher et al 2000). As noted earlier, groups of disabled people have long since recognised this need and attempted to resolve the problem through the formation of their own organisations.

THE SHIFT TOWARDS USER-CONTROLLED SERVICES

Although self-organisation and help have been a key feature of Britain's disabled people's movement since the nineteenth century with the establishment of the National League of the Blind and Disabled (NLBD) and the British Deaf Association (BDA), it really took hold in the 1960s and 1970s with the formation of organisations such as the Disablement Incomes Group (DIG) in 1965, the Union of the Physically Impaired Against Segregation (UPIAS) in 1974, the Spinal Injuries Association (SIA) in 1974, and the Disablement, Information and Advice Line (Dial) in 1977. Around this time news of the US Independent Living Movement (ILM) began to filter through to disabled people in the UK. This was particularly important because developments in the USA provided evidence of what disabled people in the UK knew already; that the barriers to their self-fulfilment were the outcome of living in a hostile physical and cultural environment, and that existing services were inhibiting rather than empowering (Campbell and Oliver 1996).

The US ILM emerged in the early 1970s, partly from within the campus culture of American universities and partly from repeated efforts by American disability organisations to influence disability legislation. During the 1960s, various 'self-help' programmes had been introduced by some US universities to enable students with 'severe' physical impairments to attend mainstream courses. But it was not until the early 1970s that the movement gained validity and momentum with the creation of the first Centre for Independent Living (CIL) in Berkeley, California (Shapiro 1993).

The Berkeley Centre was established in 1972 as a self-help group managed by disabled people. It provided a wide range of related services including peer counselling, advocacy services, transportation, training in independent living skills, attendance care referral, wheelchair repair and others. Berkeley CIL had no residential facilities and catered for people with various impairments – physical, sensory and intellectual – many of which were considered 'severe'. As other CILs developed, they responded to the needs of their local communities and therefore often provided a different range of services. Today, there are over 300 CILs operating across the USA and there are CILs in both 'developed' and 'developing' nations throughout the world (Albrecht 1992; Coleridge 1993; Charlton 1998).

Notwithstanding, user-controlled services were relatively slow to develop in the UK. This is attributable to the fact that unlike the USA and many other countries across the world, the UK has a veritable farrago of state-run services and a large and well-established voluntary sector. Most of this provision is controlled and run by non-disabled professionals of one sort or another. In several respects, therefore, the problem for the British disabled people's movement was less to do with creating services and more to do with controlling them (Oliver and Barnes 1998).

Britain's first CILs were set up in the early 1980s by two pioneering disabled people's organisations: the Derbyshire Coalition of Disabled People (DCDP) and the Hampshire Coalition of Disabled People (HCDP). The former was established in 1981 by disabled activists from DIAL Derbyshire. From the outset, the idea of setting up a CIL in Derbyshire was given the highest priority. But it was not until 1985 that the Derbyshire Centre for Integrated Living (DCIL) was registered as an independent autonomous company. The delay was due to several factors; notably, protracted discussions within the Coalition, with other disabled people's organisations, both inside and outside the UK, and with the local council on what form the new CIL should take. Since its inception, DCIL has flourished despite severe funding cutbacks in the early 1990s (Davis and Mullenders 1993). DCIL provides a range of services commensurate with the needs of local disabled people under a new name: Derbyshire Coalition for Inclusive Living. The new title was adopted in 2000 to signal the merging of the two organisations and an inclusive and county-wide approach to service delivery for disabled people and their families.

Disabled people in Hampshire adopted a different approach. 'Project 81: Consumer Directed Housing and Care' grew out of *ad-hoc* discussions among disabled people living in a Leonard Cheshire residential home, Le Court, in 1979. Drawing on the experience of disabled people in other parts of the country and overseas, especially the USA, the Project 81 group persuaded the local authority that resources used to finance 'residential care' for disabled people would be far better spent supporting them in the community. They argued that sufficient funding should be provided to cover the cost of making houses accessible for disabled individuals and to enable them to employ their own personal assistant (PA), helper or 'carer' to do the things they were unable to do for themselves.

In contrast to established professionally dominated practices, the Project 81 group maintained that the disabled person should be responsible for assessing their own support needs. These needs might include 'personal care needs': getting up, washing, using the toilet and so on; 'domestic matters': cleaning the house, laundry, shopping, cooking and so on and; 'social care'; support for employment, leisure activities and so on. These features were something that disabled people living in institutions can never hope to achieve (HCIL 1986).

The Project 81 group were also responsible for setting up the Hampshire Centre for Independent Living (HCIL) in 1985, the same year that the DCIL came into existence. From the outset HCIL endeavoured to provide a community-based resource, not only for disabled people hoping to leave institutions, but also for those already living in the community struggling to survive and under the threat of going into 'residential care'. While HCIL's primary focus revolved around peer support for established PA users including information and advocacy, it also provided training in 'independent living skills' for those new to the idea of user-controlled services (HCIL 1990). Hitherto, HCIL have published several PA user manuals and papers. HCIL was also responsible for the setting-up and distribution of a free newsletter for PA users; 'The Personal Assistance Newsletter', a responsibility that was taken on by the BCODP in 1991. There are now over 500 PA users in Hampshire, the largest number of PA users in one local authority area in the UK.

According to the 'Creating Independent Lives' survey, there are at least 15 CILs operating in different parts of the UK. Additionally, there is a further 71 user-controlled initiatives providing 'independent living' type services that do not refer to themselves as a CIL (Barnes et al 2000).

The reluctance to adopt the mantle of CIL is partly due to the organic nature of user-controlled services and the increasing confusion over what is actually meant by the phrase 'independent living'. Many user-controlled agencies were established as campaigning organisations before they evolved into service providers. Besides user-controlled services, the concept 'independent living' as espoused by the international disabled people's movement is concerned with the ongoing struggle for equality and meaningful and enforceable civil and human rights. The setting-up of CILs was considered a fundamental part of that struggle. Over recent years, however, the phrase has been adopted and potentially devalued by its use by professional service providers to refer to non-user-controlled services such as 'Independent Living Centres' previously known as Artificial Limb and Appliance Centres (ALACs). It is also the case that the concept of user-controlled services is becoming less clear-cut.

CHARACTERISTICS OF 'USER-CONTROLLED' SERVICES FOR DISABLED PEOPLE IN THE UK

Data from the 'Creating Independent Futures' project suggests that user-controlled services take a variety of forms and that this variation extends beyond simply the type of services provided but encompasses key issues such as user control, accountability, the adoption of a social model approach and campaigning.

Participating organisations were drawn from a wide geographical area including Scotland and Wales although the south-east, midlands and the north of England were the areas best represented. All the agencies surveyed had a management committee controlled by disabled people. However, in some organisations these bodies included non-disabled service users such as 'carers' and representatives of funding agencies including local authorities' social service departments and health authorities. Only 50 per cent of the organisations studied required that their management structure were comprised exclusively of disabled people (Barnes et al 2000).

One of the main justifications for user-controlled services is that they are generally far more accountable to their users than other agencies. Some agencies equate service user with membership: disabled users automatically become members. Hence, they receive newsletters, information sheets, are invited to committee meetings and have voting rights. All the organisations studied had formal mechanisms written into their constitution or mission statements to ensure high levels of accountability. Eighty per cent of the participating groups are formally answerable to their members and almost half to their service users. However, 42 per cent of the agencies studied said that they were also accountable to funding agencies such as local and health authorities and the National Lottery, often through service agreements or other forms of contract. Indeed, 39 per cent are formally attached to local authority social service departments and 21 per cent to a health authority (Barnes et al 2000).

Furthermore, all the groups surveyed work with a variety of other organisations at different levels. The majority, 93 per cent, work with local groups, generally around the provision of services or with groups representing other minority groups such as minority ethnic organisations. A significant number operate on a national level, 65 per cent, working with organisations such as the BCODP, BCODP's National Centre for Independent Living (NCIL), DIAL, the Royal Association for Disability and Rehabilitation and Mencap. Groups from Scotland and Wales were much more likely to work at a regional/national level with agencies like Disability Wales or Disability Scotland. Some even operate at the international level with organisations like the European Network on Independent Living (ENIL) or Disabled People's International (DPI) as well as with local, regional and national groups of disabled people from as far apart as Portugal and Russia.

With regard to the social model of disability, there was general agreement that this is the foundation on which all user-controlled services should operate. Like the notion of independent living, the social model involves a holistic approach to disability involving a shift away from focusing on the functional limitations of particular individuals and on to the ways in which the physical and cultural environments impose various limitations on groups of people labelled 'disabled'.

Clearly, such a transformation has important implications for the type of services. These might address the seven needs considered essential for independent living as advocated by DCIL in 1985, which are information, peer support, housing, assistive technologies, personal assistance, transport and environmental access. Subsequently, other needs have been added to this list including advocacy, individual and collective, education and employment training. This approach poses particular problems for those working within a service-provision context and particularly so for professionals, the majority of whom still work within a conventional individualistic, medical framework (Abberley 1995; Oliver and Sapey 1999).

However, user-controlled services receive funding from a variety of sources. Only 10 of the 69 organisations in the 'Creating Independent Futures' study were sole-funded. The majority was jointly financed from a variety of sources including local authority social services departments, lottery grants and voluntary agencies, membership fees, and self-generated funding from such services as Disability Equality Training (DET) for other agencies and professionals.

Most of the participant agencies received funding for developing and maintaining particular services and for administrative, staff and premises costs, including initial start-up costs. But core funding is usually provided only on a short-term basis. Just 4 per cent of participating organisations had secure finances for more than three years. The short-term nature of funding for user-controlled services means that long-term planning, service development and provision are highly precarious. For example, 47 per cent share their office space with other groups including social services departments, health authorities, other disability organisations and private organisations. Six per cent have no fixed premises at all and 4 per cent operate out of individuals' homes.

Moreover, the nature of the structure and funding of the participating organisations impacted on both the levels of staffing and their formal employment policies. The level of staffing, by both disabled and non-disabled people, varied enormously between organisations. Many organisations had no full-time, and often no part-time, members of staff. One organisation had 37 disabled people working full time and another had 21 non-disabled members of staff. A large number of volunteers were employed by the responding organisations. The vast majority of volunteers were disabled people.

All this impacts on the type of services user-controlled organisations can offer. Most of those surveyed provided a range of services, although none offered all seven of the basic needs identified by DCIL. Some struggled to provide a comprehensive range of services while others acted as a signpost to provision elsewhere. It is notable that 64 per cent provided or were in the process of developing, 8 per cent, support services for direct payment users. But while all the participating agencies sought to be inclusive in their membership and user groups, there was a general recognition that structural and cultural barriers perpetuate an under-representation of certain groups of disabled people. These included disabled people from minority ethnic groups, lesbian and gay disabled people and younger disabled people under 25 as well as people with the label of learning difficulties and 'mental health' problems (Barnes et al 2000).

All the organisations studied were engaged in campaigning on disability issues but it is important to stress that these activities took a variety of forms.

For example, 70 per cent actively campaign on disability rights issues such as service cuts, charging for services and access issues. Almost a quarter campaigned on impairment specific issues addressing the particular problems encountered by people with different impairments such as people with the label of learning difficulties or mental health problems. Sixteen per cent supported campaigns on other related issues such as gender, race/ethnicity and sexuality; the majority of these campaigns focused on inclusion. Everyone was also aware that such activity could jeopardise relations with funding agencies but considered them integral to their future development; all of which has particular significance for established service agencies both statutory and voluntary and those who work within them.

PARTNERSHIP, CONFLICT OR SOMETHING ELSE?

Clearly, there is a tension arising from reconciling the principles and ideals of the social model and independent living with the reality of operating within an environment dominated by individual, medical model type ideologies. Participants in the 'Creating Independent Futures' project expressed concern about the constant need for compromise and negotiation to establish even the most basic services.

Further, though the representatives of the funding agencies interviewed expressed a commitment in principle to the social model, many acknowledged that this was often a formal commitment at a policy or political level rather than being embedded within practice. Additionally, local authority staff recognised that the nature of statutory agency structures and procedures mean that both services and users are generally compartmentalised into rigid boxes, such as the division between adult, children and elderly services and between 'physical and sensory disabilities', 'learning disabilities' and 'mental health', and that this has obvious implications for the type and scope of services offered.

Consequently, seeking to balance a philosophical or ideological commitment to the social model of disability within the day-to-day realities of service provision produces tensions for user-controlled organisations. While the broad interpretation of the model gives organisations greater scope to reflect local diversity and priorities, this broadness also allows for confusion and misinterpretation both by user-led organisations and statutory agencies. Moreover, despite the acknowledged need for user-controlled support mechanisms, there is evidence that many direct payments users are not receiving the assistance they need. The introduction of direct payments is complex. Within a social services context, it warrants important practical operational changes. This means a fundamental shift in concepts of risk and control and a challenge to the culture of direct service provision and established ways of working (Dawson 1999).

This re-emphasis is something many local authorities are reluctant or unable to address. Charlotte Pearson (2000) argues that direct payments can be interpreted as a wider market discourse for restructuring welfare. Hence, a growing culture of localised 'care' markets with increasingly ideological diversity threatens to erode the already fragile shift towards user-control. Indeed, successive studies show that user-controlled initiatives find it increasingly difficult to survive due to funding and resource difficulties (Hasler et al 1999). In two audits by the Social Services Inspectorate, several local authorities said that they had tried to identify user-controlled agencies to take on a peer support role but were unable to find any willing or able to do so (Fruin 2000). It has also been reported that local authorities are using social workers to advise disabled people rather than organisations controlled and run by disabled people (McCurry 1999). In the 'Creating Independent Futures' project less than half the user participants were referred to user-controlled services by social workers (Morgan et al 2001).

It is evident therefore that if user-controlled services are to develop further, there needs to be a fundamental reorganisation of provision at the local level, which has obvious implications for professionals and established ways of working. Indeed, in recognition that few disabled people make a distinction between health and social support, recent research funded by the Department of Health indicated that disabled people need a holistic approach that supersedes separate notions of 'health and social care'. The researchers concluded that current organisational, budgetary and professional divisions between health and social services 'still apparently fail to recognise and respond appropriately to the realities of disabled people's lives' (Glendinning et al 2000: 47). The government have also announced their intention to bring together health and social provision as 'care trusts' (DoH 2001). When and how these trusts are to develop is currently unclear. What is known is that hitherto professionals, and 'health care' professionals in particular, have shown little interest in the social model of disability, independent living or user-controlled initiatives.

What is needed therefore is a new breed of professional, one who is not allied to traditional individualistic approaches to disability and conventional ways of working but, instead, is allied to the local disabled community and committed to a more holistic and flexible approach to service delivery (Finkelstein 1998). Conventional disciplinary policies and practices must be abolished in favour of a broad-based social model approach. The aim is to enable these workers to put their expertise and skills at the disposal of disabled people and their organisations in order to address and remove the various institutional barriers, economic, political, cultural and professional, to meaningful independent living for disabled people and their families. This is something that the established 'health care' professions have, as yet, failed to do.

CONCLUSION

This chapter has documented disabled people's ongoing struggle to influence and control the services on which they have to depend in order to achieve an independent lifestyle within the local community. One important outcome of this development has been a radical reappraisal of policy-making in the general area of health and social support services for disabled people. The gradual but intensifying growth of user-controlled initiatives over the last couple of decades has had a significant impact on policy-makers at the national level culminating with the introduction of the 1996 Community Care (Direct Payments) Act and the 2001 Health and Social Care Act. There can be little doubt that these developments have important ramifications for all those involved in local provision whether they work in the statutory or the voluntary sector. Established ideologies, policies and practices will inevitably have to change. This chapter has suggested a means by which this process of change might begin. How and in what ways professionals and their organisations might respond has yet to be determined.

REFERENCES

Abberley, P. (1995) 'Disabling ideology in health and welfare: the case of occupational therapy', *Disability and Society* 10 (4) 221–32.

Albrecht, G. (1992) *The Disability Business: Rehabilitation in America*, London: Sage.

Barnes, C. (1991) *Disabled People in Britain and Discrimination: A Case for Anti-discrimination Legislation*, London: Hurst and Co. in Association with the British Council of Organisations of Disabled People.

Barnes, C. (1994) 'Institutional discrimination, disabled people and interprofessional care', *Journal of Interprofessional Care* 8 (2) 203–12.

Barnes, C., Mercer, G. and Morgan, H. (2000) *Creating Independent Futures: Stage 1 Report*, Leeds: The Disability Press.

Barton, L. (2001) *Disability Politics and the Struggle for Change*, London, David Fulton.

Campbell, J. and Oliver, M. (1996) *Disability Politics: Understanding Our Past, Changing Our Future*, London: Routledge.

Charlton, J. (1998) *Nothing About Us Without Us: Disability Oppression and Empowerment*, Berkeley: University of California Press.

Coleridge, P. (1993) *Disability, Liberation and Development*, Oxford: Oxfam Publications.

Davis, L. and Mullenders, A. (1993) *Ten Turbulent Years: A Review of the Work of the Derbyshire Coalition of Disabled People*, Nottingham: Nottingham University Centre for Social Action.

Dawson, C. (1999) *Implementing Successes: Implementing Direct Payments*, York: Joseph Rowntree Foundation.

DoH (2001) *Explanatory Notes to Health and Social Care Act 2001* (www.legislation.hmso.gov.uk/acts/en/2001en15.htm).

Drake, R. (1999) *Understanding Disability Policy*, Basingstoke: Macmillan.

Finkelstein, V. (1998) *Rethinking Care in a Society Providing Equal Opportunities for All* (www.leeds.ac.uk/disability-studies/archiveuk/index.html).

Fruin, D. (2000) *New Directions for Independent Living*, London: Department of Health.

Glendinning, C., Haliwell, S. Jacobs, K. and Tyrer, J. (2000) *Buying Independence: Using Direct Payments to Integrate Health and Social Services*, Bristol: The Policy Press.

Hasler, F., Campbell, J. and Zarb, G. (1999) *Direct Routes to Independence*, London: Policy Studies Institute.

HCIL (1986) *'Project 81: One Step On' Consumer Directed Housing and Care for Disabled People*, Hampshire: Hampshire Centre for Independent Living.

HCIL (1990) *HCIL Papers*, Hampshire: Hampshire Centre for Independent Living.

McCurry, P. (1999) 'The direct route', *Community Care* 20–21 September: 9–15.

Morgan, H., Barnes, C. and Mercer, G. (2001) *Creating Independent Futures: Stage 3 Report*, Leeds: The Disability Press.

Morris, J. (1993) *Independent Lives*, Basingstoke: Palgrave Macmillan.

Oliver, M. (1991) 'Multispecialist and multidiciplinary – a recipe for confusion: too many cooks spoil the broth', *Disability, Handicap and Society* 6 (1) 66–8.

Oliver, M. and Barnes, C. (1998) *From Exclusion to Inclusion: Social Policy and Disabled People*, London: Longman.

Oliver, M. and Sapey, B. (1999) *Social Work with Disabled People*, 2nd edn., Basingstoke: Macmillan.

Patten, C. (1990) *7th Annual Goodman Lecture: Big Battalions and Little Platoons*, delivered 7 June 1990, Charities Aid Foundation.

Pearson, C. (2000) 'Money talks? Competing discourses on the implementation of direct payments', *Critical Social Policy* 20 (4) 459–77.

SE (Scottish Executive) (2001) *Chisholm Announces £530,000 to Promote Direct Payments, Scottish Executive Press Release SE0940/2001, 06/04/2001*, Edinburgh: Scottish Executive.

Shapiro, J. (1993) *No Pity: People with Disabilities Forging a New Civil Rights Movement*, New York: Times Books.

Wilding, P. (1982) *Professional Power and Social Welfare*, London: Routledge and Kegan Paul.

Witcher, S., Stalker, K., Roadberg, M. and Jones, C. (2000) *Direct Payments: The Impact of Choice and Control for Disabled People*, Edinburgh: Scottish Executive Central Research Unit.

Zarb, G. and Nadash, P. (1995) *Cashing in on Independence: Comparing the Costs and Benefits of Cash and Services*, Derby: The British Council of Disabled People.

Chapter 15

Mental health in interprofessional contexts

Tony Leiba

SUMMARY

As a part of a commitment to a modern, decent and inclusive society, the government has set out clear proposals to modernise the National Health Service (NHS) and social services, requiring these agencies to work collaboratively and in partnership with users, carers, the private and the voluntary sectors, to provide integrated services that will improve the quality of life for all citizens.

The National Service Framework for Mental Health (DoH 1999a) presents the government's intentions for mental health services. The concern here is with the interprofessional opportunities and challenges that users, carers, nurses, support workers, psychiatrists, social workers, occupational therapists, psychologists, workers in the private and the volunteer sectors, managers and administrators will face in the delivery of an integrated interprofessional mental health service.

INTRODUCTION

In *The new NHS: Modern, Dependable*, the Secretary of State for Health (1997) calls for an NHS based on partnerships, driven by performance, and replacing the inequalities and inefficiencies of internal markets by integrated care. In *The NHS Plan: A Plan for Investment, A Plan for Reform*, the Secretary of State for Health (2000) stresses the need for the health and social care systems to be built on partnership with users, carers, families, the voluntary and the private sectors.

A National Service Framework for Mental Health (DoH 1999a) sets out the way mental health services will be delivered to working age adults up to 65 years of age, which covers health promotion, assessment and diagnosis, treatment and rehabilitation and care, and includes primary and specialist care. The Framework embraces the needs of children and young people, for example the interface between services for 16 and 18 year olds. Similarly, the needs of older people with mental health problems are addressed as a part of the *National Service Framework for Older People* (DoH 2001a).

The interprofessional initiatives put forward by the National Service Framework for Mental Health are presented and discussed by looking at the implications for the delivery of care. This chapter addresses the issues relevant to users, carers, mental health and social services professionals, the private and the voluntary sectors.

PROVIDING INTEGRATED SERVICES

In *The NHS Plan*, the Secretary of State for Health (2000) states that if users are to receive the best care, then the old divisions between health and social care must be overcome. Thus, facilitating effective partnerships in care, users are intended to have access to seamless services that are tailored to their particular needs.

The Health Act (1999) swept away the legal obstacles to joint working by allowing the use of pooled budgets, which involves local health and social services to put money into a single dedicated budget to fund a wide range of care services; lead commissioning, where one of the service providers, the trust, the local authority or the primary care group takes the lead in commissioning services on behalf of each other; and integrated providers, where local authorities and trusts merge their services to deliver a one-stop package of care. The 1999 Act also proposed new care trusts to provide even closer integration of mental health services and social services. Care trusts will be able to commission primary and community health and social care to all client groups including the mentally ill. Furthermore, where mental health and social services organisations have failed to establish effective joint partnerships, or where joint inspection or reviews have shown that services are failing, the government could take powers to establish integrated arrangements through new care trusts.

These changes will remove the outdated institutional barriers between the mental health services and social services that have prevented people from obtaining the care they need and when they need it. However, the management and control of such a diverse set of organisations is difficult because these organisations are not accustomed to working together in a coordinated way. These organisations have developed and sustained policies and procedures that serve their own culture and interests. Their internal procedures and systems have usually been developed in isolation. Eaton (1998) argues that in mental health services, coordination between mental health and social services is notoriously poor.

Owens (1998) suggested that the nature of the health service and a local authority body such as social services may be a source of conflict. Local authorities are answerable to their local electorate and so subject to political control. If a local authority is controlled by politicians not in government, there could be policy differences that might differ from the government's approach to a particular issue. How would such a dispute be resolved within the context of a partnership duty?

THE CARE PLANNING APPROACH

The National Service Framework for Mental Health states clearly that the Care Planning Approach must be fully integrated into mental health services, so that mental health and social services are integrated to minimise the distress and confusion experienced by users, carers and their families. Furthermore, that the Care Planning Approach would enable a seamless service to be achieved through an integrated approach to care coordination, the coordination of the respective roles and responsibilities of each agency in the system and access through a single process, to the support and resources of both mental health services and social services. These processes should ensure that access to services provided by the NHS or local authority social services are based on the assessment of needs, the prevention of duplication and provide an agreed plan of action. It must always be remembered that mental illness places demands on services that no one discipline or agency can meet alone. Therefore, a system of effective care coordination is required if all services are to work in harmony for the benefit of the service user.

Other features of a truly integrated system of the Care Planning Approach include: a single operational policy; joint training for mental health and social services professionals; one 'lead officer' for care coordination across mental health services and social services; common and agreed risk assessment and risk management processes; a shared information system across mental health and social services; a single complaints procedure; agreement on the allocation of resources and, where possible, developed budgets; a joint serious incident process; and one point of access for mental health and social services assessments. Essential to the achievement of integration is the role of a 'lead officer' with authority to work across all agencies, to ensure that audit of practice is undertaken and that feedback is provided to practitioners and managers alike (DoH 2000a).

Effective joint working projects between health and social services have been operating throughout the UK since the early 1990s. According to Eaton (1998), joint working between general practitioners and social workers in Solihull has resulted in having a social worker attached to the practice, which has led to general practitioners, users and carers who can give and receive a quicker service; the social worker can obtain more information, with the outcome of the development of a better understanding of each other's roles. Another example cited by Eaton (1998) is a joint mental health risk team in Hertfordshire between the health authority, social services, police, probation and psychiatrists. This team shared information on individual cases to inform the ways the professionals work together, to monitor action and provide appropriate support. Before, there would have been heavy reliance on individual social workers or the psychiatrists, which would have been *ad hoc*. Now asserts Eaton (1998), the team members have a better grasp of what each agency can offer, what the constraints are and what their common concerns are.

However, there are reports and evidence suggesting that the coordination being achieved in the Care Planning Approach is very patchy (Audit Commission 1994; Shepherd 1995). Some of the reasons relate to inadequate coordination and integration of mental health services and social services. Evaluation of the Care Planning Approach in use might benefit from the following analysis: to examine the degree to which the respective organisations are aligned to the needs of the users, carers and the professionals involved; the ability of organisations to address the concepts of users first; and to adhere to the corporate goals as well as to work with others. Further, in view of the fact that the internal procedures and systems of health and social services have been developed separately, there remains the need for the organisations involved to show evidence of procedural alignment. Two further relevant factors are the cultural differences between the organisations in their procedures, practices and administration along with the systems of information technology used. Overall, if internal procedures and systems have usually been developed in isolation, this background makes the benefits of integration more difficult to realise.

Addressing user and carer issues

No current social policy document on mental health fails to mention the need to involve users, carers and their families in collaboration and partnerships within service development and delivery (Secretary of State for Health 1997; DoH 1999b, 2000b).

The National Service Framework for Mental Health (DoH 1999a) demands that local mental health services must listen to the users' and carers' voice, in order to involve both groups in the decision-making process, to enable users and carers to be trained with professionals and to become involved in projects and research. Furthermore, while achieving these goals the mental health service must work in partnership with services in the private and the voluntary sectors, so as to provide culturally appropriate support for ethnic group service users.

Carers receive special acknowledgement: health and social care service providers are asked to ensure that provision is made for the needs of carers who give regular and substantial care for those with mental illnesses (DoH 1999b, 1999c). All carers supporting users on a Care Planning Approach should be assessed as to their caring, the physical and mental health needs on an annual basis, as well as to have their own care plan (DoH 1999b).

Users and carers are keen to develop opportunities for collaboration and partnerships to influence policy formation and to contribute to the planning of appropriate services that reflect their perceived needs. Users and carers are now more organised, articulate, informed and challenging to the mental health system. The question now for user groups is whether they should attempt to influence existing services and participate in collaboration and in partnership or work independently to establish alternatives (Edwards 2000).

To start the processes of collaboration and partnership, mental health and social care professionals must put aside all attitudes that suggest 'we know best' and 'we should not be questioned', but to start listening and to provide care in a sensitive manner with users as an active participant in their own care. Millar and Rose (1986) suggested that devising therapeutic schemes in which clients had a share in their own care had better outcomes than those schemes that did not have this outlook. Mental health and social care professionals must realise that users emphasise the importance of the context of their lifestyle that relates to poverty through shortage of money, poor accommodation, unemployment and loneliness that require change. On the other hand, users see the medical diagnosis and mental illnesses as taking a back seat to the issues relating to everyday living and the isolation experienced through stigma and lack of opportunity. The Audit Commission (1994) reported that poverty and inadequate housing are particularly common among people with mental health problems. These matters, which are high priorities for users, are often overlooked by mental health and social care professionals, who focus on treatments and therapy while ignoring the users' social and economic needs.

To take a step further in collaboration and partnership with users, Shields (1985) suggested questions that are still relevant today. Shields (1985) asks mental health and social care professionals to ask themselves how much the professionals actually know about users' views of the mental health and social care services they provide; whether the professionals want to know and can be flexible enough to admit that the user may know better than the professional about what is best for themselves. The views of users, Shields (1985) argues, must be sought. Users are usually a vulnerable group, often frightened, unassertive and inarticulate. In order to provide the most effective interventions and treatments, their views provide one measure of usefulness, hence such views could lead to an improvement in the services and give better value for money. In a democracy it is right that mental health and social care services, which are publicly supported services, are accountable to users. A way to achieve accountability is by participation. Such participation could help reduce the feelings of alienation that service users often experience and help to negate the 'us and them' resentment that is often present.

According to Hickey and Kipping (1998), the concept of user involvement in mental health and social care is difficult to define. The common terms used include negotiated care, collaborative care, partnership, person-centred care and user participation, all of which refer to varying degrees of user participation. The understanding that the user, the carer, the family and the health and social care professionals have of these terms will determine the relationships and the resulting interprofessional behaviours and activities employed. An important starting point is whether there is a shared set of assumptions between mental health services, social services and users (Melville 1997). User participation may extend to the sharing of information; to take part in decision-making; the involvement of carers and families; and the rejection by users of the passive acceptance of information and treatment. The outcome may lead to users who become assertive in requesting explanations and making joint decisions in the planning of their treatment and care; as well as users who take control of their circumstances and achieving their own goals (Glenister 1994).

However, there are inhibitors that may result in variations in participation. Different perspectives on user involvement may possibly exist because of the different contexts in which health and social care take place and thus, while sharing some common themes, definitions may vary in the specific focus and emphasis of concern (Glenister 1994). Cultures, structures, organisational systems and bureaucracy may constrain participation, as might confusion in terminology, communication and understanding of user involvement between professional disciplines, as well as the beliefs each professional brings to the care interface, coupled with the service users' beliefs, perceptions and prior experience of the care services (Nyatanga 1997; Playle and Keeley 1998).

McDermott's (1998) study of the Care Planning Approach revealed that users found the approach difficult to understand, were unfamiliar with their treatment programmes, had little knowledge regarding their care and felt that their opinions regarding care planning and decision-making were less valued than those of their relatives and the health and social care professionals. Anthony and Crawford (2000) argue that there are factors such as limited resources, debilitating mental state, lack of motivation, negative staff attitudes, conflicting responsibilities and duties, which may inhibit user involvement. Anthony and Crawford (2000) also consider limited resources, which encompass inadequate staffing, lack of time and a chaotic care environment, to be major inhibiting factors.

The old order within mental health services, characterised by hierarchies, authoritarian structures and social control are breaking down. The seeking of collaboration and partnership relationships with users and carers is an expression of the new emerging reality. The mental health user and carer movements are endeavouring to deconstruct the knowledge of medicine and are challenging the very power base of psychiatry that doctors know best. The people using the mental health services are contributing their perspectives to the health and social care arena; it would be foolish to ignore their perception of their reality. There is a need for true partnership with those that use the mental health services, as well as a need to re-educate professionals in a way that takes cognisance of the user perspective.

The interprofessional team

If mental health and social service professionals are to plan and deliver the most effective user and carer sensitive services, both groups must begin to celebrate collective endeavours, in which the whole effort is greater than the sum of the individual contributions. Mental health and social service professionals must also honour teams more, but aggressive leaders and maverick geniuses less (Reich 1987).

Major changes are continually occurring in the mental health and social care services. These changes involve new forms of services and service delivery, a rise in user and carer expectations, staff shortages and the increased need for cost reduction. Furthermore, government documents require integration, collaboration and partnerships to be at the very heart of the provision and delivery of care for and with users and carers (Secretary of State for Health 1997; DoH 1998, 1999a, 2000a, 2000c).

The *Oxford English Dictionary* provides definitions of teamwork; one definition offers that teamwork is like two or more beasts of burdens harnessed together. This description might feel appropriate to many mental health and social care workers; nevertheless, the opportunity for discussion, sociability and the chance to shift the load occasionally is implicit even in this type of team. Therefore, even if mental health and social care workers are working as beasts of burden, life might be pleasanter if both groups work together towards common aims than alone. Another definition presents teamwork as a set of players on one side in a game such as football. The football analogy adds to our understanding of the attributes of a team. The team has a captain or leader, the players have distinct functions and can take over the functions of other players when necessary. These definitions refer to combined efforts and organised cooperation, that is a group of people coming together to get things done (Firth-Cozens 1992).

There is evidence that working in teams enhances the organisation's effectiveness (Kallerberg and Moody 1994). Teamworking produces better user care in terms of improved mental health and social care services delivery and staff motivation (Wood et al 1994). Claims are also made that multidisciplinary teams allow a more efficient use of staff and service planning (Ovretveit 1988). Effective teamworking will welcome diversity and opposing views while working towards unity and managing conflict (Tjosvold 1991). Firth-Cozens (1992) suggested that the characteristics of teamwork are common goals, diversity of skills and knowledge, support for team members, acceptance and management of conflict, development of individuals and working towards unity. Furthermore, a team composed of similar individuals who hold common beliefs and have similar abilities are likely to view a task from a single perspective. Although solidarity can be useful, it can also lead to an absence of the critical thought necessary for evaluating complex problems and for decision-making. Therefore, the team needs users and carers to inform the professionals of their needs and to contribute to planning, innovation and change, in order to realise collaboration and partnership between the service users and the service providers. Furthermore, the team needs questioners, as well as sometimes team members who act as devil's advocates to put forward difficult and uncomfortable questions that require attention.

When teams are not functioning well, the following are signs of trouble: members cannot easily describe the team's mission, they have lost the focus of the task at hand; the meetings are formal, stuffy and tense, with absenteeism and drop-out rate at a high level; there appears to be a great deal of participation and activities but very little is accomplished; there is talk but not much communication, so decisions are constantly being put off; disagreements are aired in private conversations after meetings, differences, critiques and conflicts are not managed; when decisions are made they tend to be made formally by the leader with little meaningful involvement of other team members; members are not open with each other because trust is low; there is disagreement about roles, responsibilities, boundaries and work assignments; cooperation between team members is low and there may even be sabotage; the team is overloaded with people who have the same team player style; the team members have always been there, there is a need for change; and the team has never assessed its functioning and effectiveness. There are also some paradoxes that haunt teams: the fear of taking risks that may result in separation from one other; the members who feel out of the team who cannot bring up their concerns because of the myth that everyone else is in; people reject exclusivity and covet inclusiveness, being needed, being involved, being cared about and the fear of being left out of interactions.

Mental health and social care professionals may refuse to work in teams for various reasons; some professionals may find a particular team threatening. Others may feel that there is unfairness in the team such as, who has the easiest service users or who does not do their fair share of work or fair share of out-of-hours' work. Although diversity of skills is essential in tackling the complexity of mental health service users' needs, it is usually the case that staff are more comfortable mixing with those who are similar to themselves. Not only may nurses prefer to communicate with other nurses, or psychiatrists with other psychiatrists, but also team members may prefer to make alliances with those that are similar to avoid those who approach life differently (Firth-Cozens 1998).

Interprofessional teams in mental health may exert social control over users and carers. In some circumstances the mere construction of a team may limit the choices available, which makes it more difficult to challenge the decisions of professionals, who now represent a collective rather than an individual wisdom. The team may also facilitate control through the presentation of a united front, with the nurse or social worker who does not express their differing professional views in order to maintain good team and interprofessional relationships, as well as to allow participants to look good, which can reduce the options to users and carers (Mackay 1995).

To be effective, interprofessional mental health and social care teams must be integrated and it must be realised that they will need ongoing support. Freeth (2001) makes the point that interprofessional collaboration and teamworking are well promoted but less funding and energy goes into making sure that initiatives are sustained.

Training

The delivery of an integrated mental health and social care service require agencies to collaborate. To achieve this goal, it is important that health and social care professionals are participating in the promotion and implementation of interprofessional education and training. Whatever the reservations there may be about interprofessional education and training, the Department of Health is pressing ahead with its commitment to accelerate the development of such education and training for health and social care staff, as one of its key requirements for improving standards and quality of user and carer care (DoH 1999c, 2000a, 2000b, 2001b).

There is now a fair amount of literature on the benefits of multidisciplinary and interprofessional education and training. Nevertheless, little seems to have been rigorously evaluated. The few evaluations undertaken show benefits for attitudes towards user care and collaborative practice rather than outcomes such as improved patient care (Carpenter 1995). Harden (1998) argues that the interprofessional education experience of learning with other professional groups benefits working together effectively as a team by:

• Enhancing personal and professional confidence
• Promoting mutual understanding between health and social care workers
• Achieving intraprofessional and interprofessional communication
• Encouraging reflection in and on practice

For mental health and social care services, the Care Planning Approach is at the core of the government's policy on mental health (DoH 1995), which emphasises user and carer participation. In order to achieve an integrated Care Planning Approach, joint and interprofessional training in the workplace must be encouraged. Members of the team should train together, to ensure that the potential keyworkers from different professional backgrounds develop a shared approach to the keyworker's role. The Social Services Inspectorate Report (DoH/SSI 1995) recommended that social services departments should identify areas where joint training would be appropriate.

In the development of education and training for mental health and social care professionals, training should be based in the practice area and be provided at both team and agency levels. Users, carers, managers, administrators, receptionists and secretaries should be involved, as their perceptions and expectations will inform the professionals, which will in turn enable a greater understanding of the different professionals' roles and functions. According to Beresford and Trevillion (1995), the move to a more collaborative approach can amount to no less than a cultural revolution. Managers and administrators require management and continuous training development in this area, to assist them in the task of reshaping their agencies in order to release the potential of their staff. The planning, content and presentation of training should include shared learning, interprofessional learning and interagency learning. There is no clear separation between these teaching and learning approaches and many issues will overlap in the teaching processes. The shared element is concerned with the exchange of information, which is relevant to all the mental health and social care professionals, for example documents emanating from the Department of Health. The interprofessional element is concerned with the issues that arise when two or more professions learn with, from and about each other to facilitate collaboration and to improve the quality of practice (CAIPE 2001). Finally, the provision of interagency training is needed to enable the professionals, users and carers to gain insights into the culture and administration of each other's organisation.

CONCLUSION

It is expected that in the new NHS, mental health and social services providers will work together and collaborate with users, carers, the voluntary and the private sectors. If users are to receive the best care then the old divisions between mental health and social services providers must be overcome. If this pathway is not achieved, users will continue to be denied access to seamless services that are tailored to their needs. These changes will remove the outdated institutional barriers between mental health and social services, which have prevented users from obtaining the care they need, when and where they need it.

In *A National Service Framework for Mental Health* (DoH 1999a), a service is requested that is sensitive to the needs of users, carers and their families, committed to meeting ethnic and cultural needs and engaged in initiatives to reduce the stigma attached to mental health problems. In the planning and delivery of services, it is expected that the Care Planning Approach to care management will be used and that teamwork will be developed and sustained as an essential part of working together. Finally, all the professional staff, users, carers and managers must engage in continuous educational and training opportunities so that interprofessional and interagency insights can be shared.

REFERENCES

Anthony, P. and Crawford, P. (2000) 'Service user involvement in care planning: the mental health nurse's perspective', *Journal of Psychiatric and Mental Health Nursing* 7, 425–34.

Audit Commission (1994) *Finding a Place: A Review of Mental Health Services for Adults*, London: HMSO.

Beresford, P. and Trevillion, S. (1995) *Developing Skills for Community Care: A Collaborative Approach*, Aldershot: Arena.

CAIPE (2001) *Resource Pack for Teachers and Trainers*, London: CAIPE.

Carpenter, J. (1995) 'Interprofessional education for medical and nursing students; evaluation of a programme', *Medical Education* 29, 265–72.

DoH (Department of Health) (1995) *Building Bridges: A Guide to Arrangements for Inter-agency Working for the Care and Protection of Severely Mentally Ill People*, London: HMSO.

DoH (1998) *Partnership in Action*, London: HMSO.

DoH (1999a) *A National Service Framework for Mental Health*, London: HMSO.

DoH (1999b) *Caring for Carers: A National Strategy for Carers*, London: HMSO.

DoH (1999c) *Making a Difference Strengthening the Nursing and Health Visiting Contribution to Health and Healthcare*, London: HMSO.

DoH (2000a) *Effective Care Co-ordination in Mental Health Services: Modernising the Care Programme Approach*, A Policy Booklet, London: HMSO.

DoH (2000b) *Meeting the Challenge: A Strategy for the Allied Health Professions*, London: HMSO.

DoH (2000c) *A Health Service of all Talents*, London: HMSO.

DoH (2001a) *National Service Framework for Older People*, London: HMSO.

DoH (2001b) *Investment and Reform for NHS staff – Taking Forward the NHS Plan*, London: HMSO.

DoH/SSI (1995) *Social Services Departments and the Care Programme Approach: An Inspection*, London: HMSO.

Eaton, J. (1998) 'Arranged marriages', *Health Service Journal* 108 (5627) 24–6.

Edwards, K. (2000), 'Service users and mental health nursing', *Journal of Psychiatric and Mental Health Nursing* 7, 555–65.

Firth-Cozens, J. (1992) 'Building teams for effective audit', *Quality in Health Care* 1, 252–3.

Firth-Cozens, J. (1998) 'Celebrating teamwork', *Quality in Health Care* 7, 3–7.

Freeth, D. (2001) 'Sustaining interprofessional collaboration', *Journal of Interprofessional Care* 15 (1) 36–7.

Glenister, D. (1994) 'Patient participation in psychiatric services: a literature review and proposal for a research strategy', *Journal of Advanced Nursing* 19, 802–11.

Harden, R. (1998) 'AMEE guide no.12: multiprofessional education: part 1 – effective multiprofessional education: a three dimensional perspective', *Medical Teacher* 20 (5) 402–16.

Hickey, G. and Kipping, C. (1998) 'Exploring the concept of user involvement in mental health through participation continuum', *Journal of Clinical Nursing* 7, 83–9.

Kallerberg, A. and Moody, J. (1994) 'Human resource management and organisational performance', *American Behavioral Science* 37, 948–62.

Mackay, L. (1995) 'The patient as pawn in interprofessional relationships', in K. Soothill, L. Mackay and C. Webb (eds), *Interprofessional Relations in Health Care*, London: Edward Arnold.

McDermott, G. (1998) 'The Care Programme Approach: a patient perspective', *Nursing Times Research* 3 47–63.

Melville, M. (1997) 'Consumerism: do patients have power in health care'? *British Journal of Nursing* 6, 337–9.

Millar, P. and Rose, N. (1986) *The Power of Psychiatry*, Cambridge: Polity Press.

Nyatanga, B. (1997) 'Psychosocial theories of patient non-compliance', *Professional Nurse* 12, 331–4.

Ovretveit, J. (1988) *Essentials of Multidisciplinary Team Organisation*, Uxbridge: Brunel University.

Owens, D. (1998) 'Dual carriageway', *Health Service Journal* 108 (5672) 29.

Playle, J. and Keeley, P. (1998) 'Non-compliance and professional power', *Journal of Advanced Nursing* 27, 304–11.

Reich, R. (1987) Entrepreneurship reconsidered: the team as hero, *Harvard Business Review* 65, 77–83.

Secretary of State for Health (1997) *The new NHS: Modern, Dependable*, London: HMSO.

Secretary of State for Health (2000) *The NHS Plan: A Plan for Investment, A Plan for Reform*, London: HMSO.

Shepherd, D. (1995) *Learning the Lessons: Mental Health Inquiry Reports Published in England and Wales between 1969–1994 and their Recommendations for Improving Practice*, London: The Zito Trust.

Shields, P. (1985) 'The consumer view of psychiatry', *Hospital and Health Services Review*, May 117–19.

The Health Act (1999) Section 22 (1) (2).

Tjosvold, D. (1991) *Team Organisation: An Enduring Competitive Advantage*, Chichester: Wiley & Sons.

Wood, N., Farrow, S. and Elliott, B. (1994) 'A review of primary health care organisations', *Journal of Clinical Nursing* 3, 243–50.

Chapter 16

Under One Roof

An experimental interagency service for homeless people in south London

Graham Park

SUMMARY

The origins of the Under One Roof project are described. Two models of approach are then discussed and assessed: (1) casework: six agencies working together to provide a one-day service at each of two day centres for homeless people; (2) multiagency discussion panels that met at a total of five locations. Some key issues are then reviewed: the relationship between statutory and voluntary agency workers; exchanging information about clients; the place of language; confidentiality; techniques and methods for chairing and minuting meetings; and responding to geographical distance between agencies alongside the demands on time when supporting homeless people. The conclusion lists key actions to take for the future where interagency issues are involved.

THE ORIGIN AND START OF THE PROJECT: A MULTIAGENCY CASEWORK SERVICE

Under One Roof ran from 1997 to 2000 as an interagency project aiming to provide better integrated services to homeless single people in two neighbouring London boroughs, which brought together a partnership of a dozen statutory and voluntary organisations. The programme was commissioned by the King's Fund, their interest generated by the report *Health and Homelessness in London: A Review* (Pleace and Quilgars 1996), which *inter alia* commented on the poor information exchange and limited collaboration between services. Despite strong recent encouragement for joint assessment – defined as assessing all an individual's needs and involving all necessary services from the outset – Pleace and Quilgars (1996) could find no examples of joint assessment occurring beyond isolated individuals or projects. Key agencies were sometimes even unaware of each other's existence. Although many agencies could claim good links with health, or housing, or social services, and sometimes two of these, sound relationships with all three were rare. *Health and Homelessness* (Pleace and Quilgars 1996) considered all manifestations of homelessness, but Under One Roof chose to address the most severe and visible form of this – rough sleeping.

In parallel with the King's Fund's interest, core members of the project's steering group had been impressed by The Hub, a multiagency project in Bristol for people with housing problems (The Hub 1997), and wondered if such a service might be developed for central London.

Under One Roof began as a multiagency casework service based in two day centres for homeless people: North Lambeth Day Centre and the service provided by St Giles Trust in the London Boroughs of Lambeth and Southwark, respectively. In common with similar voluntary sector services elsewhere, these day centres provide shelter and food, access to washing facilities, recreational activities, assistance with accommodation and other problems and, partly through existing arrangements with visiting agencies, help with health problems, training and guidance on employment.

Alongside the host day centres, voluntary sector agencies included, in Southwark, Shelter's Piccadilly Advice Centre and, in Lambeth, Thames Reach that provides, among other services, outreach on the street to people sleeping rough. Statutory staff came from the Benefits Agency, local authority social services and housing departments, the Three Boroughs' Primary Health Care Team (a community nursing team for homeless people) and START, a mental health team with a similar client brief.

It was argued that, with this new collaborative structure, the service would particularly be able to meet the needs of rough sleepers who had such complex problems that existing methods of assistance had so far failed to work (Under One Roof 1997: 3). In an ideal case, a referring agency would identify a rough sleeper and bring him or her to an Under One Roof session. The day centre would provide a comfortable waiting environment, while the various professionals would conduct an assessment and plan a response to the client's needs, which was immediately likely to include restarting their benefit claim and placement in temporary accommodation, followed by a more extensive response by participating agencies' mainstream services over the coming weeks. Any spare capacity could be made available to people with less severe difficulties.

It was also expected that the exercise in itself would be instrumental in bringing the participant agencies closer together, variously through day-to-day practice, through the management groups, and as a result of a series of facilitated planning and review days involving a wide network of agencies (Under One Roof 1997: 4).

The effectiveness of Under One Roof's initial model – a multiagency casework service located in day centres – can be considered in service delivery and organisational terms:

1 *Service delivery*
   In practice, client interventions of the kind described above rarely

occurred. On one morning a week, the service was offered on an absurdly limited scale: people repeatedly acknowledged to be 'chaotic' could not be expected to arrive within such a narrow time band for any assessment, let alone one involving two or more agencies. For those that did use the service, queuing problems were created by having one worker from each discipline, while other staff were idle for long periods. Too many features seemed to match the list of factors likely to make an interagency project fail offered by Øvretveit (1993: 100): a part-time service; a temporary office; key client decisions made elsewhere; and others. It was also questionable whether there ever was a large number of people for whom such a response was likely to be more effective than existing services; we feared we may simply have added to the number of agencies that promise much to homeless people but deliver considerably less. Although there was some difference between sites – St Giles Trust, with a larger staff team of its own and a stronger commitment from management, managed to maintain an almost adequate flow of cases, while North Lambeth Day Centre did not – the mid-term evaluation (Randall 1999) concluded that this model was unlikely to deliver a more effective response than existing services provided.

2 *Interagency development*

Interagency development was, perhaps unsurprisingly, more effective. Early on, staff could be observed telling each other in detail about how they worked. For some of the voluntary agencies – notably the day centres – the principal relationship development was from one of suspicion, with indirectly reported concerns that staff felt in some way 'deskilled' by others' presence, to one of cooperation; but the mature relationship of felt equality was rare until the next phase, which is discussed in the following section. There were parallel developments within the managers' steering group. For example, initial voluntary sector hopes that the Benefits Agency and, in Southwark, the local authority homelessness service could assess and then act on client needs while at the day centres were accepted as unrealistic. Over a series of meetings, voluntary sector staff came to understand that what seemed a single event in fact involved a series of actions, some of which must inevitably occur at the agency's own office.

This first phase lasted almost a year, with closure delayed by attempts to make it work – for example by mail shots to potential external referrers and by improved links with the day centres – and because a reasonable period was needed to evaluate the project as commissioned.

Changing to panels

For its next phase, first in February 1999 in Lambeth and shortly afterwards in Southwark, Under One Roof overcame its principal problem – getting target clients to attend at all in the narrow time slot available – by eliminating that aspect of the service. Instead, the same staff group as before would discuss in detail clients put forward by the host day centre and later by other agencies, and minutes would be provided. This was far more effective, though there was considerable variation between locations.

In Lambeth, panel meetings were held at North Lambeth Day Centre, followed by a series of 18 cases at a hostel for people with high-support needs managed by Thames Reach. Finally, four clients were discussed at a hostel managed by St Mungo's, the largest hostel provider in London, in an exercise involving that agency's employment worker.

In Southwark, meetings were held at St Giles Trust, this time in parallel with the continuing and moderately successful casework service, and in the winter of 1999/2000, at a cold weather shelter run by Crisis, another homelessness charity. The latter was a temporary service for people known to have slept rough over a long period, almost all of whom had severe problems with mental illness, alcohol or drugs, which in itself was a collaborative arrangement between agencies including specialist resettlement and substance misuse services.

These experiences allowed detailed scrutiny of each agency's practices and needs and allowed the following observations:

1   Often while claiming otherwise, some agencies have insufficient professional and administrative backing to allow proper participation in interagency practice. At day centre meetings in Lambeth, for example, most early panel meetings felt shallow, consisting of little more than participants agreeing to check agency records and report back, and with day centre staff offering little information or opinion about their own clients. As time went on the project became confident about some individuals' practice, but not about the agency as a whole.

2   Despite wide differences in discipline and depth of training, there was a developing sense in most settings that all present were participating as equals. While personal qualities of participants should not be overlooked, the speed with which this sense of collaboration developed is also likely to be structural – all participants were in some way homelessness specialists within their own disciplines. Such felt equality is to be valued: participants sometimes complained of its absence elsewhere with, for example, qualified and experienced homelessness specialists feeling like junior partners in mainstream medical, psychiatric or social work meetings, and were sometimes not being invited at all when their presence was in their view essential.

3   The project found its systems generally working better if the Under One

Roof panel was faced with a specific task. At the cold weather shelter, for example, the need to assess and find placements for all clients by the temporary shelter's closing date provided a focus that the generic services at other locations lacked, so that in many ways this was the best manifestation of the exercise.

4 Although the generic service at, for example, the St Giles Trust was eventually not thought cost-effective as a permanent service, the project was a valued contribution to that agency's development. Close observation of statutory practice generated rapid improvement in their assessment procedures, detailed discussion with practitioners reduced the number of inappropriate referrals in both directions and firmer links with key agencies were formed (Currie 2001).

THE FINAL PHASE: MEETINGS FOR CONTACT AND ASSESSMENT TEAMS

In Under One Roof's final phase, the lessons learned and networks established were applied to a currently unmet demand for high quality interagency practice. The government had in 1998 set up the Rough Sleepers Unit to respond to the large numbers of people sleeping rough in London and elsewhere. Among other developments, the Unit reorganised voluntary sector outreach services into Contact and Assessment Teams (CATs) (Rough Sleepers Unit 1999: 12) charged with encouraging rough sleepers to move into hostels where further assistance could be provided. Under One Roof administered and chaired a series of case conferences for CATs, involving agencies including Westminster Social Services, two central London day centres for homeless people, voluntary sector drugs agencies and the Metropolitan Police. Features of these meetings that were particularly appreciated were a formal structure usually overlain by an informal style, and chairing and minuting practices that drew on a wide technical knowledge of social work, housing, health and homelessness services and, following experience earlier in the project, was sensitive to variation in the range and depth of participants' technical knowledge so that, for example, conscious efforts were made to probe for a clear explanation of procedures and the meaning of technical terms.

Meetings of this kind are commonplace in mental illness or child protection services (and procedures were consciously borrowed from them here). It can be argued that the gravity of the situation faced by some homeless people requires a response of equal seriousness.

As well as these eventual positive practical outcomes, Under One Roof provided an opportunity to reflect on the special nature of rough sleeping and the agencies charged with responding to it, to comment on some of the obstacles to interagency cooperation and to make some observations about professional practice in this setting.

ROUGH SLEEPING AND SERVICES FOR ROUGH SLEEPERS: A SPECIAL CASE

Although rough sleeping is commonly presented as an issue subject to technical and administrative responses much in the manner of, say, substandard housing or poor health, there is something exceptional about this problem. First, chronic rough sleeping lies so far outside most people's social experience that it is hard for otherwise sympathetic people properly to understand, even if they are directly engaged in providing services (Wiseman 1970: 242). Second, it is a situation of extreme and unusual failure. The client group might be defined as people for whom all taken-for-granted social support systems that normally sustain people in their own accommodation – individual resources, the family, the market and welfare services – have failed (Pleace 1998: 57; Stern et al 2000: 11), and it follows that a simple reapplication of mainstream services and practices is likely to have limited success. Organising appropriate services is made particularly difficult – especially in London – by the need to contend with a continually changing network of agencies as the client forms and abandons contact with agencies as he or she moves between boroughs – usually by accidents of geography such as the availability of hostel vacancies or of safe sleeping-out sites rather than by wilfulness on the homeless person's part.

Although not unique to homelessness services, there are also problems with responses to the issue. The limited statutory response can be hard to negotiate even for people with undoubted rights to housing by their local authority (Robinson 1998), and although voluntary agencies are often described as having particular expertise, their provision is often residual to a need that the state has traditionally regarded as unimportant. While some voluntary agencies reach a high standard of service, staff are often younger and less qualified than in equivalent statutory services, and managers will often have been promoted from within the service without the training considered necessary elsewhere (Timms 1998: 74). There is something more to negotiate than professional difference; wide variations in agency approach, resources and competence – often unacknowledged – will be there also.

COMMUNICATION BETWEEN AGENCIES

Participation in Under One Roof permitted reflection about what exactly it was that agencies knew and did not know about each other and what some of the obstacles to understanding and communication might be. While there is an extensive literature to draw on, immediate observation focused on the differing depth of practitioner knowledge of other organisations – described here as inventory and operational knowledge – and some problems arising from language and from physical distance.

INVENTORY KNOWLEDGE: KNOWING WHICH ORGANISATIONS EXIST

Despite the frustration expressed in *Health and Homelessness in London* (Pleace and Quilgars 1996) about locating appropriate services, ignorance of agencies' existence was not a problem experienced directly at Under One Roof. The sector is well served by Resource Information Service's (1998: 2001) directories of Day Centres and London hostels respectively and their web site (www.homelesspages.org.uk) lists over 30 other directories. Unsurprisingly, the project did encounter practitioners elsewhere (hospital discharge managers for example) who had only occasional contacts with homeless people and did not know these publications. Agencies were often good at answering enquiries from people unfamiliar with homelessness services, but a reminder may nevertheless be needed that, in order properly to respond to enquirers who may understandably mentally group all homelessness services together, organisations familiarise themselves with services they do not themselves offer – in this case perhaps those for families or refugees – so that agencies can redirect people quickly and appropriately.

OPERATIONAL KNOWLEDGE: UNDERSTANDING HOW ORGANISATIONS WORK

Under One Roof became increasingly convinced that it was detailed information about the functioning and processes of agencies that practitioners lacked. At the start, there were many occasions when staff could be observed explaining in some detail how their own agency worked, their own role within it and the amount of discretion that was open to them. Similar processes occurred when considering outside agencies, with practitioners with detailed knowledge of, say, a specialist hostel, enabling placements to be made with a sensitivity unavailable if only directory information were available.

Although comparatively easy to overcome in this setting – Under One Roof was clearly *about* interagency cooperation, with questioning encouraged – it was also evident how hard it can sometimes be for staff to articulate what they do not know about other organisations and, equally, to identify what outsiders need to know about their own. During the series of review days, group exercises asking agencies to explain or ask questions about each other's practice mostly generated exchanges that, while not valueless, were often shallow and despite conscientious minuting were hard to record. This is not unusual: understanding and describing the physical and organisational contexts in which services for homeless people are set are essential but, because of their unfamiliarity, often difficult to achieve (Knowles 2000: 17). For clients, contexts that matter might include aspects such as the entrance to a hostel, day centre or office: its appearance, accessibility and clarity of purpose; who will meet the client and what they will ask, tell and know about the visitor; where they will be spoken to or interviewed; and whether other clients are likely to be present whose behaviour may cause concern. For staff, contexts will include spatial matters such as office premises – whether, for example, an agency has separate areas for reception, formal and informal interaction with clients, and paperwork, or is using a room in a hostel for all these activities – but will more often be structural: agency responsibilities, the technical knowledge of staff, how paperwork is processed, how decisions are made and who you need to speak to in a given situation.

Understanding how agencies work at this level of detail matters both for reducing practitioner stress and error and for delivering an acceptable service. As a recently homeless man commented at a review day:

> It would help if people assessing our needs could take more care with it. It takes time for me to explain what I want and find out if that is what I am getting. Sometimes I wish people would explain *what is actually going to happen*. [My emphasis.]

Too often, practitioners do not *know* what is going to happen, but consider the act of referral to another agency as sufficient and assume that responsibility for smoothing the process lies with the other party. Agencies and practitioners need to be prepared to *explain* in some detail how their agency and associated systems work; practitioners need to be prepared to *ask* for service details and if necessary ask apparently naive questions; and homelessness agencies need to remind themselves that other practitioners with irregular contact with homeless people may not know about these services or almost as importantly, not understand what they are like.

DIFFICULTIES WITH LANGUAGE

The project encountered instances of misunderstanding created by the imprecision of language among services that, while seemingly directed to a specific social problem, lack a shared professional technology. It proved difficult, for example, to discover what was meant locally by 'resettlement', a key service for homeless people that should properly involve the successful establishment of a home and consist of much more than a move to new accommodation (Deacon 1999). For some 'resettlement' indeed implied a comprehensive service that included frequent home visits offering guidance and practical help, but for others it meant rather less, with no contact at home once the client had moved in (see also Randall and Brown 1999: 57), and for some it simply meant obtaining a bed for the night. It often required careful questioning to establish precisely what was on offer.

'Keyworker' caused similar uncertainty, with some agencies using its original meaning developed in residential social work – 'a member of staff with *prime* responsibility for ensuring that a resident is looked after in all aspects' (Centre for Policy on Ageing 1996: 5; my emphasis); others mean the client's *only* worker; and others use it to indicate responsibility while failing clearly to define where that responsibility begins and ends. Even terms for concrete facilities such as 'day centre' or 'hostel' had a wide range of meanings depending on how they are managed, in a way that more established services such as 'hospital', 'surgery' and even 'residential care' do not.

An amalgam of practices lacking the coherence of an established discipline cannot reasonably be expected to agree on what their terms mean, particularly given the variation of standards and resources between agencies and a reminder – especially to managers and to those chairing meetings – that closer attention be paid to what terms mean locally is perhaps all that can be suggested.

PHYSICAL DISTANCE

Although the original proposal to bring agencies together Under One Roof indicated an awareness of problems with the physical distance between services, and although this must often be a problem for clients and staff, it was hard to stimulate discussion about it; one might guess because of the considerable change in staff deployment that a proper response might imply. Under One Roof brought up these issues, pointing out a need for more services to escort fragile clients between locations and trying out ways for staff to overcome distance by using telephone conferences in place of physical meetings, but there was little lasting progress with this: an area for further discussion.

EXCHANGING INFORMATION: CLIENT RECORDS

The project offered an opportunity to examine the client recording systems of most participant agencies. Unsurprisingly, statutory and other well-established agencies usually – though not always – had stationery better designed for the task and had superior systems for processing records, having had years to revise practice in the light of experience.

Standards were more variable in the voluntary agencies – one having a particularly inadequate recording system – with the choice of style and depth, and indeed of making a permanent record at all, left to individual staff. External communication was poor simply because they had little to communicate about.

A more common problem was the design of some voluntary organisations' recording stationery which, in effect, assumed that paperwork would remain internal, displaying no name or logo to identify its origin should it be passed on – often no doubt a simple oversight but also indicating the limited attention paid to interagency practice.

CONFIDENTIALITY AND INFORMATION EXCHANGE

The Under One Roof project was asked to start by negotiating a detailed interagency confidentiality policy but quickly decided against this, aware that trying to do so could have a fatal effect on interagency initiatives and that the right time to do so was later (Greenberg et al 1992). Instead, a simple policy was drafted that began with first principles – the reasons why confidentiality matters to clients – and went on to outline the essentials of good practice. In contrast to many other such policies, an approach addressing both confidentiality and exchange of information was taken. A form was also designed for use with clients which, rather than presenting a simple agreement to release information, separately identified the main categories of contact: the immediate Under One Roof group, other agencies and because of their special status medical contacts. There was also an option for the client to give instructions about specific agencies or situations. Most clients gave general agreement; a few wanted some kind of restriction but, with very few exceptions, this did not obstruct progress.

Although useful internally, the policy did not feel sufficiently comprehensive to offer as a model for others to follow. Equally, despite a search, no model from elsewhere was found that felt entirely satisfying; but it seems rapidly achievable to produce documents that are both ethically sound and provide helpful practice guidance. This experience needs to be placed in a historical context. Even a few years ago the default position of many voluntary agencies in this field was to withhold information from others, a result one suspects of diffidence about transmitting agencies' own practice, unfamiliarity with receiving agencies' roles and procedures, and a dependence within the sector on training in counselling as a way to learn interviewing techniques – training in which confidentiality has a centrality absent from most other social welfare practices.

JOINT ASSESSMENT

One of Under One Roof's planned outcomes was 'progress towards joint assessment of clients across agencies' (Under One Roof 1997), although the project quickly found itself struggling with what joint assessment actually meant.

The simplest interpretation – two agencies interviewing the client together and reaching a shared conclusion – occurred on too few occasions to establish anything like a routine joint interview. As a housing officer put it:

234 From policy to practice

> Doing a joint interview with the social worker is interesting – I am pick-ing up more and more about how she works – but because we ask differ-ent questions and in a different order, we usually end up interviewing the client twice: I sit through her bit, then she sits through mine.

Later, with the development of multi-agency panels, participants wondered if this was the joint assessment that was sought. Some agencies (The Scottish Office 1998) use this definition, regarding joint assessment as a multidiscipli-nary meeting, though that report also speaks of 'social work coordinated joint assessments' where the social worker considers housing, health and social care together when assessing someone's needs. The detailed documents produced during the period working with Thames Reach's Stamford Street hostel probably matched the latter interpretation.

Some excellent examples of stationery were seen that invited several discip-lines to complete their own sections for assembly into a comprehensive analy-sis. Under One Roof considered devising something similar, but it was later recognised that, while this may suit a well-defined sector such as acute mental health, it was unlikely to be routinely useful in a field where needs, combin-ations of necessary disciplines and agency responsibilities and skills varied so widely from client to client.

It was eventually decided that the notion of 'joint assessment' was less helpful than it might seem. The meaning of 'assessment' differed according to the discipline concerned, and 'joint' implied a degree of collaboration that was rarely achieved or, usually, needed. What really mattered was, first, that the nature of these various assessments were understood and their values recognised; and second, that practitioners conducting assessments of any complexity had access to information and advice from all the agencies and disciplines that had a bearing on their clients' needs. Because, due to differ-ences in status and training within the voluntary sector, the latter is far from guaranteed, the King's Fund commissioned further work on this aspect of Under One Roof, nominally about assessment but also examining the manner in which information is gathered from the disparate agencies involved and subsequently distributed (Park 2002).

CONCLUSION

While a 'one-stop' client service is an attractive concept and sometimes works well, it was ineffective here, partly because such services need to run on a considerable scale if queuing problems are to be avoided, and partly because of the administrative complexity created by a mobile client group in a large city. Other techniques, in this instance offering case conferences about homeless people whose severe and lasting difficulties necessarily involved several agencies, supported by an experienced chair and technical minute taker, can be more effective in bringing agencies together to address a complex task.

Even widely dissimilar agencies can work together effectively, but leadership by someone charged with making it happen in day-to-day practice is required (Goodwin and Shapiro 2001: 27). Effective leaders need to respond to the limited depth of understanding that participants are likely to have about each other's agencies, encouraging explanation about administrative processes as seen by practitioners and clients, and ensuring through enquiry and explanation that misunderstandings do not arise through different interpretations of seemingly shared technical terms. A chairing style that enables case meeting participants to feel that they are taking part as equals is recommended which, given that non-professional members will often know the client best, is fortunately easy to achieve in this field. When contacting outside agencies that are not primarily set up for homeless people, more than usual care will often be needed when describing clients' problems and the specialist services available to the users if misunderstanding and stereotyping are to be avoided.

Case meetings of the kind that evolved in this example offer no response to homeless clients' (and also staff) needs to deal with the physical distance between agencies, but although the project pointed this problem out, it generated little interest. On the other hand, the sometimes inquisitory chairing style recommended allows such unresolved problems to be readdressed from time to time.

Even time-limited projects of this kind can have lasting effects on interagency relationships (Harries et al 1999: 42), and there are indications that this is the case here: an interagency practitioners' group, now involving a wider group of organisations, has followed on to discuss policy, explain agency practices and, through case examples, resolve problems. Managers have reported greater satisfaction with the performance of partner agencies. A more extensive presentation of these arguments can be found in Under One Roof's final report (Park and Barrington 2001).

ACKNOWLEDGEMENTS

My thanks to Liz Barrington for comments on earlier drafts of this chapter. My thanks are also extended to the London Borough of Lambeth, the London Borough of Southwark, St Giles Trust, North Lambeth Day Centre and St Mungo Community Housing Association, who have agreed to the use of their names in this chapter.

REFERENCES

Centre for Policy on Ageing (1996) *A Better Home Life: A Code of Good Practice for Residential and Nursing Home Care*, London: Centre for Policy on Ageing.

Currie, D. (2001) Personal communication at St Giles Trust.

Deacon, A. (1999) 'The resettlement of single homeless people: what works and for whom?' in F. Spears (ed.), *Housing and Social Exclusion*, London and Philadelphia: Jessica Kingsley.

Goodwin, N. and Shapiro, J. (2001) *The Road to Integrated Care Working*, Research Report 39, Birmingham Health Service Management Centre.

Greenberg, M., Levy, J. and Palaich, R. (1992) *Confidentiality and Collaboration: Information Sharing in Inter-agency Efforts*, Washington, DC: American Public Welfare Association.

Harries, J., Gordon, P., Plamping, D. and Fischer, M. (1999) *Elephant Problems and Fixes that Fail: The Story of a Search for New Approaches to Inter-agency Working*, London: King's Fund Publishing.

Knowles, C. (2000) *Bedlam on the Streets*, London and New York: Routledge.

Øvretveit, J. (1993) *Coordinating Community Care: Multidisciplinary Teams and Care Management*, Buckingham: Open University Press.

Park, G. (2002) *Someone and Anyone: Assessment Practice in Voluntary Sector Services for Homeless People in London*, London: King's Fund/Homeless Link.

Park, G. and Barrington, L. (2001) *Loose Connections: Bringing Together Agencies Working with Single Homeless People*, London: King's Fund Publishing.

Pleace, N. and Quilgars, D. (1996) *Health and Homelessness in London: A Review*, London: King's Fund Publishing.

Pleace, N. (1998) 'Single homeless as social exclusion: the unique and extreme', *Social Policy and Administration* 32 (1) 46–59.

Randall, G. (1999) *Evaluation of Under One Roof: Report on Stage Two*, unpublished report, King's Fund/Research and Information Service.

Randall, G. and Brown, S. (1999) *Homes for Street Homeless People: An Evaluation of the Rough Sleepers Initiative*, London: DETR.

Resource Information Service (1998) *London Day Centres Directory: Services for Homeless People*, London: Resource Information Service.

Resource Information Service (2001) *London Hostels Directory*, London: Resource Information Service.

Robinson, D. (1998) 'Health selection in the housing system: access to council housing for homeless people with health problems', *Housing Studies* 13 (1) 23–41.

Rough Sleepers Unit (1999) *Coming in from the Cold: The Government's Strategy*, London: DETR.

Stern, R., Warner, D., O'Neill, E., Park, G. and Barrington, L. (2000) *Joined-up Working with Single Homeless People: Reflections from the Under One Roof Project*, London: King's Fund Publishing.

The Hub (1997) *Annual Report 1996/97*, Bristol: Bristol City Council.

The Scottish Office (1998) *Modernising Community Care: Guidance on the Housing Contribution – a Consultation Draft*, Edinburgh and London: The Scottish Office.

Timms, P. (1998) 'Partnership and conflict: working relationships between voluntary and statutory agencies providing services for homeless people', in D. Cowan (ed.), *Housing: Participation and Exclusion*, Aldershot: Dartmouth.

Under One Roof (1997) *Under One Roof in Lambeth and Southwark: One Stop Assessments for Single Homeless People*, unpublished proposal to the King's Fund.

Wiseman, J. (1970) *Stations of the Lost: The Treatment of Skid Row Alcoholics*, Chicago and London: University of Chicago Press.

Chapter 17

The perspectives of users and carers

Jill Manthorpe

SUMMARY

Why should professionals and organisations work together? The answer surely has to lie in the added value that is given by this approach. Value can be interpreted economically but can also relate to the quality of life and enhancing communities. In this chapter, users' and carers' perspectives are explored, noting that while many join professional calls for increased co-operation, it is users and carers who identify some of the risks of increased integration or co-ordination. Before embarking on interprofessional activities, practitioners need to be mindful that this can be construed as a way of increasing their power. Users and carers may wish, at times, for greater abilities to control their own care and practitioners may need to accept that their models of interprofessional working do not always meet the needs or priorities of individuals. The main challenge of interprofessional care in the new century will be drawing on the perspectives of users and carers to say what works for them.

INTRODUCTION

Evidence from a variety of sources confirms that both service users and carers consider that problems with interprofessional working make a direct impact on their support. The Report of the Mental Health Foundation Committee of Inquiry (1996: 27), for example, found that people with a learning disability recommended:

> Different organisations and services need to talk to each other to give better services.

Joint working was also identified as the most important issue by carers in a recent survey (Henwood 1998) exploring their views at that most difficult juncture, discharge from hospital. However, it would be simplistic to present users and carers as having identical interests and perspectives or to see them as merely repeating professional calls for greater collaboration. This chapter explores a series of issues arising from studies in which users' and carers' experiences are centre stage.

This chapter is divided into four main sections. The first sets out the diversity of carers' experiences and gives examples of their criticisms and interpretations of 'joined-up' care. The second section addresses matters of significance raised by service users, in particular, coordination of control and rights to confidentiality. These issues present alternative perspectives to the rhetoric of coordination circulating in professional and agency circles. The third section considers future agendas for interprofessional work with carers and the final section identifies future developments from users' perspectives. In the conclusion, the potential for new fissures developing is considered.

SECTION I   CARERS – CRITICAL VOICES

During the 1990s a variety of studies and policy documents brought the needs of carers into the public domain (Twigg 2000). Indeed, the naming of carers, instead of kin, relatives or family, as participants in the delivery of community care for disabled adults was part of a process that identified carers as having their own legitimate needs for support. In the UK, this policy interest culminated in the Carers (Recognition and Services) Act 1995, the National Carers Strategy (HM Government 1999) and the Carers and Disabled Children Act 2000. The latter conferred a separate status for carers by awarding them the right to an assessment of their needs for social care even if people with a disability has refused such an assessment for themselves and also established that carers could receive services for their own needs.

Twigg (2000: 103–19) has referred to carers as a new quasi-client group and like many such groups, their needs, circumstances, problems and perceptions have been studied in respect of their relationships to services and professionals. From such studies, two key themes emerge:

- Many carers can find services a maze: support available at times is elusive or ephemeral
- Many carers act as coordinators of care and manage support in the light of particular social contexts and relationships

Examples of the first conundrum comes from a variety of studies, most notably those where parents of disabled children have articulated their frustration with lack of information, multiple but conflicting advice and apparent gaps in knowledge among those who are professionals. As one carer told the Scottish review of services for people with learning disabilities: 'You have to find out about services for yourself. No one comes to you automatically to inform you what services there are, or asks you is there anything you want to know' (Scottish Executive 2001: 30). For almost 30 years parents have asked for 'key', 'link' or coordinating practitioners to provide a familiar face, to facilitate access to specialist and general services and to avoid time-consuming and stigmatising repetition of their families' circumstances. The idea of a coordinating professional to act as a portal in the complex world of health and social care helps explain the popularity of many practitioners, such as teachers or specialist nurses, who take on or who are awarded such roles.

A picture emerges for such carers, and from other studies, of families who both understand and seek to devise their own solutions to problems of coordination and interprofessional difficulties. As Beresford (2000) has emphasised, carers are frequently resourceful and cope. In the case of families with disabled children, for example, families often turn to each other for self-help and support and many have been key to the development of voluntary sector provision that often sits astride professional role demarcations and agency boundaries.

At the other end of the life course, family carers supporting older people with dementia reveal similar resourcefulness. Like children with disabilities, at times people with dementia are buffeted between health and social care agencies and professionals. Similar policy strategies are emerging to reduce the negative impact of such artificial divides. The National Service Framework for Older People (Department of Health 2001a), for example, sees teams as important in bridging such divides in respect of dementia and also in respect of stroke care and fall prevention. For some carers, however, a plethora of teams and special services can coordinate services at one level but then expose new barriers or fissures. Cornes and Clough (2001), for example, found that some families receiving a short-term, coordinated, intensive package of rehabilitation or intermediate care, then felt cast adrift when the scheme ended and the personnel with whom they had become familiar had moved on and new arrangements and staff were introduced.

In order to navigate the welfare maze, intermediate care is just one example of a new service that looks set to make the maze more complex, carers are considered to need a map or information. Clearly identified as the first of the strategic elements of the Carers National Strategy (HM Government 1999: 6), information is seen as important in relation to:

- Health information about their own health
- Accessible information through a national helpline
- Standards and expectations about services
- Internet information

Such a heavy emphasis on information paints a picture of carers, in theory, managing services and choosing from a menu of alternatives. Here is the consumer model of coordination: the suggestion that all carers need are details of different types of support, which will be described to them, not through face-to-face conversations, but through electronic media. Carers are expected to assemble such information together, in the expectation that it will be accurate, quality-assured, available and personally relevant.

This perspective is at odds with the experience of many carers who report that services are not available, insufficiently flexible, culturally insensitive at times and that they do not communicate well with each other. This is reflected in *Valuing People* (Department of Health 2001b), the English White Paper on learning disability services, where family carers are promised investment in services to provide them with the information they have campaigned for, such as a national learning disability information centre. The family carers' working group report *Family Matters, Counting Families In* (Department of Health 2001c) acknowledged that accessing services is often experienced as stressful and resembles fighting a battle.

Such experiences make it clear that carers do not just want coordinated care but also wish to see this as appropriate to the context of their lives and family circumstances. Carers are also highly conscious of resource constraints. A third of all carers, for example, have reported that no one else helps them with their role and 59 per cent do not receive regular visits from health or social care services (Department of Health 1998). Charnley (2001) found that inadequate packages of care, no matter how well coordinated, are not able to meet people's needs. The savings (some £57 billion each year) to the public purse outlined by Carers UK (2002), the pressure group for carers, are used to argue for increased resources and it is this chorus of demands for increased support, not simply better services, which often unites carers and users.

In the next section two further issues, identified as important by users in particular, are considered. These present further challenges to practitioners in their efforts to work interprofessionally. Users and carers are not synonymous of course and users' views about interprofessional working, while often echoing carers' calls for more information and resources, need to be considered separately.

SECTION 2 USER PERSPECTIVES

Control

Increased interprofessional working is, in theory at least, viewed positively by users. However, a number of elements of users' discussions about how this is experienced relate to more ambivalent perceptions. Often these centre around control and different models of the helping relationship. Some users show a sophisticated understanding of the pressures behind interprofessional collaboration, particularly in mental health services where associations of mental illness with dangerousness have compelled greater professional integration of joint working. The development of a keyworker role in the framework of the Care Programme Approach for mental health services is linked to this policy objective to make firm connections between mental health services and other agencies, for example, over monitoring and compliance with medication. Such a perspective was illustrated in recent research on risk (Alaszewski et al 2000), where a user of mental health services set out the network of communication between professionals as it applied to him, for example, if he were to miss an appointment with his keyworker. In his experience, a nurse would call on him at home within the day:

> There's a bush telegraph in mental health. If the warning signs start, they know.
>
> (Alaszewski et al 2000)

Such a perspective acknowledges the potential of coordinated support to be helpful. However, some users fear the possibility that communication between professionals may lead to unwanted and unnecessary attention. In their study of mothers who had mental health problems, for example, Stanley et al (2001) found that nearly all the women interviewed reported fears that they might lose their children as a result of their mental health problems. A third said that this affected their relationship with those who thought they were helping them. One woman revealed:

> That's why I won't ask for help. I'm worried that they will come and take them off me.
>
> (Stanley et al 2001: 15)

These researches observed that mothers were generally able to differentiate between the many professionals involved in their support and were not confused about their roles. Some were aware that professional communications did not always operate satisfactorily. As one woman put it:

> information gets passed over and sometimes it gets confused and muddled up.
>
> (Stanley et al 2001: 18)

Other users, such as people with learning difficulties who are parents, have pointed to patchy and uncoordinated services and the negative effect this may have on their lives. Some have argued, however, that it is not simple improvements in coordination that are required. More sharing of information or suspicions may just serve to reinforce perceptions that they are deficient as parents. Booth and Booth's (1994) detailed and lengthy interviews with parents who have learning difficulties led them to conclude:

usually under close surveillance from the statutory services, families feel their every move is under scrutiny and any mistake risks punitive consequences.

(Booth and Booth 1994: 15)

Confidentiality

Many practitioners espouse confidentiality as a positive part of practice and as central to the professional–client relationship. However, in a world where information-sharing has been criticised as insufficient and where professional communication is seen as important to effective service delivery, confidentiality can assume problem status. The views of service users are important in such discussions as users value the dignity and protection associated with confidentiality. From their perspective, confidentiality provides important safeguards and a number of research studies, exploring users' views, point to their perceptions that confidentiality should be sustained and enhanced. The promotion of advocacy can be seen as a way of (re)creating a trusting relationship between a service user and a professional who is there to represent their interests and not the interests of the service or team. Many advocacy groups see confidentiality as essential to gaining and promoting trust. Henderson and Pochin (2001) have described why this approach might be beneficial:

> When an organisation believes that it 'knows all about' an individual, a terrible determinism can creep into its dealings with that person. . . . If such a person has an advocate, whose dealings with them are confidential, there is at once something 'not known' about that person, a distance which commands respect. They are seen as a person with interests: interests which do not necessarily coincide with those of their service providers.
>
> (Henderson and Pochin 2001: 77)

Confidentiality is not only relevant at an interpersonal level but increasingly arises in connection with the growing use of technology in welfare services. Practitioners may identify the increased efficiency provided by technology and reductions in their workload through, for example, decreased need for appointments for visits to check on well-being or medication. Users, however, may regret the loss of face-to-face contact and fear breaches of confidentiality when information is shared across a range of personnel and agencies (Tang et al 2000).

Such examples demonstrate that being on the receiving end of apparently rational collaborations may have its drawbacks. Telecare, for example, may appear to have advantages by maximising resources and enabling information to be shared but potential or actual users may find it presents multifaceted risks. Simplistic, one-sided presentations of the advantages of technological systems need to acknowledge user perceptions that information technology may possess insufficient safeguards for privacy or that information-sharing protocols may permit agencies to share information that increases the risk of stigma.

Bailey (2001: 71–84) provided an illustration of the myth of confidentiality as experienced by some service users in her report of a young woman who had multiple placements in care and custody settings. By the age of 17, these placements numbered 28 and Bailey and the young woman together estimated that at least one thousand professionals had heard or read the young woman's history. As Bailey (2001: 83) described it, an 'ever-growing procession of professionals . . . stepped in, questioned, stepped out and went on to discuss (the young woman's) life with professionals'.

Working together across agencies requires acknowledgement of different perceptions of confidentiality and sensitivity to whether understandings are shared. These factors will be increasingly important as agencies and practitioners face imperatives both to share information but also to respect private and family life under the Human Rights Act 1998. These compulsions have been evident in mental health work in particular, with a key finding of almost every independent inquiry into mental health tragedies calling for better communication between professionals and agencies (Stanley and Manthorpe 2001).

Children's rights to confidentiality present further challenges to professionals and have been explored to a limited extent in relation to interprofessional work and interagency services. Among the most positive developments are those that seek to involve children in developing an understanding of the issues and in contributing to their resolution. One such account, provided by Dalrymple (1999), identified local variations in the sharing of information and unnecessary exchanges. However, many of the children invited to discuss the meaning of confidentiality for them revealed that they appreciated that confidentiality could not always be guaranteed. In their view, such breaches could be justified at times but what could not was unwarranted low-level and insidious attrition of the principal. Dalrymple (1999) found that many children supported the policy developed but the children warned:

> Agency representatives should be aware of the likely negative repercussions of breaches of confidentiality through gossip.
>
> (Dalrymple 1999: 36)

The involvement of young people and children in the development of multi-agency policies and practice in the area of information-sharing seems to provide opportunities for their views and experiences to be heard. In this study, professionals seemed to be concerned with high level competing ethical priorities (protection or confidentiality) and it was helpful to hear from the young people that informal gossip was experienced as damaging and commonplace. We have much to learn from children and young people about their views of 'joined-up' working and whether and in what circumstances they see it as beneficial.

SECTION 3   FUTURE INTERPROFESSIONAL WORK WITH CARERS

What might carers' support look like in more collaborative welfare? First, it might be that the message 'think carer' could be adopted in all professional practice and broader policy. Repeatedly, carers have drawn attention to the practical barriers that make their tasks more difficult. These barriers include lack of flexibility amid service provision but also a sense that carers are taken for granted by some practitioners. Barnes and Wistow's (1993) research on carers' views of what might constitute a sensitive service found that carers wanted to be able to define their own needs and that assumptions about their circumstances could lead to inappropriate or conflicting offers of support or misinterpretations of meaning. 'Think carer' as a slogan requires professionals to consider the perspectives and experiences of carers – which may include more than a desire for greater interprofessional working.

Second, carers also emphasise that 'joined-up' support involves more than spanning the health and social care divide. In developing a geographical model of what a carer friendly city might look like, carers in one group proposed:

- Chairs in shops
- Attention to transport systems
- Help with pushing wheelchairs
- Details of parking provision for disabled drivers and passengers
- Development of family-friendly employment policies in the city's businesses

In rural areas, the needs of carers for support, which does not entail excessive travelling, have also drawn attention to caring in place issues. There may be negative aspects of coordinating and centralising services in rural areas.

Third, in reviewing evidence for the Royal Commission on Long Term Care of Older People (Sutherland 1999), Parker (1999: 62) has observed that 'the "carer support" agenda has largely failed to take root in the health service'. Parker (1999) ascribes this missed opportunity partly due to the impact of radical changes in the NHS, noting that some of these changes have probably contributed to extra stress on carers by emphasising rapid hospital discharge for instance. In the context of integration and developments in primary care services, Parker (1999) warns that carers' issues may be sidelined. It is difficult to both contain expenditure and to provide carer support.

SECTION 4   FUTURE FORWARD: USER PREDICTIONS ON COLLABORATION

Organisational and professional barriers can present users of services with additional difficulties in accessing appropriate support. Despite this, many people persist and manage to negotiate the complex world of welfare services. They build on their own experience and communicate with each other to learn the quick cuts and safest routes. This approach reflects a consumer model of welfare and, in particular, a 'do-it-yourself' form of consumerism (Gilliatt et al 2000) where individuals and families are seen as increasingly responsible for taking up appropriate services and paying for them. If this pathway is difficult then more advice and information are seen to be the solution, packaged in different ways to meet different circumstances and capacities. *The NHS Plan* (Department of Health 2000), presented a series of commitments to community pharmacies, telephone advice lines and walk-in clinics, all of which may fragment rather than necessarily integrate services. From user perspectives, the advantages of such services are that they are accessible (in theory) and reduce waiting times and demand on primary care. However, not all users can make use of such services or find the provision appropriate. User circumstances may be difficult or users may be part of a newly defined social group, the 'information poor, which is increasingly excluded from such initiatives' (NCCSDO 2001: 79). Furthermore, the voices of those who are excluded from services are not heard. This perspective is little recognised in the policy objectives to target coordinated services on those who present greatest risk or with the highest needs.

More positively, what might support for users look like in a more collaborative world? First, the demand 'nothing about us without us' might be more evident. Such a call, made initially by the disabled people's movement, is increasingly heard in debates about learning disability, older people's services and dementia support. It is axiomatic to consultation but requires a greater transfer of power and control.

Second, we may witness further individual coordination of services through increasing use of direct payments systems that provide service users (and in some cases carers) with cash to purchase their own support. While at a low level initially, these forms of service provision appear to have the capacity to respond to users' calls for highly individualised packages of support. New practitioner roles may have to evolve to help develop and sustain such initiatives.

Both these developments focus on adults and so one final comment about users' needs is to note children's relatively quiet voices in debates about 'joined-up' thinking and practice. This will require greater collaboration with children's services such as education but also with new services such as Connexions that have been explicitly designed to bridge service divides. One prediction for the future, therefore, may be that interprofessional work will have to encompass more than the familiar families of health and social care. The issues identified and discussed in this chapter also set an agenda for including users' and carers' perspectives when identifying the outcomes of interprofessional working.

REFERENCES

Alaszewski, A., Alaszewski, H., Ayer, S. and Manthorpe, J. (eds) (2000) *Managing Risk in Community Practice*, London: Ballière Tindall.

Bailey, S. (2001) 'Confidentiality and young people: myths and realities', in C. Cordess (ed.), *Confidentiality and Mental Health*, London: Jessica Kingsley.

Barnes, M. and Wistow, G. (1993) *Gaining Influence, Gaining Support: Working with Carers in Research and Practice*, Leeds: Nuffield Institute for Health, University of Leeds.

Beresford, P. (2000) *Our Voice in Our Future: Mental Health Issues*, Shaping our Lives, London: National Institute for Social Work.

Booth, T. and Booth, W. (1994) *Parenting Under Pressure: Mothers and Fathers with Learning Difficulties*, Buckingham: Open University Press.

Carers UK (2002) *Without Us*, London: Carers UK.

Charnley, H. (2001) 'Promoting independence: a partnership approach to supporting older people in the community', in S. Balloch and M. Taylor (eds), *Partnership Working: Policy and Practice*, Bristol: The Policy Press.

Cornes, M. and Clough, R. (2001) 'The continuum of care: older people's experiences of intermediate care', *Education and Ageing* 16 (2) 197–202.

Dalrymple, J. (1999) 'What is confidentiality? Developing practice relating to young people', *Practice* 11 (3) 27–38.

Department of Health (1998) *Patients' and Carers' Social Needs*, London: NHS Executive.

Department of Health (2000) *The NHS Plan: A Plan for Investment, A Plan for Reform*, London: The Stationery Office.

Department of Health (2001a) *National Service Framework for Older People*, London: The Stationery Office.

Department of Health (2001b) *Valuing People: A New Strategy for Learning Disability for the 21st Century*, London: The Stationery Office.

Department of Health (2001c) *Family Matters: Counting Families In*, London: Department of Health.

Gilliatt, S., Fenwick, J. and Alford, D. (2000) 'Public services and the consumer: empowerment or control?', *Social Policy and Administration* 34 (3) 333–49.

Henderson, R. and Pochin, M. (2001) *A Right Result? Advocacy, Justice and Empowerment*, Bristol: The Policy Press.

Henwood, M. (1998) *Ignored and Invisible? Carers' Experiences of the NHS*, London: Carers National Association.

HM Government (1999) *Caring for the Carers, National Carers Strategy*, London: The Stationery Office.

Mental Health Foundation (1996) *Building Expectations: Opportunities and Services for People with a Learning Disability – Report of the Mental Health Foundation Committee of Inquiry*, London: Mental Health Foundation.

NCCSDO (National Coordinating Centre for NHS Service Delivery and Organisation) R&D (2001) *Access to Health Care*, London: Department of Health.

Parker, G. (1999) 'Impact of the NHS and Community Care Act (1990) on Informal Carers', in S. Sutherland (ed.), *With Respect to Old Age: Long Term Care: Rights and Responsibilities: A Report by the Royal Commission on Long Term Care of the Elderly*, Chapter 4, Research Volume 3, 51–67, London: The Stationery Office.

Scottish Executive (2001) *The Same as You? A Review of Services for People with Learning Disabilities*, Edinburgh: The Scottish Executive.

Stanley, N. and Manthorpe, J. (2001) 'Reading mental health inquiries: messages for social work', *Journal of Social Work* 1 (1) 77–99.

Stanley, N., Penhale, B., Riordan, D., Holden, S. and Barbour, R. (2001) *Mental Health Services and Child Protection: Responding Effectively to the Needs of Mothers*, Hull: University of Hull, Department of Social Work.

Sutherland, S. (1999) *With Respect to Old Age: Long Term Care: Rights and Responsibilities: A Report by the Royal Commission on Long Term Care*, Cm. 4192–2, London: The Stationery Office.

Tang, P., Gann, D. and Curry, R. (2000) *Telecare, New Ideas for Care and Support at Home*, Bristol: The Policy Press.

Twigg, J. (2000) 'The changing role of users and carers', in B. Hudson (ed.), *The Changing Role of Social Care*, London: Jessica Kingsley.

Chapter 18

Master and servant

The myth of equal partnership between the voluntary and statutory sectors

Jenny Weinstein

SUMMARY

Five key interfaces between the statutory and voluntary sectors are explored: purchasing/providing, service development, culture and values, volunteers, quality assurance and regulation. The contract culture has undermined voluntary sector independence so that voluntary income and labour now subsidise many essential public services. Although there are voluntary agencies who thrive on a firmer financial footing, some staff and volunteers find traditional values have been eroded by the business/regulation ethos. New relationships can offer potential for some creative service developments as long as the voices and needs of service users are not forgotten by purchasers concentrating on cost rather than quality.

THE POLICY CONTEXT

It is interesting to see how the wheel turns full circle. Throughout the Victorian era and until 1945, it was the responsibility of charities and the Church to look after the 'deserving poor' while the local government Poor Law Guardians provided minimal 'relief' or punitive workhouses for the undeserving (Marshall 1975). It was a significant shift during the twentieth century for the state to assume full responsibility for the health, welfare and education of all its citizens, but one which only lasted for three and a half decades until consensus about the role of the welfare state ended during Mrs Thatcher's reign in the 1980s. By the beginning of the twenty-first century, the voluntary or 'independent', as it is sometimes called (including private or not for profit), sector is set to resume the role of delivering all except the very 'hard end' of welfare services. Malcolm Dean (2001a: 7) aptly quotes Tony Blair who divided the twentieth century into two: 'in the first half the country learned it could not achieve its aims without the help of government; in the second, that government could not achieve the nation's aims without the help of the voluntary movement'.

During the heyday of the welfare state in the 1960s and 1970s, the voluntary sector was vibrant and active – able to concentrate on campaigning or providing specialist services that complemented or provided innovative alternatives to those provided by the state (Wolfendon Committee 1978). At that time, government and local authorities gave grants to charities, leaving the voluntary organisations' leaders to manage as they chose. However, the relationship between the voluntary and the statutory sector fundamentally changed following the implementation of the National Health Service and Community Care Act (1990). The resulting contract culture meant that voluntary sector managers were left to feel 'like "junior partners" in the new era of welfare pluralism and, at worst, helpless supplicants' (Harris et al 2001: 3).

The National Health Service and Community Care Act (1990) adroitly addressed criticisms of the welfare state from both Left and Right. By claiming to be 'needs-led' with the service user at the centre, it seemed to be responsive to the growing anti-professional movement, often led by voluntary sector organisations such as Family Rights Group, Age Concern and the Disability lobby. On the other hand, it was no secret that the real driving force behind the legislation was finance and the Conservative government's determination to curb the 'bottomless pit' of welfare spending (Ridley 1988), especially on the growing elderly population. It is ironic that the resulting 'market' made it more rather than less difficult for some voluntary agencies to provide real choice for their constituents. Although the income of the voluntary sector increased by a quarter in real terms during the 1990s, it is the larger organisations that have tended to benefit. Others have been squeezed because local authorities, grant-making bodies and trusts became far less likely to fund infrastructure or revenue costs, preferring to provide seed money or short-term pump priming for new initiatives with carefully specified targets and outcomes.

Although the New Labour government retained a commitment to welfare pluralism, it tried to distance itself from the previous regime (the Conservative government 1992–7) in a number of ways. New Labour abandoned the requirement on local authorities to undertake compulsory competitive tendering and asserted a change of emphasis from competition to collaboration. Two key initiatives within this new policy framework addressed relationships with the voluntary sector. The 'best value' regime required local authorities to review all their services on a five yearly cycle with a view to ensuring optimum quality and cost-effectiveness. More directly, the government published a *Compact* (Home Office 1998) with the voluntary sector. This publication recognised the valuable role played by the voluntary sector, acknowledged the right of the sector to campaign and innovate, committed the government to consult the sector on key policy developments and exhorted local authorities and health authorities to work constructively in partnership with voluntary and community groups.

This chapter begins to explore the degree to which the new rhetoric of partnership is a reality from the perspective of the voluntary sector. It is based on a review of the literature supported by case examples gleaned from the author's membership of a network of London-based voluntary organisations. Five key interfaces with the statutory sector are explored:

- Purchasing/providing
- Service development
- Culture and values
- Volunteers
- Quality assurance and regulation

The above list is by no means exhaustive but may provide some useful indicators of how well the *Compact* is working.

The voluntary sector at the beginning of the twenty-first century is extremely diverse in size, origins, aims, income and structure. There are approximately 136,000 registered voluntary and community organisations in the UK (Voluntary Sector National Training Organisation 2001) and the voluntary sector paid workforce increased by 60 per cent between 1990 and 1997 (NCVO 2000). There are national and regional variations; large national charities, local and national umbrella organisations, local initiatives run entirely by volunteers and organisations run by only one or more paid workers. It is therefore impossible to generalise or to cover all the different aspects in one short chapter.

PURCHASING/PROVIDING

A key feature of the mixed economy of welfare was the creation of a market through contracts and tendering. The problem at the beginning was that few staff on either side of the divide – local authority staff who had been trained as social workers or voluntary sector staff who were campaigners, fundraisers and informal providers of services – had the required skills, or the will to engage in these market procedures. Clients became 'consumers' who, allegedly, could 'choose' their care package but in reality found themselves endlessly waiting for funding and having to pay for services that previously came free of charge. While some senior managers on both sides of the divide saw exciting career opportunities in the new way of working, many middle managers lost their jobs and grass roots staff lost their sense of purpose and their enthusiasm for the job (Deakin 2001).

The dangers inherent in this phenomenon are summed up by Stevenson (2000: 10) who warns that:

> Years of discouragement and frustration among professionals working in the public sector have led to widespread cynicism, even negativism . . . it

is important . . . not to get sucked into the vortex of angry helplessness which has characterised so much professional debate in recent years

The impact on the morale of those working in the voluntary sector does not appear to be as severe as it is in the statutory sector, although the voluntary sector is not immune. For example, social workers in an ethnic minority agency who act as a gateway for clients into its home care, day care and residential services, used to be able to work directly with service users to decide on the best care package to meet their needs. Their organisation's funding has now changed from a grant to a fee per care package. This means that the social workers, depending on where they work, either act as assessors on behalf of local authorities and present cases for funding to those agencies' panels, or they have to refer clients to the relevant local authority for an assessment. Although the voluntary agency undertakes a significant number of assessments on behalf of local authorities, the charity is not remunerated for doing this work.

The clients do not really understand the relationship with the local author-ity so that being turned down from the agency's services because there is no local authority funding can result in complaints about the social workers and detracts from the reputation of the agency within its own community.

Nevertheless, these social workers do have other opportunities for job satis-faction. They hold manageable caseloads and can still offer a degree of coun-selling, support and follow-up that would be less possible for a local authority assessor. They have certain services available within the agency that do not require local authority funding and, ultimately, voluntary agency staff do not carry the same statutory responsibility or pressure as local authority colleagues.

Contracting and best value impact on partnership working at all levels. A voluntary sector provider of residential and special day care places has to negotiate prices with the local authority on an annual basis. Inevitably, the local authority wants to keep the price down below inflation while the volun-tary agency, which has inflation-linked outgoings, does not want to increase the subsidy they already pay. A national survey of contracts undertaken in 1997 identified a significant number where the fee paid to the voluntary sector did not by any means cover the cost of the service. Voluntary organisations' fund-raising activities and use of volunteers mean that local authorities gain far more in value for their purchases (Scott and Russell 2001). Russell et al (1996) found that for every £1 invested by the state a further £1 in charitable funding or voluntary effort was generated. In some circumstances there is no fee whatsoever. A voluntary agency that provides day care, outreach and sheltered employment to people with severe and enduring mental health problems may receive virtually no funding for care packages for individuals who use these services.

An explanation for this situation was suggested by Kendall (2000) who formed a view that voluntary sector providers were motivated more by a desire to provide a service than those in the private sector. They suggested that the cost-effectiveness of voluntary sector day care provision may be due to the informal atmosphere and lower burden of management that attracts comparatively large numbers of volunteers and therefore reduces labour costs. In one successful day centre in North London, 200 volunteers support a staff of 10 to provide a service for 500 older people each week.

In any event, there is no question about who has the power in negotiations about charges and fees. Voluntary organisations depend on the continuation of contracts to remain in business and know, ultimately, that the statutory agency may choose to go elsewhere. This can have a knock-on effect on relationships between voluntary agencies that provide similar services in that they may close ranks if they find themselves in competition and thus lose out on the advantages of collaboration.

Some agencies are able to persuade authorities to block purchase, ensuring some security about annual income. However, spot purchasing is more common and this leaves voluntary agencies vulnerable when local authority funds dry up completely, especially towards the end of the financial year. With a spot purchasing process, the decision-making within the local authority is often devolved down to the care manager. In best practice scenarios this really does enable a service user to 'choose' the most appropriate placement but more often than not the care manager is too constrained by cost to facilitate this.

Research undertaken by Taylor (1997) identified positive outcomes for voluntary agencies from the changes in financial arrangements, especially during the period before the Special Transitional Grant (transferred from central to local government to expedite the community care reforms) began to run out. Russell and Scott (1997) found agencies who reported overall increases in funding and Kumar (1997) found that contracts made with two large national charities were negotiated through dialogue rather than imposed. Kumar also mentioned managers who had moved between sectors and spoke the same language – professionals on both sides of the divide sharing the same high aspirations for service users and wanting to work together.

Unfortunately, no commitment by individuals can overcome the powerlessness of the voluntary sector in the face of inadequate community care budgets or local authorities that are too short staffed to process assessments and release funds within reasonable time scales. In these situations, statutory agency representatives may cover their own discomfort and defensiveness through bullish, patronising or even hostile attitudes towards voluntary sector colleagues.

At a conference held by the National Council for Voluntary Organisations in February 2000, voluntary organisations of all sizes and types raised a large number of problems that they had experienced since the introduction of best value. For example:

- Larger voluntary agencies contracting with many local authorities were faced with different performance indicators and targets and different monitoring systems
- Small grant-funded organisations were concerned about their functions being subject to review within the local authority timetable
- Medium-sized organisations feared that they may be squeezed between very large providers and local organisations
- Some voluntary agencies thought that their wider role was not understood by statutory employees who viewed them as an 'extension of the council'
- There were general concerns that the focus of best value was more and more about cutting costs than promoting quality

In response to these issues, the National Council for Voluntary Organisations (NCVO) and the Improvement and Development Agency (I&DEA) (representing local authorities) both produced publications for their constituencies on working in partnership for best value (NCVO 2001; I&DEA 2001).

The introduction of the contract culture fundamentally affected the relationships between the sectors, the ethos of service delivery and the nature of services provided to users. Some of these changes are explored further in the rest of the chapter.

USER-LED SERVICE DEVELOPMENT

One of the key clauses of the *Compact* is about the need for government at national and local levels to consult with the voluntary sector (Home Office 1998). However, few representatives of voluntary agencies encountered within the author's network recalled being consulted on local authority service development plans, nor are they invited to participate actively in best value reviews. Their experience was that local authorities tend to rely on token representation from a small number of umbrella bodies or from the best known national charities, paying minimal lip service to involving community-based voluntary organisations in high level planning or policy development. Involvement of service users at these levels is similarly tokenistic.

Away from the funding and resource allocation issues, the situation at the grass roots is much better. There are many examples of good practice on the ground where, for example, voluntary agency home care providers are invited to local authority run training sessions and the local authority organises network meetings for voluntary and independent home care providers. There is often excellent professional support from care managers or registration and inspection officers to support voluntary agencies who encounter adult abuse or complex complaints. Voluntary agencies are invited to interagency training

on key issues such as child protection. Most significantly, where good relationships and trust had been developed between the operational professionals
on both sides, genuine partnership working enhances the development of
services to users.

Although voluntary sector staff are as likely to be patronising and paternalistic towards service users as staff from other sectors (Oliver 1996), it is
often the voluntary sector that will seek the views of service users: children
(Gardner 1987), people with dementia (Killick 1997), survivors of mental
illness (Faulkener et al 1998) and people with learning disabilities (Flynn
1999). Voluntary sector campaigning around users' views and aspirations
have influenced the development of mainstream services for example:

- The direct payments that people with disabilities now receive to purchase
  their own packages of care
- Improved coordination between social services, education and health in
  the best interests of looked-after children
- The extension of social services' responsibilities to continue to assist
  children after they have left care
- Improved crisis care for people suffering from episodes of acute mental
  illness
- Involvement of service users and carers in care planning
- Rights of carers to receive an assessment of need

This is a constructive and creative model of service development between the
voluntary and statutory sectors. The voluntary sector actively seeks and
records the views of service users and helps them to campaign for new ways
of delivering services. The statutory sector responds by introducing new funding arrangements, new requirements or even new legislation in order to meet
identified needs. The two sectors then work in partnership to deliver the
evolving services. Initiatives currently being developed such as Supporting
People – to provide sheltered housing with support for vulnerable groups and
Step Down – to provide intermediate care between home and hospital will
undoubtedly benefit from this kind of partnership working.

CULTURE AND VALUES

A constant issue for voluntary agencies is managing the tensions between
internal values and aims and the imperatives of the external policy context.
Even if an organisation has the capacity to respond to statutory initiatives,
the demands on the agency may involve an ill-considered speedy and
opportunistic response that takes the organisation away from its original
mission and values (Joseph Rowntree Foundation 2000).

The 'market' environment has inevitably affected the culture of many voluntary sector organisations that have had to adopt professional and managerial approaches to replace the previous informal ways of working. There have been both advantages and disadvantages from these developments.

In one organisation studied by Scott et al (2000), the introduction of a corporate structure and system of business planning made it better able to develop new services and monitor existing ones. It also enabled the improvement of communication systems and better targeting of scarce resources. On the negative side, the development of vertical structures and horizontal hierarchies made it more difficult to continue to provide a really responsive seamless service to the user. Demarcations between departments meant that it took longer to refer service users to the right person where before they would have been dealt with by whoever they met first. The new bureaucracy can be difficult to cope with for long-term staff and volunteers in established voluntary agencies and hard to explain to the agency's constituents.

A symbolic manifestation of this pressure on large voluntary organisations has been their increased use of marketing strategies. The volunteers rattling their tins in the shopping centre or visiting house to house have been replaced by expensive advertising hoardings. While charities such as Barnardos and the NSPCC have been criticised for these sorts of campaigns, their representatives argue that it pays both in terms of fund-raising and in getting a message across about children's needs.

Equal opportunities and the importance of meeting the needs of ethnic minority communities is a fundamental value to which all social care agencies are expected to aspire. The National Health Service and Community Care Act (1990) and its accompanying guidance specifically emphasise the importance of considering the particular needs of ethnic minority groups and consulting ethnic minority communities. However, in reality, local authorities vary in their commitment to supporting ethnic minority voluntary organisations. The services provided by these agencies, for a variety of reasons, can be more costly than mainstream services. Some black organisations have no extra sources of funding so the fee for service must cover all infrastructure, capital and revenue costs. Numerous specialist black agencies have been unable to keep afloat because of financial pressures.

While local authorities may pay lip service to provide ethnically sensitive services, this aspect will fly out of the window when money is tight. One relative complained bitterly that her very orthodox Jewish mother had been refused funding for a Jewish residential home by the local authority because 'funding had run out'. The local authority placed her mother in a Jewish unit in one of their own resources. The only 'Jewish' aspect was kosher food brought in cartons by an outside contractor. In a different local authority, relatives of older people with dementia who attended a Jewish special day centre were constantly pressured by their local authority to transfer their loved ones to a less expensive in-house resource that did not cater for ethnic needs.

A more controversial variation is the US government's support for faith-based and community initiatives that now have their own office within the White House (Dean 2001b: 7). Interestingly, these developments have not only been attacked from the Left – who fear the imposition of moral imperatives – but also from the Right who fear the interference of a potentially Liberal state in their religious values and ethics. It will be interesting to monitor their progress in the UK.

IMPACT ON VOLUNTEERS

In his 2001 budget, Gordon Brown invested an additional £180 million for the training and management of volunteers. Fears expressed by some in the statutory sector that the government intended to replace paid workers with volunteers were denied but not allayed. In spite of this initiative some organisations are struggling to recruit the volunteers they need because the evolving context makes volunteering a more complex and demanding role than before.

There has been a significant impact on volunteers from the top to the bottom of voluntary organisations. Boards of trustees or management committees have had to adapt to the changing social policy environment. Where previously any good-hearted person with time to spare was welcome into the group, voluntary organisations are now seeking individuals with specific skills in management, finance and so on in order to ensure that the organisation stays on track.

Boards have to spend a great deal of time thinking about fund-raising and seeking different sources of funding (Harris 2001a). For example, the Family Centre established in 1977 to run a crèche, youth club, play group, summer play scheme, luncheon club and counselling service saw its social services grant eroded over the years. The different projects are now fragmented and those that have survived have only done so by seeking alternative sources of funding. The small local management committee has to contend with numerous funding bodies and the previously thriving centre constantly struggles with the threat of closure.

Boards and trustees carry increasingly heavy responsibilities for ensuring appropriate use of resources, meeting specific targets, adhering to new legislation on issues such as human rights, data protection and health and safety and meeting local and national standards or service frameworks.

The impact of all these pressures make it increasingly difficult for boards to maintain their independent role of promoting the values and mission of their agency and the needs of their user group. The complex demands on trustees and directors also militate against any more than tokenistic involvement of service users at board level.

The profile of volunteers across the sector generally is fairly elderly because the previous pool of women at home has virtually dried up since this group entered the workplace. However, the importance of gaining practical experience for young people's CVs means that they may well see a spell of volunteering as useful for career development. There is also a growing army of healthy, active, retired people looking for ways of making a useful contribution. These new recruits are more comfortable than established volunteers with the more professional approach to selecting and developing volunteers and procedures such as police checks for those volunteering to work with children or vulnerable people.

Longer standing volunteers often do not see the point of training or having their roles reviewed. A local day centre for older people that had been run by volunteers for 10 years had to appoint a professional manager because the volunteers were struggling to cope. The first thing the manager did was to replace the volunteers who had provided lunches with a professional catering firm because health and safety standards were not being met. The volunteers were mortally offended.

REGULATION AND QUALITY ASSURANCE

Another problematic development for older volunteers is the increasing prominence of quality assurance, audit and regulation in all aspects of the health and care sectors. As with parallel developments described above, these new approaches have brought both advantages and disadvantages for organisations and service users. Contrary perhaps to its responsive and innovative image, much of the charitable sector has been as conservative, paternalistic and patronising towards service users as any other parts of the care sector. Quality assurance processes inevitably ruffle feathers but can lead to positive change.

In response to cries for help from below and requirements from above, the NCVO established a special task group to promote quality in the voluntary sector. The group aims to act as a bridge between the voluntary sector and various models and approaches to quality assurance being developed in other sectors. The business excellence model has been adapted to meet the requirements of the voluntary sector and a range of self-assessment tools for small organisations are popular within the sector. Many charities have achieved investors in people status or alternative recognition via external accreditation. Some organisations have appointed quality professionals while others have integrated responsibility for quality into the job descriptions of all managers.

The advantage of introducing quality systems is that they always involve reviewing current arrangements and ways of doing things. This often means questioning practices that have continued unchallenged for many years. In an article in *Guardian Society* (Jackson 2001), the chief executive of a Christian-based organisation in the Midlands describes the pain involved in having to close down a 'flagship' residential drug project that simply was not economical. Lessons learned from the closure led to a system of regularly reviewing all projects against an audit checklist of published standards. This process ensures that projects continue to meet identified needs and that they are cost-effective. Successful projects continue to change and develop as an outcome of the reviews.

While the development of internal quality systems has been fairly gradual in the voluntary sector, the impact of external regulation has been far more dramatic. One of the most unpopular outcomes for staff has been the significant increase in paperwork, as procedures have to be written, records maintained and forms completed and processed. Many staff in the sector still regard this as something that has to be done to meet regulation requirements and do not see any improvements for the service user. Problems are compounded when registration and inspection officers spend much more time poring over paperwork when they visit registered resources than they do speaking with service users and grass roots staff.

A plethora of regulations and inspection systems developed during the 1990s led to overload and inconsistency. The Care Standards Act 2000, the establishment of a Care Standards Commission, National Minimum Standards and National Service Frameworks were introduced to rationalise the quality framework and minimise duplication. On the downside, many smaller voluntary agencies believe that the demands of the new standards reduce user choice because smaller providers offering specialist personalised care to service users are put out of business by requirements on room sizes, national minimum wage, training requirements and so on. Although there was wide consultation about the standards, many voluntary agencies may feel that their views have been ignored.

CONCLUSION

The Chancellor of the Exchequer, Gordon Brown, told the NCVO annual conference in 2000: 'Voluntary organisations are at the heart of Britain's civic renewal and represent the better Britain we want to build in the twenty-first century'. If this aspiration is to become a reality, the current trend of the voluntary sector being 'incorporated' (Harris 2001b: 215) into the public or business sectors through tight contracting and rigorous regulation has to be reversed. Malcolm Dean (2001a: 5) suggests that the *Compact* should be made mandatory – with closer parliamentary monitoring of ministers and advisers and more use by voluntary organisations of the complaints' procedures and the Ombudsman.

Both national and local government must facilitate a genuinely independent third sector that can respond effectively to the whole range of service user groups, including minority ethnic groups and others with special needs. An equal partnership, which enables the sector to promote its own values, develops its local communities and, in response to identified need, find new and improved ways of doing things, will be much more productive than a master/slave relationship totally tied into statutory preoccupations, targets and budgets.

REFERENCES

Deakin, N. (2001) 'Public policy, social policy and voluntary organisations', in M. Harris and C. Rochester (eds), *Voluntary Organisations and Social Policy in Britain: Perspectives on Change and Choice*, Hampshire: Palgrave.

Dean, M. (2001a) 'Evolution not revolution', *Guardian Society*, Wednesday, 21 March, 7.

Dean, M. (2001b) 'The iron hand that feeds them', *Guardian Society*, Wednesday, 15 August, 5.

Faulkener, A., Wallcroft, J., Nicholls, V., Blaxdell, D. and Treitel, R. (1998) 'The right to ask questions', *Open Mind* 91, 14.

Flynn, M. (1999) 'Involving users at all levels', in K. Billingham, M. Flynn and J. Weinstein (eds), *Making a World of Difference: Developing Primary Health Care*, London: RCGP.

Gardner, R. (1987) *Who Says? Choice and Control in Care*, London: National Children's Bureau.

Harris, M., Rochester, C. and Halfpenny, P. (2001) 'Voluntary organisations and social policy: twenty years of change', in M. Harris and C. Rochester (eds), *Voluntary Organisations and Social Policy in Britain: Perspectives on Change and Choice*, Hampshire: Palgrave, Chapter 1.

Harris, M. (2001a) 'Boards: just subsidiaries of the state?', in M. Harris and C. Rochester (eds), *Voluntary Organisations and Social Policy in Britain: Perspectives on Change and Choice*, Hampshire: Palgrave.

Harris, M. (2001b) 'Voluntary organisations in a changing social policy environment', in M. Harris and C. Rochester (eds), *Voluntary Organisations and Social Policy in Britain: Perspectives on Change and Choice*, Hampshire: Palgrave.

Home Office (1998) *Consultation and Policy Appraisal: A Code of Good Practice*, London: Home Office. Active Community Unit, Room 235, Horseferry House, Dean Ryle Street, London SW1P 2AW.

Home Office (1998) *Compact – Getting it Right Together – A Compact on Relations between Government and the Voluntary and Community Sector in England*, London: Home Office.

I&DEA (Improvement and Development Agency) (2001) *Partnerships for Best Value – Working with the Voluntary Sector*, London: I&DEA.

Jackson, L. (2001) 'Shut or Bust', *Guardian Society*, Wednesday, 18 April.

Joseph Rowntree Foundation (2000) 'Critical issues for voluntary action', *Findings*, May, York: Joseph Rowntree Foundation.

Kendall, J. (2000) 'The voluntary sector and social care for older people', in B. Hudson (ed.), *The Changing Role of Social Care*, London: Jessica Kingsley.

Killick, J. (1997) 'Communication a matter of life and death of the mind', *Journal of Dementia Care* 90, 14–15.

Kumar, S. (1997) *Accountability Relationships between Voluntary Sector 'Providers', Local Government 'Purchasers' and Service Users in the Contracting State*, York: York Publishing Services.

Marshall, T. (1975) *Social Policy*, London: Hutchinson University Library.

NCVO (National Council for Voluntary Organisations) (2000) *UK Voluntary Sector Almanac 2000*, London: NCVO.

NCVO (National Council for Voluntary Organisations) (2001) *Best Value – a Guide for Voluntary Organisations*, London: NCVO.

Oliver, M. (1996) 'User involvement in the voluntary sector – a view from the disability movement', in Commission on the Future of the Voluntary sector, *Meeting the Challenge of Change: Voluntary Action into the 21st Century Summary of Evidence and Selected Papers*, London: Directory of Social Change and the Media Trust.

Ridley, N. (1988) *The Local Right*, London: Centre for Policy Studies.

Russell, J., Scott, D. and Wilding, P. (1996) *Mixed Fortunes: The Funding of the Local Voluntary Sector*, Manchester: University of Manchester.

Russell, J. and Scott, R. (1997) *Very Active Citizens? The Impact of the Contract Culture on Volunteers*, Manchester: University of Manchester Department of Social Policy and Social Work (SP119).

Scott, D., Alcock, P., Russell, L. and Macmillan, R. (2000) *Moving Pictures: Realities of Voluntary Action*, York: Joseph Rowntree Foundation.

Scott, D. and Russell, L. (2001) 'Contracting: the experience of service delivery agencies', in C. Rochester (ed.), *Voluntary Organisations and Social Policy in Britain: Perspectives on Change and Choice*, Hampshire: Palgrave.

Stevenson, O. (2000) 'The mandate for interagency and interprofessional training: legal, practical, professional and social factors', in N. Charles and M. Charles (eds), *Training Together to Safeguard Children*, Leicester: NSPCC, Chapter 2.

Taylor, M. (1997) *The Best of Both Worlds: The Voluntary Sector and Local Government*, York: Joseph Rowntree Foundation.

Voluntary Sector National Training Organisation (2001) *Workforce Development Plan 2001*, London: NCVO, Regent's Wharf, 8 All Saints Street, London N1 9RK.

Wolfendon Committee (1978) *The Future of Voluntary Organisations*, London: Croom Helm.

Part III

From policy to practice

Learning together

Chapter 19

Unpacking interprofessional education

Hugh Barr

SUMMARY

Professions work better together when they learn together thereby improving the quality of care for service users. That is the proposition, a proposition as seductive as it is simple. The reality is more complex. Interprofessional education can have a direct and positive impact on the quality of care, but its benefits can also be diffuse and indirect defying easy evaluation. It takes many forms with many objectives, mostly interim, that may, under favourable conditions, contribute towards better care.

Much has been learned about different types of interprofessional education and their outcomes during the 30 years since it took root (Barr 1994, 2002; Barr et al 1999; Freeth et al 2002). Much has also been demanded which, depending on your point of view, complements or competes with the original proposition.

This chapter unpacks interprofessional education, selecting examples, each with a different objective and making a different contribution.

THE WORLD HEALTH ORGANIZATION

A seminal report from a World Health Organization workshop advocated shared learning to complement profession specific programmes. The report stated that students from different health professions should learn together during certain periods of their education to acquire the skills necessary for solving the priority health problems of individuals and communities known to be particularly amenable to teamwork. Emphasis should be put on learning how to interact with one another, community orientation to ensure relevance to the health needs of the people and team competence (WHO 1988).

Deliberations in Geneva were informed by those in Copenhagen where delegates at a previous WHO workshop had argued that students from health professions with complementary roles in teams should share learning to discover the value of working together as they defined and solved problems within a common frame of reference. Delegates argued that such learning should employ participatory learning methods to modify reciprocal attitudes, foster team spirit, identify and value respective roles, while effecting change in both practice and the professions. This approach would support the development of integrated health care, based on common values, knowledge and skills (d'Ivernois and Vodoratski 1988).

These reports set seven expectations for interprofessional education:

- To modify reciprocal attitudes
- To establish common values, knowledge and skills
- To build teams
- To solve problems
- To respond to community needs
- To change practice
- To change the professions

Each of the following examples focuses on one of these expectations.

Modifying reciprocal attitudes

Teachers at Moray House in Edinburgh found that students entering community work, social work and primary school teaching were more prejudiced by the end of their courses than at the beginning. The college tried to modify those attitudes by helping students to bypass the need for stereotyping as the means by which each group defined the others. More contact, providing opportunities to identify similar attitudes, would, teachers believed, lead to mutual approval. To that end, three shared learning programmes were put to the test, each with different students.

The first offered placements to student teachers in community or social work settings, and to student community and social workers in schools. This programme was not evaluated. The second comprised a common course in social psychology organised around small and large groups. Workshops created opportunities for interaction. Each required the students to complete a questionnaire, repertory grid or rating scale to expose their thoughts to each other. They discussed ethical issues, competed in games and engaged in role play. Comparing before and after responses to questionnaires found that student teachers became more favourably disposed to the student community and social workers, but that this was not reciprocated. The third programme also comprised a series of workshops, including tutorial groups with between two and four students from each profession. Groups discussed a case study and videos about communication problems and the management of conflict. Members also took part in an exercise on work priorities and a do-it-yourself collaborative project. Again, student teachers changed most, showing greater awareness of how social workers could help them in their work, although this did not extend to community workers. For their part, student community and social workers remained critical of primary education, but became more alive to some of the teachers' frustrations.

(McMichael and Gilloran 1984; Barr and Shaw 1995)

Other early initiatives in interprofessional education also focused on modifying reciprocal attitudes and perceptions (Hasler and Klinger 1976; Jones 1986; Carpenter 1995a, 1995b; Carpenter and Hewstone 1996) in the belief that overcoming ignorance, countering prejudice and correcting negative stereotypes would overcome resistance to collaboration.

Some, like Moray House, invoked the 'contact hypothesis' (Tajfel 1981), which holds, in its simplest form, that contact enhances mutual respect and understanding. This hypothesis was applied in the USA to test whether contact between members of different ethnic groups improved race relations. Findings were disappointing. Familiarity alone, it seemed, did not necessarily lead to liking (Zajonc 1968). Much depended on the quality of the interaction. Even then, other factors may negate positive influence (Berkowitz 1980).

The implication for interprofessional education is clear. The learning needs, according to Hewstone and Brown (1986), to create opportunities for rewarding interaction between students in their respective professional roles with equality of status, positive expectations and a cooperative atmosphere, if mutual understanding is to result.

The risk remains that exposing one group to another may serve only to confirm prejudices and stereotypes. Attitudes and behaviour unacceptable to others, deficits in knowledge and skill, weaknesses in professional codes and disciplinary process, all or any of these may be exposed with implications for the governance of the professions, their regulation and education, which students and teachers can do little or nothing to resolve.

Nor can there be any certainty that removal of prejudices and negative stereotypes, if and when achieved, will unlock the door to better collaboration. Much depends on whether the working climate is conducive and whether the student has been equipped with the necessary knowledge and skills.

Establishing common values, knowledge and skills

The University of Birmingham launched a part-time mental health programme in 1997 open to community psychiatric nurses, occupational therapists, psychologists, psychiatrists, social workers and others. Students are encouraged to come in pairs or small teams from health and social service districts in the region. The programme leads to a postgraduate certificate or diploma after one year, and to a master's degree following a further year of supervised research.

The aim is to give practitioners from all these professions a common skill, knowledge and value base. The curriculum includes modules on the philosophy, policy, practice and ethical and legal framework for community care, training in psychosocial interventions and interagency working. The focus is on severe and enduring mental health problems with an emphasis on user participation. Values taught include anti-racist and anti-oppressive practice, user-centred decision-making, social inclusion and support for families and peers.

Service users have taken part in the appointment of staff, including the programme director, curriculum development, teaching and participation as students.

Early findings from the evaluation focus on the impact of the programme on attitudes to community care for people with mental health problems and professional stereotypes (the latter being the more interesting in this context).

Students in the first two cohorts identified strongly with their own professions, although less so over time. But they identified more strongly with their teams than with their professions. Reciprocal perceptions were revealing. Psychiatrists and psychologists received significantly higher scores from other groups for academic rigour and leadership skills, and social workers for interpersonal skills. Community psychiatric nurses (CPNs) and occupational therapists (OTs) were rated significantly lower for leadership and academic rigour. CPNs, however, scored relatively high on interpersonal and practical skills and OTs highest on practical skills.

No significant changes in attitude were noted during the programme, from which the researchers concluded that the programme had had no effect on professional stereotypes. They offered two explanations. Either stereotypes were reinforced in day-to-day contact with colleagues in the workplace, or conditions necessary for disconfirmation of stereotypes were not sufficiently present in the programme. Other findings add credence to the latter. The atmosphere had indeed been conducive to co-operative rather than competitive learning, and students

> had worked together as equals, but opportunities had been lacking to explore differences as well as similarities between professions. Conditions necessary for the contact hypothesis to take effect had not therefore been fully met.
>
> (Barnes et al 2000a, 2000b)

These findings highlight the risk that programmes designed to reinforce common values, knowledge and skills may inadvertently underplay differences, limiting opportunities for interactive learning and missing opportunities to effect attitudinal change. The programme was postgraduate, but the findings have major implications for undergraduate studies in the UK where much emphasis is currently put on common rather than comparative curricula (Department of Health 2000).

Common learning introduces common concepts employing a common language, which can lay foundations for collaborative practice, yet fail to obviate the barriers. Value is added, according to leading exponents of interprofessional education, when learning is also comparative and interactive (Barr 1994).

Team-building

> The University of British Columbia piloted a two-day interprofessional team experience for senior students from nine different undergraduate health care and human service programmes. Content included the purpose of interprofessional teams, group dynamics, team communications, multiple professional paradigms, and team management. Methods were interactive, emphasising reflection upon insights gained from the learning experience rather than the acquisition of programmed knowledge and focusing upon professional roles and expertise, communication, conflict resolution and team issues.
>
> The first of two exercises was a competition between four teams of mixed professions to build a model from Lego blocks. Lest that seem too easy, the model that they had to copy was abstract and each team given the necessary parts, but in different colours from the original. The object was to provide students with a common experience base in applying teamwork concepts and tools. Each team member was assigned a different role. 'Project managers' were given different instructions (unbeknown to each other), based upon different organisational design philosophies. This enabled lessons to be learned during the debriefing about the different approaches taken from different theoretical perspectives. The learning-based team outperformed the traditional, value and process-based teams. Flexibility proved to be the key to success.

The second method developed team responses to needs identified in two half-page case studies chosen to create opportunities to demonstrate the effectiveness of interprofessional team working. Members were assigned to roles and expected to assess team performance and clarify delegation through 'responsibility charting'. Teams were more comfortable, and exchange of ideas more efficient, during the second case study.

The workshops were oversubscribed, helped no doubt by the decision to pay $100 to students who participated on both Saturdays (chosen to avoid time tabling problems), but feedback suggested that many would have attended anyway. Recruiting teachers (with no extra pay) was more difficult. Students were unanimous in their praise for the workshops and the relevance of learning to practice, although all made suggestions for improvement. Follow up six months later confirmed that students had found the workshops helpful, notably in demonstrating the value of interprofessional collaboration and understanding the roles of other professions, although some had had a hard time implementing what they had learned.

(Gilbert et al 2000)

Few examples of team-building *per se* can be found in the interprofessional education literature for health and social care. Some question whether skills training is necessary for teamworking, believing that once autonomy, equity and mutual respect is established between professions, a team will develop its own way of working and learning effectively together (SCOPME 1999). That view seems to be reflected in a preference for team development rather than team-building, where teamwork is reinforced as members engage in activities designed to improve services or resolve problems (Barr 1994).

Undergraduate education for the health professions has been criticised in the UK for failing to prepare students for teamwork (Miller et al 1999). Rectifying that omission is a high priority, but collaboration cannot be wholly contained within teamwork. It also includes co-working and networking beyond the bounds of a team, however defined, as well as collaboration within and between organisations and with service users, their carers and communities (Secretary of State for Health 2000). Teamwork may have once been a sufficient organisational framework for interprofessional education, but no longer.

Solving problems

Undergraduate programmes in physiotherapy, prosethics, orthotics and diagnostic radiography at Salford University incorporated three inter-professional modules. One of these entitled 'People in Society' had three themes: social structure, health and the NHS. Problems were presented for students to discuss, for example:

'The population's mean age is increasing and changing the pattern of health and illness in the community. Explain the phenomenon in terms of healthcare delivery.'

Each assignment followed the seven stages of problem-based learning:

- clarifying terms and concepts
- defining the problem
- analysing the problem
- making a systematic inventory of the explanations that emerge from the analysis
- formulating targets for learning objectives
- acquiring knowledge in relation to the learning need
- synthesising and checking the newly acquired information and knowledge

The students identified areas in which they lacked information and understanding, and decided how these deficits could best be made good. They then engaged in a variety of independent learning activities, which helped them to explore the constructs, issues, theories and mech-anisms involved. The results were brought back to the group for further discussion to elaborate the problem and its implications.

Ninety percent of students agreed that interprofessional learning objectives had been met during the problem-based learning. These covered: interaction, co-operation, sharing of knowledge, appreciation of values, effective communication, listening to others, reflection and respect for others' contributions.

(Hughes and Lucas 1997)

Problem-based learning (Barrows and Tamblin 1980) is perhaps the most widely used interprofessional learning method, drawing on its worldwide application in community-based medical education, but it is one of many (Barr 1996). Other learning methods also involve participants in joint investi-gation to effect change, such as collaborative enquiry developed by Reason

(1988, 1994); as applied to interprofessional learning by Glennie and Cosier (1994); and continuous quality improvements (see below).

Practice-based learning is held to be essential (Bartholomew et al 1996) and can take many forms: observational study (Likierman 1997), shadowing (Reeves 2000), cross-professional placements (Anderson et al 1992) and experience on training wards (Freeth and Reeves 2002: 116–38; Reeves and Freeth 2002).

There is much that teachers can do in the classroom to complement practice-based learning by stimulating exchange between the professions (debates and case studies) and simulating collaboration in practice through role play and games. Skills labs simulate practice (Nicol and de Saintonge 2002). So, in a very different way, do experiential groups, like those during the 'Pride and Prejudice' workshop organised by the University of Westminster in conjunction with the Tavistock Institute that approximate to interprofessional, interagency and intersector work settings (University of Westminster 2001).

Opting for just one method is needlessly restrictive. Imaginative teachers ring the changes to enliven learning and to respond to different needs in different ways. Methods can also be combined, as the next example illustrates.

Responding to communities

Groups of pre-registration medical, nursing and social work students in Leicester interviewed patients in deprived neighbourhoods, and representatives of three key agencies involved in their care. The aims were to enable students to understand health in the wider context of society, to appreciate the range of professions involved, to develop practical understanding of inequalities in health and to learn about the diversity of common health problems seen in primary care. Objectives included the application of sociological concepts and theories, the analysis of user-centred care and the assessment of models of health care, taking into account strategies adopted by the Leicester Health Action Zone.

Students assessed not only patients' medical problems, but also the impact of physical, emotional, social and economic factors. They then returned to their study base to discuss and interpret their learning with tutors, followed by an interview with a front-line worker involved with the case before visiting the selected agencies in a subsequent session. Each group presented its case to an invited audience of community workers, health and social care workers, public sector managers, policy makers and fellow students where members are questioned and challenged.

The learning leant heavily upon shared problem-solving strategies as a means to increase understanding of roles and responsibilities of other professions and to highlight the need for teamwork.

Eighty-six percent of the students who completed a follow-up questionnaire said that they had found the experience enabled them to understand the importance of inter-agency collaboration for regeneration.

(Leicester Warwick Medical School 2001)

This project had been introduced initially for medical students and drew on the development of community-based learning in medical education (see, for example, Thistlewaite 2000).

The methodology generates a practice-led curriculum that incorporates team development, observational study and problem-based learning building to acquire individual and team competencies (Barr 1998; Allen and Pickering 2001).

Changing practice

The NHS funded three projects in the south west of England to develop new models of interprofessional teaching and learning intended to improve education, practice and patient care. The projects operated as a collaborative, exchanging experience, working together to resolve problems and accounting to the same Board.

In Avon, Somerset and Wiltshire experienced practitioners joined action learning sets to make care for people with cancer more sensitive and more responsive by understanding the lived experience of service users, employing a continuous quality improvement cycle.

Bournemouth University co-ordinated a programme that placed service users at the centre of health improvement in three locations. In Andover, the focus was upon improving support for parents of young children, in Dorchester upon improving care for acutely ill elderly people in hospital and in Salisbury upon improving community mental health care. All comprised action learning sets, employed continuous quality improvement and involved service users.

In Plymouth, the project focused upon skills required to work interprofessionally with people who had severe, enduring mental health problems, with particular reference to their primary care. Developed around taught modules, the curriculum applied principles of interprofessional learning to collaboration while teaching evidence based practice.

(Annandale et al 2000; NHS South West 2001)

Developments in south-west England, notably in Bournemouth, enjoy close links with the Interdisciplinary Professional Education Collaborative in the USA, which is dedicated to the introduction of continuous quality improvement (CQI) into interprofessional education (Schmitt 2000). Numerous CQI projects have been introduced in the USA as a grass roots response to the pressing need to improve services following the collapse of health care reforms proposed by the Clinton administration.

Where the CQI process entails learning between the participant professions, it is increasingly treated as interprofessional education – interprofessional education with direct impact on the quality of practice (Berman and Brobst 1996; Freeth et al 2002). Some may cry foul, suspecting sleight of hand to redraw the boundaries of interprofessional education to 'prove' that it benefits practice. Others may see the redefinition as critical to put quality improvement at the heart of interprofessional education. Viewed thus, the challenge lies in building CQI into other models of interprofessional education. Bournemouth University, for example, places undergraduate students in teams employing CQI so that they can learn how to effect service improvements (Annandale et al 2000), although the general application of the CQI model may be constrained by the number of suitable placements (Barr 2000).

Changing the professions

Six courses in England prepare students for joint qualification as social workers and learning disability nurses. The impetus at South Bank University came from local learning disability service managers who believed that neither qualifying system, on its own, would equip staff adequately for the new community services being set up following the closure of a large hospital. The South Bank programme lasts three years and confers qualifications in learning disability nursing (RNMH) and social work (DipSW) as well as a BSc in Nursing and Social Work Studies.

The programme reportedly gains from combining two professional cultures, meeting the requirements of two regulatory bodies, the English National Board for Nursing, Midwifery and Health Visiting (ENB) and the Central Council for Education and Training in Social Work (CCETSW), and their commitment to partnership between education and practice. Partnership also includes people with learning disabilities who contribute to teaching on their own terms.

Two long placements follow a common foundation programme. The second of these is carried out, so far as possible, in a practice setting involving interprofessional teamwork. Weekly tutorials encourage reflection on practice – interprofessional practice – while regular seminars explore the concept of 'joint practitioner'. Service users help to determine objectives and as teachers. Students are assessed against eight core competencies, which integrate requirements made by the regulatory bodies.

Students valued the way in which the course had helped them to make assessments holistically, work in multidisciplinary teams and establish a broad knowledge base for their practice. Learning from people with learning disabilities prompted students to reflect upon their own power and enhanced understanding of the user perspective. Service managers welcomed students' capacity to embrace both health and social needs. Of the first 15 students to graduate, 13 provided information about their subsequent employment. Seven had taken nursing posts (six in learning disability posts), five had taken social work posts (one in a learning disability post) and one had become a care manager.

(Davis et al 1999; Sims 2002)

These joint programmes came about indirectly from the Jay Committee (1979), which was intent on replacing a medical model by a social model for the learning disabilities field. The Committee recommended that the nursing qualification be replaced by a social care qualification. Nurses, parents and pressure groups were implacably opposed. Relationships between nursing and social care deteriorated as a result, frustrating efforts to establish closer collaboration in education and practice, and forcing government to reject the Jay recommendation. It called instead on the then General Nursing Councils and CCETSW to convene a joint working group to find a way forward, which they duly did with recommendations for joint training and dual qualifications (GNCs/CCETSW 1982).

Interprofessional education, as hitherto conceived, was a means to cultivate collaboration between discrete professions, based on mutual respect for boundaries, functions and values. Could it, at the same time, be an instrument of 'educational engineering' to change designations, roles and qualifications? Or would tension generated compound collaboration, as it did, at least in the short term, in learning disabilities? That tension may have been resolved in those learning disability services where dual qualification holders have been deployed, although numbers are few, impact on practice correspondingly small and independent evaluation lacking.

Dual qualifications and combined professions sit uncomfortably within interprofessional education as understood in other fields. Experience gained in learning disabilities must, however, be taken into account now that NHS workforce policies expect education, not only to promote collaboration, but also a more flexible and mobile workforce (Department of Health 2000).

Was this what the WHO meant by changing practice and the professions through education? Perhaps, for it too was frustrated by restrictions that threatened its health promotion strategies (WHO 1976, 1978). National or international, arguments for joint studies to cultivate collaboration and create a more flexible workforce must be reconciled.

Integrating the approaches

Modifying reciprocal attitudes may under favourable conditions help to surmount barriers to collaboration, yet fail to provide the knowledge and skills necessary to work intelligently and competently with other professions and organisations. Acquiring common values, knowledge and skills may secure common foundations for collaborative practice, yet fail to surmount the attitudinal barriers to collaboration for lack of opportunity to address professional differences.

Team-building may prepare students for teamwork, yet neglect more diffuse and more diverse collaboration across agency boundaries and with communities, involving service users and carers. Problem-based learning may often be the preferred interprofessional learning method, but it is not the only one and may be more effective when used in combination with others. Community-based enquiry may ensure that learning is practice-led, but its effectiveness depends on a responsive college curriculum.

Continuous quality improvement may be the one interprofessional learning method with direct impact on practice, but its application will remain limited to locally based learning unless and until constraints can be overcome to apply it in combination with other interprofessional learning methods. Interprofessional education may be employed to remodel professions, redistributing responsibilities, redrawing boundaries and lowering barriers, and so help to implement workforce reforms, but may generate discord and frustrate collaboration. No one approach has all the answers; together they offer a promising repertoire.

Given that interprofessional education is typically short and work-based (Barr and Waterton 1996), teachers and trainers must set realistic objectives within the constraints of time and place (Barr 1996). Students and workers need to be discriminating in choosing the interprofessional learning opportunity best suited to their immediate learning needs, but with an eye to their continuing personal and professional development plan, which may include a variety of interprofessional learning experiences with different but complementary objectives. Similarly, teams need to decide which members should take advantage of which interprofessional learning opportunity in the interest of overall competence.

Longer and more complex interprofessional education programmes are being introduced in the UK, notably at undergraduate level, with time, space and resources to include diverse approaches such as those explored in this chapter. Successful integration will entail more than mixing and matching, which presupposes an agreed and coherent theoretical rationale, based on a critical and comparative evaluation of selected approaches grounded in the evidence. Systematic reviews can help, but sources are too few and too limited to permit such analysis (Barr et al 2000; Freeth et al 2002). Prospective research will have to be undertaken, evaluating different approaches and employing consistent research methodology within a single conceptual framework. That is the next challenge.

REFERENCES

Allen, M. and Pickering, C. (2001) *Core Competencies of Clinical Teams: Draft 8*, Leeds: West Yorkshire Workforce Development Confederation.

Anderson, D., Bell, L., Eno, S., Littleford, E. and Walters, P. (1992) 'Common ground: an experience of transdisciplinary practice learning', *Journal of Interprofessional Care* 6 (3) 243–52.

Annandale, S., McCann, S., Nattrass, H., Regan de Bere, S., Williams, S. and Evans, D. (2000) 'Achieving health improvement through interprofessional learning in south west England', *Journal of Interprofessional Care* 14 (2) 161–74.

Barnes, D., Carpenter, J. and Bailey, D. (2000a) 'Participation with service users in interprofessional education for community mental health', *Journal of Interprofessional Care* 14 (2) 189–200.

Barnes, D., Carpenter, J. and Dickinson, C. (2000b) 'Interprofessional education for community mental health: attitude to community care and professional stereotypes', *Social Work Education* 19 (6) 565–83.

Barr, H. (1994) *Perspectives on Shared Learning*, London: CAIPE.

Barr, H. (1996) 'Ends and means in interprofessional education: towards a typology', *Education for Health* 9 (3) 341–52.

Barr, H. (1998) 'Competent to collaborate: towards a competency-based model for interprofessional education', *Journal of Interprofessional Care* 12 (2) 181–8.

Barr, H. (2000) 'Working together to learn together: learning together to work together', *Journal of Interprofessional Care* 14 (2) 177–80.

Barr, H. (2002) *Interprofessional Education: Today, Yesterday and Tomorrow*, London: The Learning and Teaching Support Network for Health Sciences and Practice.

Barr, H. and Shaw, I. (1995) *Shared Learning: Selected Examples from the Literature*, London: CAIPE.

Barr, H. and Waterton, S. (1996) *Interprofessional Education in Health and Social Care in the United Kingdom: A CAIPE Survey*, London: CAIPE.

Barr, H., Hammick, M., Koppel, I. and Reeves, S. (1999) 'Evaluating interprofessional education: two systematic reviews for health and social care', *British Educational Research Journal* 15 (4) 533–44.

Barr, H., Freeth, D., Hammick, M., Koppel, I. and Reeves, S. (2000) *Evaluations of Interprofessional Education: A United Kingdom Review for Health and Social Care*, London: CAIPE and the British Educational Research Association (www.caipe.org.uk).

Barrows, H. and Tamblin, R. (1980) *Problem Based Learning*, New York: Springer.

Bartholomew, A., Davis, J. and Weinstein, J. (1996) *Interprofessional Education and Training: Developing New Models. Report of the Joint Practice Teaching Initiative*, London: CCETSW.

Berkowitz, L. (1980) *A Survey of Social Psychology*, New York: Holt, Rhinehart & Winston.

Berman, S. and Brobst, K. (1996) (eds) 'Collaboration for change in health professions education', *Journal of Quality Improvement* 22 (3) Special Issue.

Carpenter, J. (1995a) 'Interprofessional education for medical and nursing students', *Medical Education* 29 265–72.

Carpenter, J. (1995b) 'Doctors and nurses: stereotypes and stereotype change in interprofessional education', *Journal of Interprofessional Care* 9 (2) 151–62.

Carpenter, J. and Hewstone, M. (1996) 'Shared learning for doctors and social workers', *British Journal of Social Work* 26 239–57.

Davis, J., Rendell, P. and Sims, D. (1999) 'The joint practitioner – a new concept in professional training', *Journal of Interprofessional Care* 13 (4) 395–404.

Department of Health (2000) *A Health Service for All the Talents: Developing the NHS Workforce*, London: Department of Health.

d'Ivernois, J-F. and Vodoratski, V. (1988) *Multiprofessional Education of Health Personnel in the European Region*, Copenhagen: World Health Organization.

Freeth, D. and Reeves, S. (2002) 'Evaluation of an interprofessional training ward: pilot phase', in S. Glen and T. Leiba (eds), *Multiprofessional Learning for Nurses – Breaking the Boundaries*, Basingstoke: Macmillan.

Freeth, D., Hammick, M., Koppel, I., Reeves, S. and Barr, H. (2002) *A Critical Review of Evaluations of Interprofessional Education*, London: The Learning and Teaching Support Network for Health Sciences and Practice.

Gilbert, J., Camp, R., Cole, C., Bruce, C., Fielding, D. and Stanton, S. (2000) 'Preparing students for interprofessional teamwork in health care', *Journal of Interprofessional Care* 14 (3) 223–35.

Glennie, S. and Closier, J. (1994) 'Collaborative inquiry: developing multidisciplinary learning for action', *Journal of Interprofessional Care* 8 (3) 255–64.

GNCs/CCETSW (General Nursing Councils/Central Council for Education and Training in Social Work) (1982) *Co-operation in Training: Part 1. Qualifying Training*, London: General Nursing Councils for England & Wales, Scotland and Northern Ireland and the Central Council for Education and Training in Social Work.

Hasler, J. and Klinger, M. (1976) 'Common ground in general practitioner and health visitor training: an experimental course', *Journal of the Royal College of General Practice* 26, 266–76.

Hewstone, M. and Brown, R. (1986) 'Contact is not enough: an intergroup perspective on the contact hypothesis', in M. Hewstone and R. Brown (eds), *Contact and Conflict in Intergroup Encounters*, Oxford: Blackwell.

Hughes, L. and Lucas, J. (1997) 'An evaluation of problem based learning in the multiprofessional education curriculum for health professions', *Journal of Interprofessional Care* 11 (1) 77–88.

Jay Committee (1979) *Report of the Committee of Enquiry into Mental Handicap Nursing and Care*, London: HMSO.

Jones, R. (1986) *Working Together – Learning Together*, Occasional Paper 33, London: Royal College of General Practitioners.

Leicester Warwick Medical School (2001) *Community-based Multi-agency Learning: Evaluation Report*, Leicester: Leicester Warwick Medical School.

Likierman, M. (1997) 'Psychoanalytic observation in community and primary health care', *Psychoanalytic Psychotherapy* 11 (2) 147–57.

McMichael, P. and Gilloran, A. (1984) *Pathways to the Professions: Research Report*, Edinburgh: Moray House College of Education.

Miller, C., Ross, N. and Freeman, M. (1999) *Shared Learning and Clinical Teamwork: New Directions in Education for Multiprofessional Practice*, London: English National Board for Nursing, Midwifery and Health Visiting.

NHS South West (2001) *Interprofessional Education*, Bristol: NHS Education Development Team in the South West.

Nicol, M. and de Saintonge, M. (2002) 'Learning clinical skills: an inter-professional approach', in S. Glen and T. Leiba (eds), *Multiprofessional Learning for Nurses – Breaking the Boundaries*, Basingstoke: Macmillan, 84–96.

Reason, P. (1988) *Human Inquiry in Action: Developments in New Paradigm Research*, London: Sage.

Reason, P. (1994) *Participation in Human Inquiry*, London: Sage.

Reeves, S. (2000) 'Community-based interprofessional education for medical, nursing and dental students', *Health and Social Care in the Community* 8, 269–76.

Reeves, S. and Freeth, D. (2002) 'The London training ward: an innovative interprofessional learning initiative', *Journal of Interprofessional Care* 16 (1) 41–52.

Schmitt, M. (2000) 'Continuous quality improvement in health professions education. Editorial', *Journal of Interprofessional Care* 14 (20) 109–10.

Secretary of State for Health (2000) *The NHS Plan: A Plan for Investment, A Plan for Reform*, London: The Stationery Office.

SCOPME (Standing Committee on Postgraduate Medical Education) (1999) *Equity and Exchange: Multiprofessional Working and Learning*, Wetherby: Standing Committee on Postgraduate Medical and Dental Education.

Sims, D. (2002) 'Joint training for integrated care', in S. Glenn and T. Leiba (eds), *Multi-professional Learning for Nursing: Breaking the Boundaries*, Basingstoke: Macmillan.

Tajfel, H. (1981) *Human Groups and Social Categories*, Cambridge: Cambridge University Press.

Thistlewaite, J. (2000) 'Introducing community-based teaching of third year medical students: outcomes of a pilot project one year later and implications for managing change', *Education for Health* 13 (1) 53–62.

University of Westminster (2001) *Pride and Prejudice in Interprofessional Work: An Experiential Workshop*, London: University of Westminster School of Integrated Health.

WHO (World Health Organization) (1976) *Health Manpower Development* Doc/A29/15 (unpublished), presented at the 29th World Health Assembly.

WHO (1978) *Primary Health Care: Report of the International Conference on Primary Health Care, The Alma Ata Declaration*, Geneva: World Health Organization.

WHO (1988) *Learning Together to Work Together for Health*, Geneva: World Health Organization.

Zajonc, R. (1968) 'Attitudinal effects of mere exposure', *Journal of Personality and Social Psychology*, Monograph Supplement 9 Part 2, 1–27.

Chapter 20

Canada – interprofessional education and collaboration

Theoretical challenges, practical solutions

John Gilbert and Lesley Bainbridge

SUMMARY

Structural changes need to be made within universities such that interprofessional education and collaboration (IPE/C) becomes a responsibility that crosses faculty jurisdictions. In communities, the patient or client is the centre of professional attention requiring care that goes beyond the skill and scope of any one profession. Notions about collaboration inform and drive IPE/C and should lead to testable hypotheses that lend credence and acceptability to the IPE/C process. A College of Health Disciplines has been developed at the University of British Columbia, which conforms to the university statute while at the same time allowing for IPE to cross traditional faculty boundaries.

The College of Health Disciplines of the University of British Columbia is not the only institution that is trying to foster collaboration between the health professions, but it is unique in its concentrated effort to work through some of the problems and to initiate some of the changes that appear to be necessary for the creation of an atmosphere in which planning, testing and eventual implementation of interprofessional educational programmes, leading to a lowering of barriers between professions, may take place (Szasz 1969). Multiprofessional education does not replace but complements the part of a curriculum concerned essentially with one particular profession (WHO Study Group 1987).

INTRODUCTION

It is 33 years since Szasz (1969) described efforts at the University of British Columbia (UBC) to promote interprofessional education (Gilbert et al 2000). It was only two years ago that educators in the health and human service programmes at UBC presented an account of an interprofessional module on teamwork, which provided opportunities for students to learn from and with each other about health and human service-related professions and their approaches to patient or client care. In 33 years, much has changed in health care, but the problems identified by Szasz (1969) still persist.

Much that has been written about IPE/C has concentrated on two or at most three professions, for example, primarily medicine, nursing and social work (Carpenter 1995a, 1995b; Pryce and Reeves 1997; Freeth and Nichol 1998). Educational programmes described in the literature tend to focus on activities involving students and/or practitioners. Very little has been written, however, about the *structural changes* that need to be made within universities and colleges in order that IPE/C is considered a joint responsibility across a number of faculty jurisdictions that may subsequently impact institutional practice.

These university-oriented structural changes are needed because it is clear that community health and human services correctly view the patient or client as the centre of professional attention. By extension, this implies interprofessional collaboration in practice, since it is clear that client-centred service is beyond the competencies and scope of practice of any *one* profession.

It was clear from the work undertaken at UBC that quantifying teamwork learning is a most difficult matter. Ideally, interprofessional education (IPE) should accompany interprofessional collaboration (IPC), hereafter IPE/C (The Standing Committee on Postgraduate Medical and Dental Education (SCOPME 1997; Zungolo 1994)). In addition, determining whether skills acquired in IPE/C are actually translated into practice is a complicated and complex exercise. It requires that we develop models of clinical reasoning that allow us to measure change, and to relate that change to collaborative (teamwork) experience.

In this chapter we explore notions about collaboration that inform and drive IPE/C. We attempt to show how and why such notions should allow for testable hypotheses that lend credence and acceptability to the IPE/C process. We conclude by linking these ideas with a description of a new cross-faculties, interprofessional, college that will focus on IPE/C through unique structural changes within the UBC.

THEORETICAL CHALLENGES

Barriers to implementation

IPE/C is not easy to implement for a number of structural and philosophical reasons. Structural barriers include: differences in prerequisites for admission to professional programmes; the length of professional education; the extent and nature of the utilisation of community and hospital resources for field-work (clinical) education; students' freedom, or lack of, in the selection of professional courses; timetabling differences and conflicts across professional programmes; faculty teaching loads; research interests of faculty; methods of administration within the various programmes; and the powers vested in deans of faculties through statutory legislation, for example, through the power to appoint faculty members, and to develop curricula. Philosophical barriers include: attitudes of faculty to IPE with respect to its value; resistance to changes in learning models; and reluctance of students to step beyond professional boundaries.

As Freeth (2000), Drinka and Clark (2000) and others have pointed out, IPE/C faces some particular challenges, which seriously impede efforts to sustain it. These challenges include, for example: structural differences between organisations; conflicting organisational and professional agendas; resource requirements; complex communication demands; rotation and replacement of team members; and lack of regular evaluation of the team's stated goals and programmes.

Providing interprofessional learning experiences through IPE/C that would help promote teamwork and collaboration is therefore difficult. Finding space in diverse curricula, and times at which students may engage in joint activities, needs creative rethinking of structural obstacles inherent in the research university.

Time and space are needed as well as academically acceptable mechanisms for measuring the effectiveness of such IPE/C activities. Changing attitudes of students, faculty and administration in order to make IPE effective is both a challenge and an opportunity. To promote IPE/C and to measure its effectiveness, there is a need to ensure that students' attitudes to such work are clearly assessed: on entry to their professional programme of study; on completion of their clinical/fieldwork experiences; on completion of their professional education; and finally (and most difficult), once they are in practice. These structural and philosophical issues are addressed through student and faculty surveys conducted by Gilbert et al (2002).

Convincing both faculty and students about the value of IPE/C is a major barrier to overcome. The barrier requires that a fundamental issue be addressed, that is, the need for a robust *theory of collaboration*, which allows us to test hypotheses about IPE/C.

As generally understood, a theory is an explanation *independent* of the phenomenon being studied. A theory is based on principles that are coherent, generalisable and transferable, and of continuing applicability.

Without the use of theory, any discoveries about collaboration and understanding of its operational power remain moot, hence a body of knowledge that might better inform the practice of IPE/C simply does not grow.

IPE/C remains at the mercy of fashion and expediency unless a coherent body of knowledge develops in which practice and teaching can be based, assessed and evaluated. A suitable theory must therefore recognise and include some fundamental concepts.

Possible theoretical approaches to IPE/C

Parsell and Bligh (1999) have proposed that a reasonable theory of collaboration should provide conceptual opportunities to test assumptions that at the very least provide data on the relationship between different professional groups as expressed in the values and beliefs that their practitioners hold. The data would include, for example: an understanding of the knowledge and skills needed to collaborate and work in teams; an understanding of the roles and responsibilities of other health and human service professionals in a team, that is, what those professionals actually do in their work lives; and an understanding of the benefits of IPE/C to patients or clients, to the practice of a profession, to an individual's professional growth and to general health outcomes.

Each of these concepts is clearly open to investigation, that is, they provide the bases for stating hypotheses that allow tests on a theory of collaboration. What evidence (data) do we have that would allow us to talk in a more informed fashion about IPE/C? To date, however, the data to support IPE/C is sparse and confusing.

Using the guidelines for systematic review developed by the Cochrane Collaboration, Zwarenstein et al (1999) concluded that no rigorous quantitative evidence exists on the effects of interprofessional education. As these authors point out: 'The chain connecting IPE, improved educational efficacy, closer teamwork, better care and improved outcomes seems appealingly logical and theoretically coherent, and is often asserted. But there is not widely accepted evidence on which to base the belief that they are linked at all, let alone causally'. Zwarenstein et al (1999: 418–19) continue: 'Although IPE is unlikely to cause mortal harm, it may have other negative effects *and could use up resources that might have been used for proven interventions* (our italics), and so rigorous evaluation of its effectiveness is advisable before widespread implementation'.

It is important to note that while the study by Zwarenstein et al (1999) did not find evidence of *effectiveness*, neither did it find evidence of *ineffectiveness*. Simply put, at the present time *no* evidence exists in either direction. Despite the caution expressed by Zwarenstein et al (1999), however, IPE/C is now widely embraced both in education and practice.

As described above, a number of barriers have been recognised that require consideration in the promotion of IPE/C. The literature would appear to show that for collaboration to be sustained, the balance of these influences must be such that each collaborator is able to identify sufficient benefit *to themselves* as to outweigh the disadvantages of interprofessional collaboration.

As so clearly articulated by Drinka and Clark (2000), IPE/C has particular needs or requirements including: shared responsibility for management; shared space and equipment for curriculum; innovations in assessment tools;

and the presence of educators from each profession represented in courses that address complex health care issues and clinical reasoning, for example HIV/Aids and palliative care.

In a thoughtful monograph: '*Collaboration in Health and Welfare*' Loxley (1997) points out that the case for IPE can be made *only* when certain conditions are met; that is:

- When IPE/C is most likely to be effective, that is when the subject matter being addressed is complex (e.g. HIV/Aids, palliative care) and requires a team approach
- When the effects of IPE/C can be clearly measured, that is, when enhanced critical reasoning skills are observable and quantifiable
- When claims for resources can be justified, that is, when support for faculty is clearly necessary for success
- When practitioners can be held accountable, that is, when the skills being taught are within the competencies expected of a particular professional team
- When skills and knowledge can be explicitly taught and are clearly transferable to other complex health care issues

When the research literature dealing with *clinical judgement* is examined, it is clear that collaboration is usually understood inductively by practitioners, that is, through reference to their own field of practice. Even though there is an extensive literature on clinical judgement, an adequate theory of clinical collaboration to complement notions about clinical judgement is still under-developed. In Loxley's (1997: 25) words, without such a theory: 'practice struggles to make sense of itself and is hampered by the lack of any dialogue with a framework of ideas leading to transferable knowledge and skills'.

Since the word 'collaboration' implies an interaction between two or more parties, what type of theory is needed? General theories of interaction hold some appeal, for example: general systems theory; social exchange theory and/or cooperative theory. Each of these theories provides us with test points that we might use to examine the effectiveness of collaborating across professional boundaries. In this chapter, for illustrative purposes, we address only the cooperative theory. Cooperative theory, for example, allows us to assess, build, manage and evaluate some key phases of the collaborative process.

Assignment of value to these phases comes about, for example, through reflection on course planning, as experienced in teaching IPE/C courses, and through literature reviews of effectiveness. Each phase of cooperative theory becomes a testable hypothesis.

By deriving values for each of these phases, we develop knowledge, skills and attitudes that are necessary, but not sufficient, conditions, for collaboration. In addition, to support a cooperative theory, we need to understand the structure, use and distribution of power associated with each player in the interprofessional team, and the purpose and effect of that player's culture and language in building (or not) purposeful collaboration. Within the frame of cooperative theory, as IPE grows, both individual and systemic changes are necessary to success.

In her paper 'Collaboration: a sociological perspective', Abuyuan (2000) pointed out that for successful collaboration, structures need to have *open boundaries* and *effective means of exchanging resources*. Collaborators need timely information and reliable services. They also need to be organised in such a fashion that they are able to take risks in assessing the balance between *costs* and *benefits* of their collaboration. In addition, the structures that facilitate collaboration need to be *sustained* and *stable*. Stability and sustainability ensure what Abuyuan (2000) terms 'the shadow of the future', that is, the reasonable expectation that the collaborating parties will meet again. Finally, collaborations need to be set up so that they reflect an inclusive process. This inclusive process provides for continuity and facilitates ongoing trust (Abuyuan 2000: 80). Open boundaries, effective means of exchanging resources, sustainability and stability are at the heart of the new College addressed in the second part of this chapter.

In addition to those already mentioned, evaluation metrics should allow us to assess long-term outcomes: for the client/patient; for the process of collaborative practice; for individual professionals; and for agencies in which collaborations are carried out. The *costs* of collaboration can be tangible and intangible (e.g. human and financial resources), the *benefits* even more so. To understand the *benefits* we have to build the culture of IPE/C. A clear understanding of benefits comes through using the language of collaboration, in order that the outcomes of IPE/C are access to a wide range of resources, to new knowledge and to new skills. Most important (and sometimes elusive) are the positive health outcomes that accrue through the shared respect, esteem and trust of all collaborating partners.

Our task is to turn the concepts of IPE/C from either mystical attitudes of faith, or pragmatic responses to gaps in service, into ideas that can be *understood intellectually, challenged experimentally* and *argued for politically*. At the same time, IPE/C must be turned into practice that addresses difficulties lying beyond the bounds of uni-professional activity. IPE/C must, when appropriate, move beyond autonomous practice. If the interprofessional education agenda is to be more than a mystical attitude, we need to be very clear about who gains, who pays, who assesses relevance and who measures outcomes.

In attempting to move this agenda forward, our theoretical framework needs to articulate some complex questions, of the following order. Why *do* people collaborate? What makes collaboration *successful*? What makes an *effective* collaborator? What drives collaborative *partnership*?

As we frame these questions within a theoretical framework, we need then to build models that contextualise the collaborating partners: the care providers; faculty; students; and patients. It is these collaborating partners who interact with and depend on each other, and who behave in ways that suit mutual expectations captured in the theoretical framework.

The decreased *costs* to client/patient and society are achieved by well-structured approaches (Katon 1995; Mullins et al 1996). However, team approaches cannot be implemented uncritically since there is little empirical research to provide strong support for the contention that team approaches provide effective means to enhance functional outcomes, reduce costs, decrease length of hospital stays or increase quality of care (Keith 1991). It is clear that much research effort still needs to be devoted to the evaluation of teams and team approaches.

The literature contains many illustrations that attempt to build effective teams. In building collaborative teams, it is clear, however, that conflicts will arise. The literature is replete with examples of methods for overcoming conflicts by changing organisational structures. So, in elaborating the organisation of teams within a theory of collaboration, the elaboration should characterise that organisation as one that attempts to optimise individual and organisational need for *satisfaction* by encouraging the formation of *stable work groups* and participation of all team members in decision-making; good *communication* and effective supervision; non-bureaucratic structures that function by the *setting of objectives* rather than through a hierarchy of authority. These characterisations are built into the concept of 'college', as discussed below.

Despite the best efforts of universities to ensure that their graduates are *practice*-ready, it is a lack of *job*-readiness about which most employers complain. Many health and human service professionals lack effective training in teamwork during their professional education; they therefore have no explicit training in either leading, or being part of, collaborative efforts. At this time, team training is done 'on the job', and often appears to be in a poorly formulated manner.

Despite a lack of quantified support, anecdotal evidence from the health care industry suggests that there is a dramatic need for a comprehensive interprofessional education of health and human service students; that waiting until students graduate and are 'on the job' is almost too late to build effective team skills. At the present time, almost all functioning teams have been built *within* the health and human service care environment, with varying degrees of success (Drinka and Clark 2000). Interprofessional *education/collaboration* should therefore be a coherent and integrated component of professional education (Barr and Waterton 1996). It should provide opportunities for students from at least two or more health and human service educational programmes, to work collaboratively in teams on matters of mutual clinical concern. We now turn our attention to how an attempt to address the matters raised thus far are being implemented at the UBC.

TURNING THEORY INTO PRACTICE

A College of Health Disciplines

And it ought to be remembered that there is nothing more difficult to take in hand, more perilous to conduct, or more uncertain in its success, than to take the lead in the introduction of a new order of things. Because the innovator has for enemies all those who have done well under the old conditions, and the lukewarm defenders in those who may do well under the new.

(Machiavelli 1515)

The development of an *interprofessional* College at UBC is in keeping with the philosophical position articulated above, and with changes occurring internationally and nationally in all health and human service professions. It is also congruent with changes in the workplace; activities in health and human service resource planning being undertaken by all levels of Canadian governments; and National, Provincial and Regional health objectives. These objectives have been set out in *Closer to Home* (Seaton et al 1991), *Toward a Healthy Future* (Health and Welfare Canada 1997) and *Inaugural Health Plan* (Vancouver/Richmond Health Board 1999), all of which have their origins in the *Royal Commission on Health Services* (Hall 1964), *A New Perspective on the Health of Canadians* (Lalonde 1974) and *Achieving Health for All* (Epp 1986).

A *Coordinating Committee for Health Sciences* at UBC was established informally in 1961; it was formalised in 1969 following publication of a report by Dean G. F. Curtis, Faculty of Law, entitled 'Administrative Structure for the Health Sciences Centre, University of British Columbia, October 1969'. The report was submitted to the New Programmes Committee of Senate, who submitted their report to Senate in 1969, where the report was approved in December 1969. The Office of the Coordinator of Health Sciences (OCHS) was established by the Board of Governors in 1970 under the provisions of the provincial University Act, Section 27(y). The Coordinating Committee for Health Sciences was renamed the Health Sciences Coordinating Committee, and its Chair (appointed by the Board of Governors) was named Coordinator, Health Sciences.

The Coordinator of Health Sciences represented the collective view of health and human service programmes on appropriate university committees; acted as the university's liaison officer with community agencies and governments; provided policy advice and analysis on a wide variety of matters affecting the health and human service faculties, schools, departments, institutes and programmes; managed and administered various support functions for the collective health and human service programmes; and gathered and disseminated information pertinent to the health and human service programmes.

In the 30 years since its establishment, the OCHS underwent a number of transitions. Most significantly, the Health Sciences Coordinating Committee voted in 1998 to reflect its broadened membership by changing its name to the Council of Health and Human Service Programmes (CHHSP), a change approved by Senate in that year.

With the publication of the UBC's vision for the twenty-first century through *TREK 2000* and the *Academic Plan (2000)*, it was clear that a propitious moment had been reached to move the OCHS beyond its role as a coordinating/service unit to a new successor academic unit. Through the Academic Plan the place of interdisciplinary and interprofessional education was now clearly established at UBC, and a very large number of faculty members are engaged in work of this nature – through teaching, research and community activities. As mentioned in the preceding section, there have been enormous changes in health care delivery, both nationally and internationally, which have led to a focus on the development of interprofessional collaboration through teamwork. The OCHS, founded on the principle of interprofessional education and learning, moved to academic programming that necessitated a more formal academic structure. A successor academic unit to the OCHS, *The College of Health Disciplines*, was proposed and approved in accord with British Columbia's University Act (1970 updated 2000), Powers of the Board, Section 27(y) and Duties of a University, Section 47 (a–c).

As a successor to the OCHS, the College of Health Disciplines is a collaboration of seven faculties (Agricultural Sciences, Applied Sciences, Arts, Dentistry, Education, Medicine and Pharmaceutical Sciences) and occupies a unique place in the University. Its constituent partners include faculty members from all health and human service programmes (HHSPs) at UBC: Audiology, Speech-Language Pathology; Clinical Psychology; Counselling Psychology; Dental Hygiene; Dentistry; Food, Nutrition and Health; Human Kinetics; Medicine; Nursing; Occupational Therapy; Pharmaceutical Sciences; Physical Therapy; Social Work and Family Studies. The College provides leadership in collectively fostering and supporting a learning environment and courses of instruction that focus on interprofessional and interdisciplinary education, in accord with the provincial University Act. Based upon notions described in the preceding section, the College also provides leadership in developing and maintaining *effective collaboration, interdisciplinary and interprofessional understanding* and *shared communication* among health and human service programmes and other units of the University, and between the external community and the University. The following description of how the College will function is in accord with the theoretical and philosophical positions espoused in the first section of this chapter.

THE COLLEGE

Effective interprofessional education: – works to improve the quality of care; focuses on the needs of service users and carers; involves service users and carers; promotes interprofessional collaboration; encourages professions to learn with, from and about one another; enhances practice within professions; respects the integrity and contribution of each profession and increases professional satisfaction.

(Barr and Waterton 1996)

Functions

The College collectively fosters, enhances and sustains a culture of interprofessional and interdisciplinary education of practitioners. These activities are directed at innovative student learning, collaborative research and best practice. Through these means the College enables the graduation of practitioners who are expected to become leaders in effectively addressing critical issues of health and human service to people in an ever-changing service delivery system. The authors have attempted to capture the essence of this collective collaboration in Figure 20.1, which includes medicine.

Figure 20.1 acknowledges the specificity of individual disciplines while weaving through them a set of more generic, interprofessional competencies resulting in enhanced interprofessional collaborative practice. The institution of the College allows for more integrated learning experiences across and among programmes in a manner that can, and will, enhance collaborative practice in the educational and practice contexts.

Through the experience of its collective faculty, the College maximises interprofessional learning and research through teamwork that facilitates and enhances interprofessional appreciation and applies collaborative planning and decision-making skills to health and human services. The College does

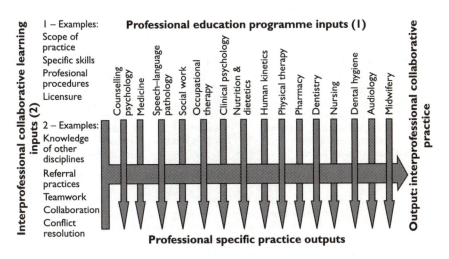

Figure 20.1 Developing interprofessional collaborative practice.

not encompass departments as normally associated with a faculty; does not hire faculty; does not provide degree programmes and does not sponsor its own courses. Rather, the College provides an innovative way of increasing collaboration through various common collaborative groupings, for example interprofessional courses, fieldwork organisation, information technology, educational support and development and collaborative work associated with its component units. The College is not 'accredited' in the sense that its constituent programmes are accredited.

The College identifies, develops and delivers collaborative educational and research experiences, both within the University and with its community partners, which include federal, provincial and municipal government ministries and all organisations that collaborate in the education of health and human service professionals. These experiences enhance the quality of existing educational programmes and respond to the changing needs of future health and human service professionals. The College also serves as a focal point for interinstitutional linkage of health and human service programmes in other universities, university colleges and community colleges.

Role

The role of the College is to maximise intellectual and facility resources by developing a sustainable educational model that incorporates creative, flexible and transferable interprofessional learning and research strategies and opportunities for students in all health and human service professional education programmes at UBC. Inasmuch as it is seen as representing common interests across a diversity of faculties, the College promotes the following collective goals and priorities as set out in the recent UBC documents *TREK 2000* and the *Academic Plan* (Figure 20.2).

In the University's Instructional Resources Centre (IRC), the College is

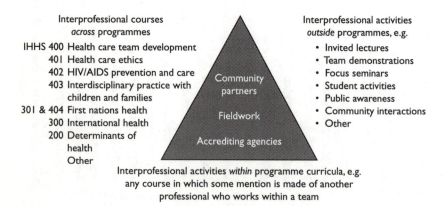

Interprofessional courses
across programmes

IHHS 400 Health care team development
    401 Health care ethics
    402 HIV/AIDS prevention and care
    403 Interdisciplinary practice with
        children and families
301 & 404 First nations health
    300 International health
    200 Determinants of
        health
    Other

Interprofessional activities
outside programmes, e.g.

- Invited lectures
- Team demonstrations
- Focus seminars
- Student activities
- Public awareness
- Community interactions
- Other

Community partners

Fieldwork

Accrediting agencies

Interprofessional activities *within* programme curricula, e.g.
any course in which some mention is made of another
professional who works within a team

Figure 20.2 Creating a culture for interprofessional collaborative learning.

developing a Learning Commons, or accessible common area, for all students in the health and human service programmes where they may easily access information resources, communication assistance, peer counselling, and so on, related to interprofessional best practice. The College, through its governing council, allocates a portion of teaching in each programme to achieve common interprofessional goals and has developed a faculty reward system that clearly credits and recognises interprofessional contributions to learning.

Surveys of students in health and human service programmes show strong and enthusiastic support for interprofessional education – from University to community (Bainbridge et al forthcoming; Gilbert et al 2000).

There is formal recognition of *interprofessional* teaching activities in the College. This recognition is by a Letter of Agreement between the heads of units about the interprofessional activities of faculty members within their units. This letter is also part of the faculty member's official record/dossier and recognised in salary, promotion and tenure decisions.

Membership in the College is for individual faculty members, although membership of the governing council will be by unit (programme). Because the focus of College activities is centred on interprofessional and inter-disciplinary work, the natural College membership comprises those faculty members who contribute either through teaching, research or committee work to the interprofessional health and human service enterprise. Recognition of faculty members through membership in the College is for peda-gogical reasons, that is, membership recognises that the professions are moving in the direction of interprofessional cooperation and collaboration, creating greater 'porosity' across professional bounds. Faculty members receive a formal, renewable appointment to the College, on the recommenda-tion of their dean, director, or head and approved by the governing council.

A collaborative working relationship of the type envisaged in a College provides clear opportunities in, for example: greater joint curricular devel-opment; husbanding of resources; the promotion of educational changes that accord with those occurring in the workplace; closer interprofessional cooperation in fieldwork placements; and the development of a new forum for promoting academic interactions. The College is confronted with a very different set of issues than those that face a faculty.

Learning across boundaries

The College has expanded opportunities for interprofessional collaborative and cohort learning across HHSPs as initiated through its support of inter-professional health and human service courses (IHHSs) (see Appendix 1). It has worked to achieve sustainable financial stability and resources to support interprofessional activities across the HHSPs. In collaboration with its con-stituent programmes represented on council, the College reviews and moni-tors the number and types of courses and credits required for undergraduate

HHSP degrees in order to ensure maximum flexibility for interprofessional learning. The College is also in the process of developing interprofessional certificate and diploma programmes as opportunities for non-degree students; and it is building interinstitutional linkages for transfer credit and other purposes. It promotes interprofessional best practice through the effective use and development of information technology by faculty, students and staff through the integration of the university libraries into the learning environment and by developing web CT courses.

The College includes a number of support units: the Division of Educational Support and Development; the Committee on Information Technology; the Media Group; and the Committee on Interprofessional Education.

Research

The College serves as a focal point for research that evaluates the parameters associated with interprofessional collaboration in education *and practice*, and that *involves a mix of health and human service professions* both within the university, and with community partners. The College is a focus for health services and policy research, for research on health human resource planning and for research on the health of Aboriginal peoples.

Community collaboration and partnerships

At UBC, the health and human service programmes have a long history of fieldwork relationships with a wide range of community agencies – hospitals, health regions and private and non-governmental agencies. In keeping with many studies of community collaboration, the College is assuming major responsibilities to support cross-faculty, collaborative health and human service activities with community partners locally and nationally, through its committee on fieldwork. The College takes a major role in interpreting to government ministries when a *collective* health and human service interest is at stake as a result of their initiatives rather than the interest of a particular faculty/school or profession. The College also encourages government ministries to initiate and/or support activities and to develop policies that foster interdisciplinary and interprofessional practices, both within educational and community institutions.

Given that the health and human service programmes have a wide variety of community partners as defined earlier, a subset of fieldwork/clinical teaching faculty members will become members of the College, particularly those engaged in a number of team-based programmes. These members might also be accorded a honorific, for example 'community fellow/associate'.

The College works closely with UBC's programme in continuing studies developing learning programmes that are action-oriented and tailored to the needs of professionals in the health and human service community. The committee on fieldwork together with continuing studies is developing a diploma programme for mentoring and preceptoring, to be offered to all fieldwork/clinical teaching faculty members.

In keeping with the University's goal to increase internationalisation, the Centre for International Health (a constituent unit of the College) fosters national and international initiatives that involve interdisciplinary, interprofessional and cross-faculty groups of researchers and educators where opportunities exist for collaborative endeavours. These include projects in South Africa, South America and Australia.

Aboriginal people

Finally, through its constituent unit – the Institute for Aboriginal Health, the College is working together with communities to increase the number of Aboriginal students in all of the health and human service programmes, and to build participatory research links with the Aboriginal community.

CONCLUSION

This chapter presents the reader with an overview of current concepts related to interprofessional education and practice. Barriers to IPE/C are identified and strategies for overcoming the barriers as well as developing and sustaining collaborative practice through interprofessional learning are offered. Cooperative theory is described as one way of testing and validating IPE/C as valuable approaches to improved health outcomes and client satisfaction. It is clear that there is much work to be done to quantify the effects of IPE/C. The authors believe that future work will support the efficacy of IPE/C and will secure both collaborative education and practice as keys to better health care.

In addition, this chapter describes a rationale for creating a new and innovative academic structure – the College of Health Disciplines. This affiliation of seven faculties promotes and supports interprofessional collaboration across curricula and practice that transcends disciplinary boundaries. The vision for this affiliation is to enhance and secure the health care of all people. Much remains to be done to secure IPE/C as an integral component of disciplinary education. We recognise the importance and complexity of evaluating IPE/C. As described by Engel and Vanclay (1997), it is imperative that close attention be focused on outcome evaluation of IPE/C in order to confirm their relevance and value in current and future health care systems.

APPENDIX 1

Existing interprofessional health and human service courses

IHHS 200	Understanding the Socio-cultural Determinants of the Health of Populations	The idea of 'population health', and the implementation and evaluation of programmes or policies to improve health. Open to all students. *Term 1 [3–0–0]*
IHHS 300	Working in International Health: A preparatory course for students planning to work in the developing world	Fully tutored, web-based course on planning/preparing for work in a developing country. Discusses causes of ill health among populations living in poverty; analyses available solutions. Health science background not essential. *Summer 2001 [3–0–0]*
IHHS 301	First Nations Health and the Traditional Role of Plants	Focuses on the traditional First Nations use of plants as medicine and food, traditional medical systems, intellectual property and the bridging of traditional ecological knowledge and modern sciences. *Term 2 [3–0–0]*
IHHS 400	Health Care Team Development	Skills, knowledge, roles and issues involved with working successfully in interprofessional health and human service teams. Intended for upper division students in any health and human service programmes. *Summer 2001 [3–0–0]*
IHHS 401	Health Care Ethics	An interprofessional approach using case studies to illustrate the application of bioethical principles and theories. Intended for students in health and human service programmes. *Term 1 [3–0–0]*
IHHS 402	HIV/AIDS Prevention and Care	Preparation for senior students to respond effectively to the HIV/AIDS epidemic and its consequences. The knowledge and skills required for interprofessional and discipline specific work are explored. Intended for students in the health and human service programmes. Permission required. Limited enrolment. *Summer 2001 [6–0–0]*
IHHS 403	Interdisciplinary Practice with Children and Families	Interprofessional perspectives, challenges and strategies. Clinical experience and some knowledge of child protection issues required. *Term 2 [3–0–0]*
IHHS 404	First Nations Health: Historical and Contemporary Issues	An epistemological approach that considers the determinants of health and spiritual–environmental–cultural perspectives. *Term 2 [3–0–0]*

ACKNOWLEDGEMENTS

We should like to thank the many colleagues who contributed to the ideas presented in this chapter, and those who were active participants in developing the College of Health Disciplines. These include the deans of the affiliated faculties, the directors, heads and faculty members of the Health and Human Service Programmes at UBC, and colleagues in the USA, the UK and Australia. We particularly thank our friends and colleagues, Hugh Barr (UK), Bud Baldwin (USA) and Mattie Schmitt (USA) for their unflagging enthusiasm and support as we moved this innovation forward. In addition, we are grateful to Maureen Phillips for her invaluable editorial and technical assistance. Any errors of omission or commission are of course our responsibility.

REFERENCES

Abuyuan, A. (2000) 'Collaboration: a sociological perspective', UNDP/Yale Collaborative Programme on the Urban Environment, Research Clinic, New Haven.

Bainbridge, L., Gilbert, J. and Pavech, G. (forthcoming) 'Give us more student perspectives on interprofessional education.'

Barr, H. and Waterton, S. (1996) *A UK Survey of Interprofessional Education in Health and Social Care*, London: CAIPE.

Carpenter, J. (1995a) 'Doctors and nurses: stereotypes and stereotype change in interprofessional education', *Journal of Interprofessional Care* 9 (2) 151–60.

Carpenter, J. (1995b) 'Interprofessional education for medical and nursing students: evaluation of a programme', *Medical Education* 29, 265–72.

Drinka, T. and Clark, P. (2000) *Health Care Teamwork*, Connecticut: Auburn House.

Engel, C. and Vanclay, L. (1997) 'Towards audit and outcome evaluation of interprofessional education for collaboration in primary health care', A CAIPE Discussion Paper, London: UK Centre for the Advancement of Interprofessional Education.

Epp, J. (1986) *Achieving Health for All: A Framework for Health Promotion*, Ottawa, ON: Health and Welfare Canada.

Freeth, D. (2000) 'Sustaining interprofessional education', in L. Meerabeau and H. Barr (eds), *All Together Better Health*, London: UK Centre for the Advancement of Interprofessional Education.

Freeth, D. and Nichol, M. (1998) 'Learning clinical skills: an interprofessional approach', *Nurse Education Today* 18, 455–61.

Gilbert, J., Camp, R., Cole, C., Bruce, C., Fielding, D. and Stanton, S. (2000) 'Preparing students for interprofessional teamwork in health care', *Journal of Interprofessional Care* 14 (3) 223–35.

Gilbert, J., Bainbridge, L. and Hawkey, C. (2002) 'Give us more – now! The views of graduating students on interprofessional education', Interdisciplinary Health Care Team Conference, Arlington, VA.

Hall, E. (1964) *Royal Commission on Health Services*, Ottawa, ON: Health and Welfare Canada.

Health and Welfare Canada (1997) *Toward a Healthy Future*, Ottawa, ON: Health and Welfare Canada.

Katon, W. (1995) 'Collaborative care: patient satisfaction, outcomes, and medical cost-offset', *Family Systems Medicine* 13 (3/4) 351–65.

Keith, R. (1991) 'The comprehensive treatment team in rehabilitation', *Archives of Physical Medicine and Rehabilitation* 72, 269–74.

Lalonde, M. (1974) *A New Perspective on the Health of Canadians: A Working Document*, Ottawa, ON: Department of National Health and Welfare.

Loxley, A. (1997) *Collaboration in Health and Welfare*, London: Jessica Kingsley.

Machiavelli, Nicollo (1515) *The Prince*, Chapter VI.

Mullins, L., Chaney, J. and Frank, R. (1996) 'Rehabilitation medicines, systems, and health: a biopsychosocial perspective', *Families, Systems, and Health* 14, 29–41.

Parsell, G. and Bligh, J. (1999) 'The development of a questionnaire to assess the readiness of health care students for interprofessional learning (RIPLS)', *Medical Education* 33, 95–100.

Pryce, A. and Reeves, S. (1997) 'An exploratory evaluation of an interprofessional education module for medical, dental and nursing students: final report for the Department of Health', London: City University.

Royal Commission on Health Services (1964) Ottawa, ON: Queen's Printer.

SCOPME (The Standing Committee on Postgraduate Medical and Dental Education) (1997) *Multiprofessional Working and Learning: Sharing the Educational Challenge*, London: SCOPME.

Seaton, B. et al (1991) *Closer to Home: The Report of the British Columbia Royal Commission on Health Care and Costs*, Victoria, BC: Royal Commission on Health Care and Costs.

Szasz, G. (1969) 'Interprofessional education in the health sciences', *The Milbank Memorial Fund Quarterly* 67 (4) 449–75.

University Act: Province of British Columbia (Updated 2000) Victoria, BC: Queen's Printer.

Vancouver/Richmond Health Board (1999) *Inaugural Health Plan*, Vancouver, BC.

WHO (World Health Organization) Study Group on Multiprofessional Education of Health Personnel (1987) *The Team Approach, Learning Together to Work Together for Health*, Geneva, October 12–16.

Zungolo, E. (1994) 'Interdisciplinary education in primary care: the challenge', *Nursing and Health Care* 15 (6) 288–92.

Zwarenstein, M., Atkins, J., Barr, H., Hammick, M., Koppel, I. and Reeves, S. (1999) 'A systematic review of interprofessional education', *Journal of Interprofessional Care* 13 (4) 417–31.

Chapter 21

Welfare and education policy – how do these factors influence interprofessional education?

The Norwegian case

Elisabeth Willumsen and Paal Breivik

SUMMARY

In Norway we consider the period after 1945 as the time for development of the professions in the welfare state. This arena is mainly influenced by the health and social policy, the education policy regarding higher education and the demand for interprofessional cooperation in practice reflected by the local authorities. The higher education system is state-financed and state-controlled, but the education institutions hold a great degree of autonomy nevertheless. This chapter illuminates the development of interprofessional education and discusses the relationship between interprofessional education and interprofessional cooperation in practice and illustrates some of the contradictions in the Norwegian case.

THE NORWEGIAN WELFARE STATE AND THE DEMAND FOR INTERPROFESSIONAL COOPERATION

In Norway the development of health and social policy after the war has to be understood in relation to the framing of the welfare state, which is based on the political and moral belief that every citizen has a right to enjoy equality of rights and opportunities. The goals of Norwegian social policy are to achieve equality in as many aspects of life as possible, to redistribute the wealth so that no one suffers from lack of material goods and to provide security and employment for all. Implementing this policy presupposes high taxes on incomes and the legitimacy of state intervention in the economic system. In Norway we have a strong dominance of public funds based on the principle of tax-financing, incorporating elements of the insurance principle mainly through employers' and individual contributions. The most basic pillar of the welfare state is the social security system, which guarantees that all of its members are provided with economic support when they are unable to provide for themselves. People falling outside this system are guaranteed social assistance from the municipality where they reside (Social Care Act 1964).

The myth of the welfare state?

While Norway has a well-developed system of social support, there are problems in living up to the promises and expectations that are created by the laws and health and social welfare programmes. During the past 25 years there have been questions raised about the legitimacy of the welfare state. There is a tough debate about priorities focusing on the costs of the welfare programmes and how ambitious the scope of the welfare systems ought to be. As a consequence ambitions concerning the National Social Security System (NSSS), for example, have become more limited in the past 15 years. Although the system will be continued as a social welfare and economic pillar of society, the breadth of NSSS scope will, however, be limited.

Occasional excesses within the bureaucracy underline the permanent need to rethink and rework health and social programmes so that the user really gets adequate service. This also stimulates the debate regarding the privatisation of public services and the reduction of state-supported provision. These discussion trends are followed by an increasing focus on the gap between 'the rich' and 'the poor' (Johannessen 1998; Birkelund 1999).

Demand for interprofessional cooperation

Regarding interprofessional cooperation, there has been a demand for cooperation from the health and social sector for the last 10–15 years. Coordination of services has been focused on and regarded as a premise for giving the users adequate help. During the last 20 years we find the first publications regarding interprofessional cooperation as a specific issue (Aarseth 1984; Jensen 1986; Askheim and Roenning 1987; Askheim 1989; Gullichsen 1989; Andersen 1992; Repstad 1993). Some authors focused on the organisation of the collaboration; others were preoccupied with projects concerning particular target groups. In the same period we find governmental publications that emphasised the welfare policy in general regarding coordination of services, increase of effectiveness in the public sector, quality protection and user perspective. We find the demand for an improved coordination of services and user participation, which implies interprofessional cooperation.

Discussion about interprofessional cooperation has also actualised the issue within the institutions for the professional training of health and social personnel, especially pointing out the professionals' role and responsibility regarding collaboration in practice to coordinate services towards the users. It seems as if there is an assumption that interprofessional education might contribute to collaboration in practice, which in consequence will give the users adequate assistance.

HEALTH AND SOCIAL WORK EDUCATION IN NORWAY

Regarding *higher education* we have four universities (Oslo, Bergen, Trondheim and Tromso) and 26 university colleges, 170,000 students in all. The three-year professional studies (undergraduate level) mostly take place at the university colleges, while medicine and psychology are sited at the universities where you also find traditional university disciplines. The basic undergraduate study programme is of three years' duration. The training of social and health personnel includes a total of eight professions in fields such as nursing, social work, child welfare, occupational therapy, physiotherapy, radiography, welfare nursing and bioengineering.

In order to promote cooperation and division of labour between universities and university colleges, a network (*Network Norway*) was set up for higher education and research. The network benefits the various academic environments by enabling them to cooperate with regard to fields of specialisation and division of labour. All available courses are reviewed and systematised and each institution is allocated specific areas. The network gives students a larger range of options and makes it easier for them to combine programmes from different institutions. The Network Norway Council has been set up as an advisory body to the Ministry in matters of a long-term, cross-sectored and national character.

The university colleges have considerable academic and administrative autonomy. The institutions have a *national curriculum* for each professional education, approved by the Department for Education. The various university colleges develop their *local curricula* themselves, and make their own decisions regarding organisational and administrative arrangements, students' practical training, pedagogical methods, teaching programmes and so on.

Professional training and vocational studies in the melting pot

Bjoerke (2000) divides the last 40 years of professional education into four different phases: establishing phase, phase of consolidation, reorientation and implementation phase. Most of the health and social studies were established during the 1960s and 1970s; *the establishing phase*. Earlier, some professional training had been run by private organisations. But during the 1970s the studies were organised as a part of 'the regional college' system. The Department for Education wanted to put pressure on establishing common curricula for all the health and social studies in their first year. This led to great dissatisfaction, but the various educational institutions started to cooperate, also with support from their unions, to prevent the Department from continuing their plans. These institutions wanted to remain in their

separate university colleges and were working on structuring their professional identity. The university colleges could continue as partly autonomous.

During the 1980s the government introduced different councils and secretariats to coordinate entrance requirements, exams and qualification standards for teachers. The coordination of these councils and secretariats gave an
opportunity for representatives from different studies to meet in mutual conferences and so on. During these years all the institutions had to make local
curricula which, in turn, showed differences and similarities, not to mention
overlaps. In this perspective we can call the 1980s the *phase of consolidation*.

In 1990 the Council for Health and Social Studies was established. The
council was a professional group, which planned a stronger connection
between the studies and started with instructed cooperation. Interprofessional education and cooperation were highlighted, including an invitation to
mutual curriculum and teaching. In 1998 the Council changed into Network
Norway Council. This phase is characterised by *reorientation*. At the end of
the 1990s we experienced that health and social studies, which assumedly had
much in common, were still unfamiliar to each other, even those that were
situated close on the same site or even in the same buildings.

Entering the first decade of 2000, we come to the *implementation phase*.
The Department of Education decided in 1994 to put forward a proposal
from the Council, regarding a mutual curriculum (10 credits) including most
of the health and the social studies, and a further 10 credits of mutual curriculum in the two social studies (social work and child welfare). The subjects
were scientific theory, ethics, communication and cooperation and scientific
methods (qualitative and quantitative). The aim was to develop common
references and cooperating skills. Only a few university colleges have actually
started this mutual curriculum.

For several decades the Department of Education has tried, in different
ways, to put pressure on the health and social studies in order to promote
interprofessional education. Obviously, there must be some obstacles since
the result is rather discouraging. This outcome might have to do with the
university colleges' autonomy, but could also be related to other factors or
resistance. The Department is not concerned about the organisation and
implementation of interprofessional education and leaves the issue to the
different university colleges to experiment. This means in practice that some
university colleges experiment, some do not. They can also continue to organise the local curriculum separately, in the specific professional studies. One
may suggest that the resistance to cooperate can be linked to what Abbott
(1988: 317) calls the fight for professional jurisdiction; the careers of the
different professionals are regarded as a competition to reign over specific
competence, clients and so forth, and we can see signs of the competition
as a resistance among the different professionals to cooperate, even at the
university colleges.

Organisation of the studies and opportunities for interprofessional education

Regarding the undergraduate studies for health and social workers, we are concerned about the degree to which we should give priority to a professional understanding versus an interprofessional understanding, or whether the interprofessional perspective should come at a later stage, that is during post-graduate education. We can imagine two models to take care of the interprofessional aspects and the particular professional aspects (Bjoerke 2000).

Model one is a traditional model based on a separate organisation of the different professional studies both at undergraduate and postgraduate levels. Cooperation between the studies may occur occasionally depending on the curricula, suitable subjects and the teacher's priorities. This model leaves predominantly interprofessional education and training as a challenge later in the practical field.

The second model emphasises mutual subjects and curricula across the different studies during the undergraduate level. Programmes at postgraduate level are all interprofessional. Model two, which is in accordance with the Department of Education's request, is quite like the existing ways of organising the interprofessional elements in health and social care studies. Several university colleges (Lillehammer, Alta, Volda and Bodoe) have implemented the model in studies for social workers, child welfare and social educators; organising the first year as a mainly mutual year and the next two years mainly separately. At the university colleges in Norway, you will find different combinations of mutual and separate curricula, from completely separate professional teaching, on the one hand, to more or less amalgamation on the other hand.

Mutual subjects – sufficient to promote interprofessional education?

The request from the Department of Education to stimulate mutual curricula is primarily concerning mutual *subjects*. The Department leaves it to the university colleges to decide how to organise and carry out the interprofessional teaching and training. It is important to concretise the content of the cooperation and ways of carrying out and implementing it in the organisations. We would like to argue for focusing on three different aspects: *physical factors, organisational factors* and *teachers competence.*

We find *physical unilocalisation* where the different forms of education are jointly localised geographically and perhaps also in the same buildings, so that teachers and students can have direct contact with each other. This approach is very positive as a starting point and presents an opportunity for interprofessional education. However, it is not a guarantee for more and better coordination between the studies and interprofessional development.

Another aspect is that the studies, which are jointly localised, provide a natural opportunity for interprofessional education. However, these students might not be the natural cooperators as professionals in the future practical field, that is medical laboratory technologists and child welfare workers. The existence of not natural cooperators as professionals challenges the possibly mutual teaching programme, and might make it difficult to see the relevance of interprofessional education and practice.

When we find *organisational coordination*, it implies the development of mutual organisation and coordination of curricula and teaching programmes. The organisational coordination does not necessarily presuppose physical unilocalisation, but naturally it would make it easier to cooperate. We can also conceive a combination of physical unilocalisation and organisational factors, which is the existing model at Stavanger University College, where we work. The studies represented are social work, child welfare work and nursing, including interprofessional postgraduate programmes, all situated in the same building and mutually organised in one department (separate institutes for each profession). This model of coordination gives a greater opportunity for interprofessional cooperation between the studies but which may not, however, be sufficient.

When we have *mutual curricula during the undergraduate education*, we presuppose organisational coordination, which represents a greater opportunity to interprofessional coordination and development, especially regarding specific subjects. But as future professionals the students will have different roles and responsibilities related to different contexts and a different legal framework; it is therefore important that the teaching methods take care of these aspects. Mutual curricula will challenge the teachers in at least two ways: first, who is most qualified regarding their profession and competence and, second, how should one construct the content in order to meet the needs of different student groups. Should teachers representing different professions be able to teach crosswise undergraduate studies? Mutual curricula also actualise questions regarding mutual examinations, adjudicators and so on that consequently lead to a more amalgamated organisation.

In the case that we implement coordination and mutual curricula, we still have to decide at *what time during the education* this is most suitable. We find arguments for starting mutual teaching emphasising interprofessional cooperation already in the first year, assuming that the students are more open-minded and interested in interprofessional cooperation before they become too professionally oriented. Contrarily, we can claim that priority has to be given to the specific professional aspects to give the students a professional identity *before* they can understand their role in interprofessional cooperation. In that case it would be more satisfactory to implement mutual curricula stimulating interprofessional education towards the end of the undergraduate level.

Most postgraduate programmes (advanced studies and master

programmes) in Norway are mutual and interprofessional. Interprofessional postgraduate programmes are requested by the Department for Education as quoted in the national curriculum for postgraduate studies. Whether the postgraduate studies are actually focusing on the development of interprofessional aspects between the studies explicitly, or just function as a physical unilocalisation with a coordinated organisation with mutual subjects, has not been examined very closely. In any case, postgraduate studies have a great potential regarding the development of interprofessional understanding and training if we give preference to these elements.

As illustrated, there are many aspects of coordination and development of interprofessional education, dependent on priorities regarding organisational factors, content of the teaching programmes and teachers' competence and choice of pedagogical methods. One variant is a type of physical coordination where the students are assembled in large lecture rooms and have mutual teaching. There is a possibility that this will stimulate interprofessional understanding, but we assume that putting the students together in the same room is not sufficient to give any interprofessional benefits. However, the effect is primarily related to resources and economical savings (rationalisation).

One way of implementing interprofessional understanding between the students from different undergraduate studies is to develop a variation of different teaching programmes implying opportunities for lecturing, practical training and group work, including possibilities to develop relations between the students. In addition, the teachers can give the students assignments, that is cases, which require mutual solutions, pointing out different angles of incidence including the importance of different professional competence. A problem-based pedagogical approach (PBL method) would seem to be most suitable.

As a conclusion, we can argue that interprofessional education implies various opportunities for combinations of physical and organisational premises, and variables related to the teachers' attitudes and pedagogical methods. We can conceive that the effect of the different combinations and development of interprofessional cooperation is so far associated with uncertainty. We also argue that it is necessary to sort out the variables more carefully when we create a research design to examine the effect.

RELATIONSHIPS BETWEEN INTERPROFESSIONAL EDUCATION AND INTERPROFESSIONAL COOPERATION IN PRACTICE

As mentioned earlier there has been a demand from the health and social sector regarding interprofessional education to improve collaboration in practice and coordination of services towards the users. However, it does not seem as if the educational institutions have taken up the challenge. Very few university colleges have actually developed and started mutual education programmes. Tromso University College started interprofessional education as an introduction in the first year of undergraduate education, including medical students (Ekeli 1992). After a few years, the medical students left the programme and now the programme has been changed to a much smaller introduction course. Oslo University College has carried out an interprofessional education programme with eight different professional studies over four years, in line with the Department of Education's suggestions (Bjoerke 2000). This programme is probably the most systematically implemented programme in Norway up to the present. Experience from this project shows that they still have two main challenges: gaining acceptance for the mutual programme from the teachers who are not participating in it and creating a natural pedagogical setting for studies sited at the same university college, which will not have a natural cooperation situation in practice (i.e. occupational therapists and laboratory technicians).

We also find some research studies related to interprofessional education and professional identity (Almaas 1996; Breivik and Willumsen 2001). Almaas (1996) compared physiotherapy and occupational therapy students and their attitudes towards interprofessional education (shared learning) and practice in Bergen and Tromso. Almaas (1996) found that students who had experienced shared learning in Tromso valued it more than those who lacked such experience in Bergen. Women expressed more positive attitudes towards shared learning than men, older students more than younger and occupational therapists more than physiotherapists. The occupational therapists were also more positive about interprofessional working. Overall, students valued interprofessional working more than shared learning.

Breivik and Willumsen (2001) examined social work, nurse and child welfare students' attitudes, strongly inspired by Almaas' (1996) research design, focusing on three main variables: attitude towards group work, attitude towards interprofessional cooperation and attitude related to the benefit of knowledge of other professions. The first two groups of students were part of the mutual curriculum suggested by the Department of Education, which the university college carried out in 1998/9. The child welfare students did not participate in the mutual curriculum, but they integrated the subjects into their ordinary first year programme. The different student groups answered the same questionnaire at the same time, in the beginning and end of the first year of their first level programmes. Between the two measuring dates, the nurse and social work students were completing the mutual curriculum. The findings showed that the nurse and social work students had developed a small change towards a more sceptical attitude regarding all three main variables; the nurse students turning more negative than the social workers. The attitudes among the child welfare students changed to a slightly more positive attitude towards all three attitude indexes during their first year.

The findings were somehow unexpected. The project was small and the tendencies need to be confirmed by similar studies. The results provoked reflection around some questions related to interprofessional education and practice. Can we assume that interprofessional education necessarily leads to a positive attitude to interprofessional cooperation? If yes, what criteria are essential to promoting good interprofessional education; factors related to organisation and implementation, composition of students, choice of subjects, pedagogical methods, like PBL, teachers' attitudes and competence and so on.

Experience shows that resistance in the teachers' group may influence factors at several levels, including implementation of the interprofessional education programme in principle. Much attention has been paid to the interprofessional part of education. How do the different factors related to the interprofessional and the specific studies promote a positive attitude to interprofessional cooperation and how do the different factors related to the interprofessional and the specific professional education correspond, from the students' point of view and from the teachers' point of view? Furthermore, what extent of interprofessional education may be sufficient to promote a positive attitude towards other professions?

There seem to be many factors influencing different aspects of interprofessional education and practice, including the relation between them. There is a need for sorting out the variables and synthesising them. Assuming that there is a connection between interprofessional education leading to interprofessional understanding, promoting interprofessional cooperation in practice, which in consequence gives the users better services, we would like to present the following draft for a theoretical approach.

As Figure 21.1 shows, we can define 'interprofessional education' as an

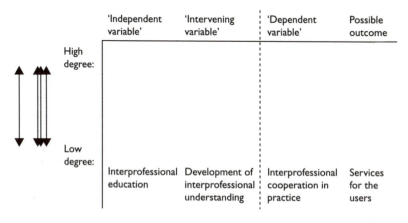

Figure 21.1 Theoretical framework showing possible connections between interprofessional education and services for the users (Breivik & Willumsen 2001).

independent variable. Indicators on this variable might be factors such as organisation and coordination of the curriculum, composition of students, degree of cooperation between the students, choice of subjects, pedagogical methods, composition of professional personnel (competence) and so on. These indicators will influence the degree of interprofessional education, either a high or low degree of interprofessionalisation. We have defined 'development of interprofessional understanding' as the intervening variable. This variable can be measured in different ways, for example through the study of the development of professional versus interprofessional identity (Almaas 1996) or through the study of the development of professional versus interprofessional understanding (Breivik and Willumsen 2001). We assume that the variable 'interprofessional understanding' may vary between a high or low degree of interprofessional understanding, reflecting the students' attitudes. The dependent variable defined as 'interprofessional cooperation in practice' we assume is influenced by the independent variable and the intervening variable.

This is not a figure to illustrate a model of causality. The intention is to make some assumptions about relations between the different variables and indicators that can illustrate possible variations and outcome. The point is to focus on different combinations and patterns that can give us various assumptions of relations and possible outcome. We might find that some combinations of indicators and variables are more essential to promote interprofessional benefits.

To measure the effect of interprofessional education on professional cooperation in practice, we have to include a variety of factors and premises related to the practical context as well. However, while not amplified here, it is important to be conscious of the need for measures to sort out the variables and to make considerations about premises for scientific methods and creating research designs. One suggestion is to use longitudinal research designs where students can be followed over several years, from their education situation and into the practical field.

CONCLUSIONS

As outlined previously, the development of interprofessional education in Norway has been influenced by the health and social policy, education policy and the demand for interprofessional cooperation in practice reflected by the local communities. In spite of the marked pressure from the Department of Education for several decades and great demand from the practical field, it seems as if most of the university colleges still choose to organise their local curricula separately.

Even if the education institutions are state-run, they still have a great degree of autonomy. This factor might be the main reason why the long-lasting pressure for more cooperation from the government has given a far more discouraging result than expected. Autonomy gives the university colleges freedom to organise their curricula according to local premises and requirements, which gives opportunities for experimenting and making the most of local potential and resources. This context is also the intention from the government's point of view. However, looking at the historical develop-ment of interprofessional education, we might assume that the government would have preferred to have the opportunity to intervene more directly into the university colleges' activities. The only way of directing the education institutions' activities, as far as we can see, is for the government to use financial strategies; either economical restrictions or economical 'carrots', which are especially designed for stimulating interprofessional education. The latter seems somehow unrealistic in today's situation. So financial restrictions might be a more suitable means, which would make the university colleges consider possible changes of organising the curricula. In consequence, this approach might effect interprofessional education, that is mutual curricula, but primarily motivated as a means of rationalisation. However, referring to our previous presentation, financial restrictions might not be the best basis for organising interprofessional education, and will not be a sufficient guar-antee as such. The government's opportunity to direct the education institu-tions regarding interprofessional education is, in other words, still rather limited.

How are we to understand the university colleges' reluctance? Even at university colleges where we find student groups being natural cooperators in the future and where there is an opportunity to coordinate curricula because of the supportive physical, organisational and administrative arrangements, we still find very little cooperation between the different professional insti-tutes. The lack of cooperation might be due to a general indolence towards changes in these systems. There are two factors to point out: teachers' resist-ance and fear of amalgamation. There seems to be a tendency to under-estimate teachers' influence on teaching programmes and students' attitudes, both in a positive and a negative way regarding interprofessional education: especially teachers, who have a professional education or vocational training previous to their higher degrees and who seem to be particularly concerned and protective regarding professional roles and boundaries. This position can partly be related to the importance of giving the students a professional identity, but it can also be related to the teachers' insecurity regarding their own competence and professional knowledge about relevant contexts, which naturally will be challenged when teaching other professions. These factors can also reinforce each other. Of course, you will find teachers with a profes-sional competence in their educational background being open-minded and inclusive towards other professions. Our point is, however, that teachers' atti-tudes, either connected to interprofessional programmes or specific profes-sional programmes, which may not have received sufficient attention so far, in relation to their influence on interprofessional education and students' attitudes.

Referring to our previous outline regarding organisational and administrative factors related to interprofessional education, we notice that blurring boundaries might be between different steps of coordination; from separate to more mutual curricula. Blurring boundaries might be conceived as confusing and also regarded as a fear of a possible amalgamation of departments or educational institutions leading to a closing down of some of them. This threat is reinforced when related to the government's education policy where the aim is more cooperation between educational institutions, and may therefore be regarded as an indirect strategy aimed at attaining the government's goal. Both teachers' attitudes and their fear of amalgamation are factors that are more or less hidden and therefore difficult to measure, but they might have an important indirect influence on the interprofessional education programmes.

There is no doubt about the demand for interprofessional cooperation in the practical field. But, as emphasised previously, the relationship between interprofessional education and interprofessional cooperation in practice is associated with uncertainty. Research projects show that the interprofessional education programmes influence the students' attitudes towards cooperation with other professions or interprofessional understanding, both in a positive and negative way. Many factors influence their attitudes; physical and organisational premises, teachers' attitudes and pedagogical methods and so on. The challenge is to find the combination of variables that produces the greatest benefits regarding students' positive attitudes towards other professions. This approach is probably the optimal contribution the education institutions are able to give to create good interprofessional education and promote interprofessional cooperation in practice. Whether this is sufficient to carry out good interprofessional cooperation in the practical field will remain to be seen, but at least it is a good starting point.

REFERENCES

Aarseth, T. (1984) *Tverretatlig samordning – i alle fall et forsoek*, hovedoppgave i offentlig administrasjon og organisasjonsvitenskap, Bergen: Universitetet i Bergen.

Abbott, A. (1988) *The Systems of Professions: An Essay on the Division of Expert Labor*, Chicago: University of Chicago Press.

Almaas, S. (1996) *Helsefaglig identitet: betingelser for at studenter skal utvikle identitet som helsearbeider*, Bergen: Det medisinske fakultet/Det psykologiske fakultet/ Senter for etter-og videreutdanning Universitet i Bergen.

Andersen, R. (1992) *Samordning under lupen*, Oslo: Tano forlag.

Askheim, O. (1989) *Samordning: ovenfra og ned eller nedenfra og opp*, Oslo: Konferanserapport, Kultur- og vitenskapsdepartementet.

Askheim, O. and Roenning. R. (1987) *Samordning av tiltak paa lokalplanet for utsatte barne og ungdomsgrupper*, Lillehammer: Oestlandsforskning.

Birkelund, G. (1999) *Sosial trygghet, marginalisering i en velferdsstat*, Fafo rapport 301, Oslo: Forskningsstiftelsen Fafo.

Bjoerke, G. (2000) '*Lille Veks*' *Ein pilotstudie av eit pilotprosjekt*, HIO-notat 2000 nr 12, Oslo: Hoegskolen i Oslo.

Breivik, P. and Willumsen, E. (2001) *Utvikling av tverrfaglig forstaaelse? En analyse av mulige konsekvenser av felles undervisning mellom sykepleieutdanningen og sosiono-mutdanningen ved Hoegskolen i Stavanger*, Stavanger: Avdeling for Helse og Sosialfag, Hoegskolen i Stavanger.

Ekeli, B. (1992) 'Tromso hoester erfaringer hele landet kan bruke', in R. Andersen (ed.), *Samordning under lupen*, Oslo: Tano.

Gullichsen, A. (1989) *Hvorfor er samarbeid saa vanskelig?*, Trondheim: Norsk voksen-pedagogisk institutt.

Jensen, B. (1986) *Samordning i helse- og sosialtjenesten*, Oslo: Universitetsforlaget.

Johannessen, A. (1998) *Fattigdom i Norge – et oekende problem?* HiO-notat 1998 nr 4, Oslo: Hoegskolen i Oslo.

Repstad, P. (ed.) (1993) *Dugnadsaand og forsvarsverker: Tverretatlig samarbeid i teori og praksis*, Oslo: Tano Forlag.

Chapter 22

Interprofessional work and education

Developments in Hong Kong

Diana Lee

SUMMARY

With the exception of some pioneering progress in the provision of community care for elderly people, the development of interprofessional work and education in Hong Kong is relatively recent. This chapter begins with a brief outline of Hong Kong's system of health and social care provision. Some of the key policy and organisational initiatives, primarily in elderly services, that have an impact on bringing health and social care professionals to learn and work together are then analysed. Finally, some major issues that need to be considered in the promotion of further developments in interprofessional work and education in Hong Kong are discussed.

BACKGROUND

The development of interprofessional work and education is relatively recent in Hong Kong. This chapter outlines and analyses some of the key policy and organisational initiatives and their impact on bringing health and social care professionals to learn and work together in an attempt to provide insights for further discussion, debate and activity in this area in Hong Kong.

Hong Kong is a small territory situated on the south China coast. Ethnic Chinese constitute 98 per cent of the total population. Provision of health and social services in the territory involves a variety of agencies. Some are in the public sector such as government departments or statutory authorities. Some are non-government organisations, which may be subsidised by the government, and some are in the private sector. The health and social care sector is enormous and includes a wide diversity of roles and functions. The Health and Welfare Bureau is the government branch responsible for the overall formulation of health and social welfare policy. It is composed of the Medical and Health Division and the Welfare Division. The former is responsible for policy matters relating to medical and health services and the latter for policy matters relating to social welfare. While the Secretary for the

Bureau oversees both divisions, the major responsibilities for health and social welfare are dealt with independently by the two divisions. As a consequence, considerable attention has to be paid to the mechanisms and collaborative activities of the two divisions in order to provide integrated health and social care services that meet the requirements of patients and other service users.

The Bureau is responsible for a number of departments related to health and social welfare, such as the Department of Health and Social Welfare. The Hospital Authority, which is a quasi-autonomous statutory body responsible for the management of all public hospitals in Hong Kong, is also accountable and subject to the directions of the Bureau.

In the following sections, the health and social service environments in Hong Kong is briefly outlined. The provision of health and social care for elderly people is then used as an example to provide a general background to understanding the nature, problems and values of interprofessionalism. In the last section, the extent and nature of interprofessional education in Hong Kong is explored.

Health care services

Health care services in Hong Kong encompass hospital medical services, public health and preventive care. A variety of agencies are involved in the provision of such services – government, private and voluntary but government-subvented. However, agencies in the public sector have the greatest influence on health service provision. Medical hospital services expanded rapidly in the 1960s and 1970s. This expansion was in accordance with government policy to provide subsidised or free medical services for all those unable to purchase or obtain care from other sources (Phillips 1998). Yet, development of public health and preventive care lagged very much behind hospital-based services (Grant and Yuen 1998).

However, in the mid-1980s, hospital medical services showed signs of considerable pressure as reflected in overcrowded wards and long waiting lists. A review of hospital medical services was therefore carried out. After a period of public consultation, the government decided in 1987 to establish the Hospital Authority as a statutory authority to oversee and manage the provision and delivery of an integrated hospital service, which would encompass all government and subvented hospitals. Provision of public health and preventive programmes was assigned as the responsibility of a government department – the Department of Health. The Hospital Authority, a major new body dealing specifically with hospital and hospital-based services, was finally established in 1992.

There has been criticism that the Hospital Authority was conceived in the absence of a clearly defined and long-term overall health policy in the territory to guide effectively the development of the health care system (Yuen

1992). The creation of such a separate body was seen as a local short-sighted response that ran counter to the trend in developed countries such as the UK, Australia and New Zealand to unify the public sector agencies dealing with health, social and community services (Grant and Yuen 1998). This trend is based on the fact that organisational, professional and financial boundaries that restrict patient movement between sectors or agencies have become recognised as important barriers to the provision of a coordinated spectrum of health and social care that is effective and efficient for service users.

Set against such criticisms, the corporate vision of the Hospital Authority was to collaborate with other service agencies in the community to create a seamless health care environment so as to ensure continuity of care provided to patients (Hospital Authority 1994). Attention has therefore been increasingly given to the consideration of interagency collaboration. New services such as the community-based geriatric assessment teams and community-based psychogeriatric teams have been developed. These teams are interdisciplinary in nature, led by either a consultant or a senior doctor who works with one or two nurses, occupational therapists and social workers. The teams work with other agencies in supporting patients and their carers at home or in the community setting, most often in residential and nursing homes (Wong 1996). New community care delivery models, such as case management, have also been piloted and evaluated (Mackenzie et al 1998).

Obviously, achievement of this corporate vision of the Hospital Authority requires agency personnel to possess skills in interprofessional collaboration and teamwork. However, interprofessional preparation of such skills is greatly lacking in Hong Kong. In addition, tensions and concerns of interprofessionalism with regard to professional territorism and rivalry have surfaced. In a pilot study of the case management model in community care, for example, community nurses were being assigned as case managers to assess, plan and coordinate the overall care delivery in the community (Mackenzie et al 1998). They continuously assessed and monitored their assigned patients in their homes and developed programmes of care to meet patient needs. They also made referrals where necessary to other agencies or service providers for integrated care delivery. The referral system that emerged required much dialogue and negotiation with different community agencies and professionals.

Social services

Social services have not been well developed in Hong Kong (Chow 1985). Before the Second World War there was a history of charitable efforts by voluntary and religious organisations. The role of the government in providing social services became significant only after the early 1960s (Kwan 1989). Chinese people tend to be self-reliant and are not actively willing to receive assistance from the government. The government has been careful not to destroy these traits and the traditional social networks such as the family. Social services policies have therefore been planned in an *ad-hoc* fashion to deal in the short term with isolated pressing needs (Ngan 1997).

The scope of social services in Hong Kong generally covers social security, family services, children and youth services, elderly services, community development, services for disabled persons, medical social services and services for offenders. These services are provided by voluntary social welfare agencies and by the government mainly through the Social Welfare Department. However, the administration of major social services is provided by voluntary agencies, which are funded mainly by the government. Indeed, apart from social security and services for offenders, two-thirds of social services provision comes through programmes run by voluntary agencies. About 80 per cent of all social services personnel are therefore working in the voluntary sector.

As can be seen, statutory provision of health and social care in Hong Kong is dealt with independently by two separate sectors – the health care sector consisting of the Hospital Authority and Department of Health and the social care sector represented by the Social Welfare Department. With the exception of the Hospital Authority, which is an autonomous statutory body but subject to the directions of the Bureau, the two sectors are administered under the Health and Welfare Bureau. Except for some of the initiatives undertaken by the Hospital Authority, which are not yet formally assessed for impact and outcome, there is little evidence of mechanisms or activities that coordinate the two sectors in the provision of integrated health and social services for the people of Hong Kong. Most of the voluntary agencies are concerned with social care provision while the private sector deals mainly with health care provision. Interprofessional working is still relatively new in Hong Kong, especially outside the health care team concept. However, some promising developments in interprofessional collaboration are evident in the recent proposed reforms in elderly services.

Elderly services

As in many other countries in the world, one of the most pressing issues in Hong Kong concerns its ageing population. In 2001 there were 747,052 elderly people aged 65 or over, representing 11.1 per cent of the total population (Census and Statistics 2001). Except for elders who live alone (9 per cent) and those who are in institutions (5.5 per cent), the majority live with their families in the community. Increasing attention is therefore being paid to issues that relate to the provision of community care for elderly people. Very often, elders have diverse and complex needs that have implications for daily life and care at home. Many times, these needs may cross-cut organisational and professional boundaries, requiring a coordinated interagency and interprofessional response (Evers et al 1994). Community care for elderly people is thus an area of constant and dynamic debate. New problems have to be addressed as new and different issues arise.

Community health and social care for elderly people

Community-based medical and health services for the elderly population are provided by the Hospital Authority and the Department of Health. The Hospital Authority supplies community nursing teams to provide services to patients through home visits, and community geriatric assessment teams to assess elders applying for long term residential placements and to provide support to care providers in the residential care homes. Outpatient clinics and day hospitals are major primary and secondary health care resources for elders living in the community. The newly established Elderly Health Centres and Visiting Health Teams are run by the Department of Health. These centres and teams are mostly located together in the general outpatient clinics to facilitate the provision of primary health care for elderly people.

There are four major types of social services available to elderly people in the community. These include home help, day care centre, multi-service centre and social centre. These services are fully subvented by the government through the Social Welfare Department and are run by non-government organisations. Home help service includes general personal care, meal service, household management, purchase and delivery of daily necessities, laundry service and escort service. Day care centres provide personal care and limited nursing service for elderly people with declining health who have no family members to look after them on a full-time basis. Multi-service centres are run on a district basis and social centres on a neighbourhood basis. These centres provide services to meet social, recreational and other day-to-day needs of elderly people in the community.

There are other social services, though limited in number, that provide support to the elderly population and their family members in the form of volunteer services, respite services, community education and holiday centre for the elders.

Policy initiatives for elderly services

The first Programme Plan to address the needs of elderly people in Hong Kong was drawn up in 1977. This Plan indicated the inadequacies of services for the elderly population in general and in particular recommended the need for policy and service coordination among government departments and between service providers. However, it was 10 years later, in 1987, that a Central Coordinating Committee on Services for the Elderly was set up to take on responsibility for regular reviews of the Programme Plan. This Committee produced a report in 1998 – recommendations of which echoed very much the earlier first Programme Plan for the Elderly. Nevertheless, the recommendations of the Committee were not implemented through any designated administrative machinery.

The need for closer attention to interprofessional relations in elderly services was highlighted when, in the early 1990s, a number of inquiries identified a lack of coordination across professions and agencies. Gaps in communication between professional groups in different organisations, resulting in either denial or duplication of service provision, were common. There was also growing concern that the services for older people were confusing to the end-users, and that service needs rather than user needs were taking priority. In 1993, the government appointed a Working Group on Care for the Elderly to review the provision of services for elderly people. An Elderly Services Division was created in 1994 under the Welfare Division to oversee policy related to social welfare, and medical and health services for older people. The Elderly Services Division liaised with other government departments to coordinate and develop programmes and consulted with non-government organisations, professional and other groups on the needs of older people (Hong Kong Government 1994). The creation of this Division was the government's initial formal attempt to encourage interprofessional and interagency collaboration.

Despite this initiative, coordination and integration of service policies were still not seriously discussed both within and across departments (Grant and Yuen 1998). Service policies at a departmental level were often made within the confines and particular expertise of a department. Unless specific requests for cross-department cooperation were made, departments generally remained isolated. As a result, coordination of interdepartmental services was very difficult to achieve. For example, community elderly long-term care clients were sometimes receiving seven or eight different types of service from different departments at the same time. Different organisations and professionals currently provide these services. Services thus provided tend to be fragmented and in many cases overlap with elders having to be assessed many times for different types of service. In addition, each organisation has its own priority in service delivery. It was therefore very difficult for the elders and their families to understand and make enquiries about their situations and even more difficult for them to participate in the planning, management and delivery of such services.

A consultancy study was therefore commissioned in 1998 to review the provision of care services for elderly people living in the community. Problems of service provision in terms of fragmentation between service providers and gaps in provision were once again highlighted. Care services were described as ineffective, with the extent and depth of problems escalating. The study recommended the introduction of an integrated long-term care system for the provision of community care services in Hong Kong (Chi et al 1998).This system proposes that a network of organisations should provide or arrange to provide a coordinated continuum of services to a defined elderly population. It is designed around home and community care with residential care being considered only for those people with a high level of impairment and limited informal care. A new long-term care office will be created for service coordination, quality monitoring and funding. There will be a central office and a number of regional offices. These offices will be staffed by the multidisciplinary teams of health and social care professionals and supporting staff involved in long-term care provision.

To achieve this integrated system, the formation of an Interprofessional Practice Council is proposed. This council will consist of representatives from health and social service professions to promote full interprofessional collaboration within the integrated system. Some of the Council's functions include:

- To assume a leadership role in facilitating and coordinating professional practice standards for all members of the interprofessional health team working in the long-term care system
- To promote full interprofessional collaboration with the long-term care system to ensure all members of the interprofessional health team are able to fulfil a full scope of professional practice
- To promote an integrated approach in the delivery of long-term service
- To accept a leadership imperative to facilitate resolution of interprofessional practice issues that may arise and effect resolution by consensus
- To provide education and consultation to the team members on interprofessional practice issues

When the consultancy report was published, the anticipated drastic changes in funding, staffing structures and staff status as a result of the new proposed system created many concerns among the different professionals involved in long-term care. Interprofessional issues, such as the criteria for service eligibility within the system, the functions of the Interprofessional Practice Council, and the role of the different professionals in the system, were especially debated.

In the proposed new integrated system, service needs' assessment and authorisation will be the responsibility of a long-term care officer. It is also proposed that comprehensive admission and discharge criteria be developed to aid the long-term care officer in decision-making. A set of such criteria has been proposed by the consultancy group. However, differences in service philosophy, principles and work approaches among the different professionals involved in long-term care provision have resulted in differing view points about the criteria. The medical professionals, for example, disagreed strongly with the use of strict criteria for evaluation of long-term care service eligibility. Heterogenicity is asserted as the rule of assessment for elderly clients. Moreover, doctors argued that expert clinical judgement should not be replaced by strict admission and discharge criteria. Medical professionals also suggested geriatricians to be the most appropriate gatekeepers to long-term care services. The social care professionals, on the other hand, supported the development of the criteria but criticised the proposed criteria heavily, as being too medically oriented and not sufficiently reflective of the social needs of elderly people.

The proposal that the Interprofessional Practice Council be responsible for professional practice standards for the different professionals involved in long-term care provision also raised major concerns. The medical profession has argued strongly that it should be the remit of the Medical Council to lead, develop and coordinate professional standards of the clinicians, rather than the responsibility of the Interprofessional Practice Council.

These debates have provided a healthy platform for interprofessional concerns to be revealed, clarified and discussed. Indeed, the discussion surrounding the provision of community care for elderly people sets a good example that demonstrates how successful interprofessional work depends on the recognition of differences, interdependence and shared objectives (Biggs 1997) in order for the unique contributions of each discipline to be enhanced and rivalry to be reduced. In the past, the divisions between health and social care professionals were shaped, not only by claims to specific knowledge, skills and values, but also by policy and organisational developments, which have reinforced the sense of separateness between professional groups. In moving forward, obstacles related to the protection of organisational and professional boundaries and the transfer of resources are to be expected. These problems may occur at different levels and in many ways (Evers et al 1994). These issues may involve senior management at the broader policy level, or may involve middle managers. The contentions may also occur in the practice context, involving fieldworkers, service users and informal carers. Finally, obstacles may also be encountered because of problems in intra-agency structures, policies, communication channels and relationships. Intervening steps have to be created at all these levels in order that any relevant policy may be translated into practice.

INTERPROFESSIONAL EDUCATION

While the need to move towards interprofessional working is acknowledged and being addressed, interprofessional learning is a relatively new concept in Hong Kong. The major health workforce consists of doctors, nurses and other allied health professionals who have statutory registration requirements, such as pharmacists, physiotherapists, occupational therapists and radiographers. Local tertiary education is available for all these categories of the professional workforce. For programmes that lead to a first qualification (pre-registration), professionals neither share common courses, nor receive mixed teaching, both academic and clinical, from other professional teachers or share seminars with students of other professions. This segregation further distances learners from their fellow health professionals.

The social welfare workforce consists mainly of social workers with various degrees of professional skill and specialisation. Proper training for social workers was introduced in the early 1960s when the role of the government in social services provision was increased. Social work education in Hong Kong is provided in local tertiary institutes but mixed learning with other professionals is not evident in the pre-registration programmes.

However, some pioneering developments were initiated a few years ago in the field of gerontological education. This is understandable given the noticeable developments of elderly policies and services in the last few years that acknowledge the need for interprofessional collaboration. Nevertheless, there are few resources available for the promotion of interprofessional education in Hong Kong. The progress that has been made in gerontological education mainly comes from self-financed continuing education and post-registration programmes run by professional bodies, research centres and tertiary institutes. Charity organisations also donate funds for these initiatives. These different programmes are outlined below.

University-based interprofessional education

The Chinese University of Hong Kong Centre for Gerontology and Geriatrics

In 1999, the Centre for Gerontology and Geriatrics was inaugurated at the Chinese University of Hong Kong. Designated as an area of excellence in the University, this interdisciplinary centre draws on the expertise of various disciplines, such as medicine, community and family medicine, psychiatry, orthopaedics and traumatology, nursing, sociology, social work and psychology. The main objectives of this Centre are to conduct interdisciplinary research on the implications of ageing for the Hong Kong population and the measures to meet the consequences and to provide undergraduate and post-graduate teaching in the areas of gerontological health and social care. In 2000 a Masters of Science in Clinical Gerontology was offered. This development aims to encourage interprofessional learning among professionals involved in the care of older people in different health and social care settings so as to promote interprofessional working. Students admitted to this programme hold a first degree in either health or social sciences. It is a two-year programme comprising taught and practical components, as well as a research project.

The theory component of this programme is taught by an interdisciplinary team of academics and practitioners. It is organised into the following five modules:

- Demography, sociology, social work and health economics
- Epidemiology, biostatistics and research methodology
- Biology of ageing and concept of successful ageing
- Services for the older population
- Clinical topics

The practical component consists of a two-hour per week attachment in an elderly health and/or social care setting for six months. A mentor is appointed in the setting to supervise students' practical learning. The research project is conducted under the supervision of a supervisor. The clinical mentors and project supervisors, who may be of a different profession to that of the students, play a key role in assisting interprofessional learning.

The students who have enrolled into this programme include medical officers, general practitioners, social workers, occupational therapists, physiotherapists and nurses. Building on the success with this programme, a diploma in clinical gerontology for health and social care professionals was implemented in 2001. Students on this programme share the same theoretical and practical components of the Master's programme, but do not need to complete a research project.

The School of Continuing Education

The School of Continuing Education at the Chinese University of Hong Kong has jointly organised a Graduate Diploma in Gerontology and a Masters of Health Science (Gerontology) with the School of Health, University of New England, Australia. These courses are offered to health and social care professionals who are already qualified in their professional roles and wish to pursue a postgraduate gerontology programme. Students may choose to exit after one and a half years to obtain a graduate diploma or continue with another year to obtain a Master's qualification. The core units in both programmes include:

- Introduction to gerontology
- Research methods in health
- Clinical gerontology
- Management issues in aged care
- Complementary therapies in the health care system
- Research topics in gerontology
- Gerontology clinical study and specialised gerontology topics

The additional units for a Master's qualification include introduction to dementia care and counselling theory.

The Open University of Hong Kong

The Open University of Hong Kong conducts a one year part-time Certificate in Gerontology for health professionals with a recognised qualification, such as nurses, physiotherapists and occupational therapists. The course consists of six modules:

- Basic theories of ageing
- Physical support in ageing I and II
- Psychosocial support in ageing
- Authenticating the discipline
- Promotion in healthy ageing

Visits to various practice settings such as nursing homes, day hospitals, community centres and rehabilitation centres are also arranged.

The University of Hong Kong Centre on Ageing

Launched in 1999 as an area of excellence in the University of Hong Kong, this Centre brings in the expertise of diverse disciplines to enhance the well-being of older persons. These disciplines include geriatrics, community medicine, family medicine, psychiatry, dentistry, nursing, psychology, sociology, social work, urban planning, architecture, statistics and actuarial science. The Centre offers short training courses and workshops for health and social care professionals. The Centre also seeks funding from the government and charity organisations to run training courses for family carers, home helpers and personal care workers who work in residential homes.

Continuing professional education

The Hong Kong Association of Gerontology

Founded in 1987, the Hong Kong Association of Gerontology is an interdisciplinary organisation that works to promote the care of elderly people in Hong Kong through encouraging cooperation among organisations and training of staff involved in gerontological care. Interprofessional input to the work of the association is reflected in the 10 council seats that represent medicine, nursing, occupational therapy/physiotherapy, social work, service administration and education. Members of the association also reflect the various different professional groups that are involved in the delivery of elderly services. The association organises a number of training courses, seminars, workshops and conferences for its members and other health and social care workers involved in elderly care. These educational forums provide valuable opportunities for the development of interprofessional relationships and learning. The annual congress of gerontology held by the Association since 1993 is perhaps the most consistent forum for exchange of research and information on collaborative practice and education.

The Hong Kong Institute of Gerontology

With support from the government and sponsorship from the Hong Kong Association of Gerontology and a charitable fund from the Hong Kong Jockey Club, the Hong Kong Institute of Gerontology was set up in 2001 to be a research and training centre in gerontology. Since its establishment, the institute has taken over most of the educational function of the Hong Kong Association of Gerontology and has conducted a variety of training courses, workshops and seminars for health and social care workers involved in gerontological care. The aim of these interprofessional educational endeavours is to strengthen the ability of health and social care professionals to work across disciplines for collaborative service delivery for elderly people.

SOME REFLECTIONS ON INTERPROFESSIONAL EDUCATION IN HONG KONG

As can be see, apart from opportunities for health and social care professionals involved in gerontological care to learn together at different post-registration levels, interprofessional education remains a new concept to promote and implement in Hong Kong. The traditional institutional or organisational segregation of the education of health and social care professionals is one of the great barriers. Although there are initial efforts for interprofessional learning in gerontological care, there is a general lack of evidence to support these types of development. The benefits of such developments in terms of patient care and change in the individual's working performance have not yet been established. Health and social care professionals might find it difficult to see it as worth while to use resources for such developments. At present, individual professionals are paying for their post-registration or continuing education. When interprofessional education starts to develop, programmes leading to pre-registration qualifications will naturally be considered. At present, these programmes are conducted and funded separately for the different professions. The current financial constraints across the health and social care sectors in Hong Kong in general will further discourage the discussion of such developments, which will obviously impact on the already scarce resources traditionally made available to the different professions. Last but not least, the preparation of teachers qualified to teach interprofessional courses or programmes is an issue that has to be well planned before any development of interprofessional education is to take place in Hong Kong.

Casto (1994) has outlined the essential elements for establishing the inter-professional education programmes. These factors include a neutral base of operation, administrative support, shared interest/commitment, credit and resources, partnership with community, training in collaborative skills, building horizontal bridges and rewards for collaborative endeavours. In looking ahead, the development of shared learning and education in Hong Kong has to consider carefully these elements. The parameters in Hong Kong may need to be extended to involve, not only the professional groups who are engaged in elderly care, but also the informal caring sector, which has all along supported the community care of elderly people. Bringing professional and informal carers together facilitates the effectiveness of interprofessional work as informal carers are expert co-workers of professionals in the care of the dependent elders (Mackenzie and Lee 1999). This form of joint working is especially relevant in a culture where Chinese elders are reluctant to share their concerns and expectations with people who are considered outside the family (Lee 1999, 2001).

CONCLUSION

In reviewing the developments of interprofessional work and education in Hong Kong, it becomes apparent that the divisions between health and social care are shaped, not only by claims to specific knowledge, skills and values, but also by policy and organisation developments, which have reinforced the sense of separateness among professional groups. If interprofessional collaboration is to develop across the whole spectrum of health and social care provision in Hong Kong, there is a need to acknowledge that such endeavours will challenge, not only individual and professional norms, but also institutional values. Formal and informal structures and opportunities for sharing of presuppositions and constraints under which professionals and institutions usually make decisions, teach and practise should be provided so that freedom exists to explore new ideas and alternatives, and possibly develop shared credit and commitment (Casto 1994). When professionals and institutions accept rather than reject challenges and opportunities of interprofessional education and practice, then interprofessional endeavours will become the norm rather than the exception.

It is also important that more should be done to demonstrate any long-term benefits of interprofessional education and work. Much of the existing reported success of interprofessional initiatives focuses on process elements of teamwork rather than on outcomes (Gerrish 1999). Research is needed to evaluate the impact of these changes and their contribution to improved health and quality of life and to demonstrate how far interprofessional and interagency collaboration actually improves the service and how far collaborative working bridges the gaps in service provision. Finally, examples of good interprofessional practice in education and work should be widely publicised.

REFERENCES

Biggs, S. (1997) 'Interprofessional collaboration: problems and prospects', in J. Ovretveit, P. Mathias and T. Thompson (eds), *Interprofessional Working for Health and Social Care*, London: Macmillan.

Casto, M. (1994) 'Inter-professional work in the USA – education and practice', in A. Leathard (ed.), *Going Inter-Professional – Working Together for Health and Welfare*, London: Routledge.

Census and Statistics Department (2001) *2001 Population Census – Summary Results*, Hong Kong: Hong Kong Special Administrative Region.

Chi, I., Lam, Z. and Chan, P. (1998) *Consultancy Study on Review of Care Services for Elderly Living in the Community*, Hong Kong: Hong Kong University.

Chow, N. (1985) 'Hong Kong', in J. Dixon and H. S. Kim (eds), *Social Welfare in Asia*, London: Croom Helm.

Evers, H., Cameron, E. and Badger, F. (1994) 'Inter-professional work with old and disabled people', in A. Leathard (ed.), *Going Inter-Professional – Working Together for Health and Welfare*, London: Routledge.

Gerrish, K. (1999) 'Teamwork in primary care: an evaluation of the contribution of integrated nursing teams', *Health and Social Care in the Community* 7 (5) 367–75.

Grant, C. and Yuen, P. (1998) *The Hong Kong Health Care System*, School of Health Services Management: University of New South Wales.

Hong Kong Government (1994) *Report of the Working Group on the Care of the Elderly*, Hong Kong: Hong Kong Government.

Hospital Authority (1994) *Annual Plan 1994–1995*, Hong Kong: Hospital Authority.

Kwan, A. (1989) 'Social welfare and services in Hong Kong', in A. Kwan (ed.), *Hong Kong Society*, Hong Kong: Writers' and Publishers' Cooperative.

Lee, D. (1999) 'Transition to residential care: experiences of elderly Chinese people in Hong Kong', *Journal of Advanced Nursing* 30 (5) 1118–26.

Lee, D. (2001) 'Perceptions of Hong Kong Chinese elders on adjustment to residential care', *Journal of Interprofessional Care* 15 (3) 235–44.

Mackenzie, A., Lee, D., Dudley-Brown, S. and Chin, M. (1998) 'The processes of case management: a review of the evaluation of a pilot study for elderly people in Hong Kong', *Journal of Nursing Management* 6, 293–301.

Mackenzie, A. and Lee, D. (1999) 'Carers and lay caring', in S. Redfern and F. Ross (eds), *Nursing Elderly People*, London: Churchill Livingstone.

Ngan, R. (1997) 'Social welfare', in J. Cheng (ed.), *The Other Hong Kong Report 1997*, Hong Kong: The Chinese University Press.

Phillips, D. (1998) *The Epidemiological Transition in Hong Kong*, Hong Kong: Centre of Asian Studies University of Hong Kong.

Wong, V. (1996) 'Medical and health', in M. K. Nyaw and S. M. Li (eds), *The Other Hong Kong Report 1996*, Hong Kong: The Chinese University Press.

Yuen, P. (1992) 'Medical and health', in J. Cheng and P. Kwong (eds), *The Other Hong Kong Report 1992*, Hong Kong: The Chinese University Press.

Chapter 23

Multiprofessional education

Global perspectives

Rita Goble

SUMMARY

Multiprofessional education has moved from a European-centred arena towards a global context. Recent developments have focused on the improvement of patient care in the community. European centres that have made a contribution to the development of multiprofessional education include the universities of Bobigny, Linkoping and Exeter. However, the changing world scene is reflected in the recent merger of the European Network for the Development of Multiprofessional Education in Health Sciences; and The Network: Community Partnerships for Health through Innovative Education, Service and Research which, in turn, may become more integrated with the Towards Unity for Health Project funded by the World Health Organization. A creative scheme in Latin America, 'Una Nova Iniciativa na Educacao dos Profissionais de Saude: Uniao a Communidade', illustrates the emphasis now placed on community-based education world-wide. This chapter highlights the global potential for the future of multiprofessional education.

BACKGROUND

Health and social care is faced with the increasing demands of an elderly population coupled with the emergence of infectious and complex diseases such as HIV/AIDS. If optimum outcomes are to be attained, ever-increasing levels of coordinated and collaborative care between the professions will be essential world-wide.

Increasing evidence suggests that collaborative learning leads to collaborative care. The advantages of collaborative work are claimed to include a greater range of professional skills, more efficient deployment of relevant skills that may or may not be highly specific, more choice for the consumer, avoidance of stereotyping, checks on procedures, mutual education, mutual support, development of high morale, cost-effective training and provision of care (Pereira Gray and Goble 1998).

However, the barriers to implementing multiprofessional education (MPE), practice and research are numerous. In the past attitudinal, organisational, political and financial problems have become cumulative. These hidden forces have even questioned the importance of 'learning together to work together' (Goble 1990). Perhaps the largest single obstacle relates to the attitudes of many health and social care professionals. Quite simply, they do not think it is important to use precious resources to promote collaborative activities. The role and relationships of the various professions are surprisingly unclear and there may even be little awareness or insight into their everyday working relationships. Another major barrier is organisational since many of the undergraduate courses that lead to qualification involve the 'segregation' of the learners into buildings and courses, which distance them from fellow students.

Multiprofessional dialogue has largely centred on pressing questions related to 'clinical irritations' (Snadden 1997). In the past it has also been *ad hoc* and depended on the formation of a critical mass of local enthusiasts who have been able to meet frequently, communicate easily and share ideas within a limited geographical area. Importantly, these enthusiasts have had to 'acquire' financial support in a variety of innovative ways (Goble 2001).

Now that multiprofessional education is becoming increasingly recognised world-wide and initiatives are emerging on a global scale, there is an urgent need to identify, document and monitor them. Importantly, it will be necessary to describe and support multiprofessional programmes, identify the qualities of the 'good' multiprofessional practitioner and document the provision of 'good' multiprofessional systems of care world-wide. This chapter now turns to key developments in multiprofessional education in Europe, which then leads on to a review of global initiatives.

EARLY ACADEMIC PROGRAMMES OF MULTIPROFESSIONAL EDUCATION (MPE) IN EUROPE

A number of MPE programmes have been pioneered in Europe. The early developments of the 1970s and 1980s influenced the formation of a European Network, dedicated solely to MPE. However, the development of MPE has also been recognised and incorporated into larger organisations with more extensive coverage of health and social care issues.

The desire of the World Health Organization (WHO) to become involved in the MPE of the health professions led to the formation of the European Network for the Development of Multiprofessional Education in Health Sciences (EMPE). The pioneers of EMPE came from Europe; namely Sweden, France and the UK. First, the University of Bobigny, Paris had introduced an innovative approach in 1984 concerned with orienting undergraduate students towards different health professions. Multiprofessional collaboration, which lasted for two years, offered students who were interested in a career in health sciences an opportunity to discover which fields suited them best.

The programme was organised around MPE core units, which were undertaken by all students. In addition, all students undertook a multidisciplinary survey. This covered an urban community wherein each student intake dealt with priority problems selected for that year by a group of community representatives, epidemiological researchers and university teachers. In addition, each student had to meet health personnel, analyse their functions and learn about the structures within which they worked, their relations with other health personnel and the problems encountered.

This initiative was intended to guide the students towards the various health care professions: medicine, dentistry, nursing, midwifery, psychology, biology, management of health establishments and so on. At the same time, significant collaboration was promoted between the professions. Indeed, the organisation of interprofessional interests and interactions between the disciplines were seen as key outcomes.

Similarly, at the University of Linkoping in Sweden, the Faculty of Health Sciences implemented radical changes related to the form and context of undergraduate medical and health care education. A stronger emphasis was placed on preventative medicine and primary care coupled with problem-based team learning, together with collaborative and interprofessional project work. Breaking down barriers between disciplines was a key concept from the start of the programme. It has concentrated on giving students a common base not only in an academic sense but also in professional skills and social perspectives. The course tries to broaden the outlook on health and social care in society and relate the students chosen profession to these concepts. Throughout the undergraduate years, these topics are reintroduced into the curriculum. Again, breaking down the barriers between the professions is a major objective of the programme. Three approaches to realising these key objectives have been employed.

First, all undergraduate students start as a unified group at the beginning of their courses. Second, problem-based learning is introduced into all the individual programmes to eliminate lines of demarcation. Last, theory and practice are integrated once the students have sufficient theoretical knowledge and practical experience to be able to determine their own occupational roles and test them within the framework of the primary care team; this enables them to make the transition from student to professional occupation (Areskog 1992, 1994).

During the final phase of the programme, the students rotate through the student training ward, an eight-bedded orthopaedic ward. Students from medicine, nursing, physiotherapy and occupational therapy operate as a team. They assume charge of the ward under the supervision of the orthopaedic surgeon, a junior doctor and a nursing sister. The students conduct daily ward rounds and provide medical treatment, nursing care, occupational therapy and physiotherapy (Wallstrom et al 1997; Richards and Saylad 2001). This learning experience is designed to prepare students for collaborative working together in the community. At the same time, postgraduate programmes of multiprofessional continuing and higher education were initiated by the Institute of General Practice at the University of Exeter in the UK (Goble 1991). The first multiprofessional initiative for the health care professions was organised in 1975 as a series of 'Evening Lectures' for the professions. These lectures established a need, brought health professionals together for the first time in a Postgraduate Medical School and encouraged multiprofessional learning and working together (Jones 1986).

Building on the success of the Evening Lecture Series, a formal Multiprofessional Continuing Education Scheme for the professions was launched. The aims of this scheme were:

- To develop interprofessional learning initiatives in order to promote multiprofessional teamwork
- To promote critical thinking, clinical problem solving and the questioning of current practice
- To introduce the principles of evaluation and research in order to promote multiprofessional practice
- To provide updating, revision and reorientation, including awareness of new advances across the professions

The success of the Continuing Education Scheme led to the development of the first Multiprofessional M.Sc. degree in health care. This development was initiated in order to improve the interprofessional standards of care provided by health professionals and to further equip the professions to question and evaluate practice. The course aimed to develop students' skills in critical thinking, research and publication coupled with the preparation of potential leaders for new responsibilities in the community. This initiative was quickly followed by a further multiprofessional MSc degree in health care for professional educators with the aim of equipping members of the health care professions with the skills, knowledge and attitudes necessary to provide a wide range of MPE programmes for the professions (Goble 1994).

It must be remembered that in the 1980s:

- Multiprofessional education as a method for preparing graduates for interprofessional cooperation during their working lives was implemented in only a few centres
- Postgraduate multiprofessional education was spread widely but thinly. In most countries it consisted of short *ad-hoc* courses only

- Continuing education, which involved established health care staff learning together, was uncommon
- Where multiprofessional education was established whether at under-graduate, postgraduate or continuing education level, it was largely due to local initiatives
- In Europe there was no national policy to encourage MPE for health professions during undergraduate, postgraduate or continuing education

EUROPEAN NETWORK FOR THE DEVELOPMENT OF MULTIPROFESSIONAL EDUCATION IN HEALTH SCIENCES

In 1987 the European Network for the Development of Multiprofessional Education in Health Sciences was formally launched to address these inadequacies. Sponsorship by the World Health Organization enabled early meetings to take place in Linkoping, Paris and Exeter. The aims were to promote the concept of multiprofessional education in health sciences through the facilitation and exchange of information, persons and experi-ences. The development of joint research and evaluation was identified as a priority. More specifically, it was decided that the main goal of the Network should be to assist educational institutions, organisations and persons to focus on multiprofessional education and research in health care. These activ-ities have always been seen in relationship to the achievement of 'Health for All' through the development of teamwork in primary and community care. Specific objectives were identified as follows (WHO 1991).

- To establish a mechanism for meeting and exchange of information and experiences
- To develop and evaluate different university or non-university models of MPE
- To develop curriculum design methods and learning tools appropriate to a MPE
- To communicate arguments, case studies and research results related to MPE to decision-makers, professionals, teachers and students
- To establish health research programmes that include basic, applied and operational research that is relevant to health and health care problems in the perspective of MPE

One of the main activities of EMPE has been to encourage the formation of a critical mass of professionals who are able to meet together to communicate results, to share ideas and to identify sources of funding for pilot pro-grammes. This has been difficult when so many members speak different languages and come from very different cultures and geographical locations.

Most particularly, the disparity between the resources of northern, southern and central Europe have made it complex in terms of organising regular meetings. However, thanks to enthusiasts in the host countries, conferences have taken place annually throughout Europe. The local venues have reflected the multiprofessional activities that are being carried out in these different countries. EMPE has always sought to have ongoing dialogue with other organisations sharing the same philosophy. One such group of like-minded individuals were those who had formed The Network: Community Partnerships for Health through Innovative Education, Service and Research.

It must be remembered that the majority of members of EMPE were non-doctors from northern Europe. Whereas the global Network consisted, in the main, of doctors from all over the world. The chief officers of both organisations acknowledged the benefits of working more closely together in order to promote and coordinate these individual strengths.

The expressed aims of The Network were to strengthen non-doctor membership and promote increased numbers of European members particularly from central Europe to become members of The Network. EMPE, on the other hand, saw the benefit in joining forces with a Network of medical schools and health sciences' institutions from around the world. Each organisation recognised that such an arrangement could help to avoid duplication of time and resources. As a result of both organisations recognising the benefits of collaboration, members of EMPE were welcomed to The Network (Goble 2000).

THE NETWORK: COMMUNITY PARTNERSHIPS FOR HEALTH THROUGH INNOVATIVE EDUCATION, SERVICE AND RESEARCH

This Network is an association of institutions for the education of health professionals; it is committed to contribute, through education, research and service, to the improvement and sustainment of health in the communities served.

Network member institutions aim:

- To collaborate with their health systems to adapt the education of health personnel to the needs of local health services
- To explore innovative educational approaches (e.g. community-based education, problem-based learning) to fulfil this mission. The Network emphasises educational research, research on priority health needs and on the efficiency of the health services. In these endeavours, The Network invites the collaboration of like-minded organisations
- To promote the creation of curricula for the education of health personnel in relationship to the priority health needs of the community (e.g.

community-oriented education) and to develop educational methods that enable students to concentrate on the acquisition of knowledge, skills and attitudes, relevant to this context (e.g. community-based education, problem-based learning)

- To establish collaboration between educational institutions for health communities, health services and related sectors in order to promote the development of model health systems and to promote their suitability for community-based basic, postgraduate and continuing education
- This global Network was established in Jamaica in 1979 at the instigation of the WHO since it was felt that medical education was no longer responsive to the health needs of large segments of the population and most particularly in rural areas and in deprived inner cities (Schmidt et al 1991).

The first meetings at which EMPE had a formal input into the global Network were held in Bahrain in 2000 and Brazil in 2001. At this time EMPE proceeded to merge with The Network to enable both organisations to promote their joint interests more effectively in multiprofessional education, practice and research.

The global Network is developing close links with yet a further like-minded organisation; the WHO Project entitled: Towards Unity for Health (TUFH). This project gives priority to improving the performance of the health service delivery system and making it more responsive to people's needs (Boelen 2000).

TOWARDS UNITY FOR HEALTH

The TUFH Project facilitates coordination and integration of a wide spectrum of interventions geared towards individual health and community health at the level of a given population. It also encourages productive and sustainable partnerships among key stakeholders; policy-makers, health managers, health professionals, academic institutions and communities. TUFH hopes to reduce fragmentation in health service delivery caused by divisions such as these between individual and community health; preventive and curative services; generalists and specialists; providers and users; private and public sectors and social and economic aspects of health. Furthermore, the Project seeks to mobilise different partners for greater social accountability and to promote continuous learning (Boelen 2001).

In the early years of The Network, activities had focused on teaching and curriculum development. However, it was acknowledged that education alone would not change health outcomes. Health Service research and development would also be needed in order to generate innovation in community health care. It was recognised that the TUFH Project could provide a powerful framework for understanding and addressing fragmented health systems. The proposed integration of The Network and TUFH was seen as an evolutionary step towards a 'Network of Networks' (Bor 2001) in the same way that the merger of EMPE and The Network provided a natural progression for the promotion and development of mutual interests.

Now that TUFH is working more closely with The Network, the first priority has been the development of a clearing house web site, addressing a number of health issues in a user-friendly and centralised facility. Currently, The Network and TUFH are looking at a partial integration of their organisations. This type of development would enable a unique organisation to be formed that could preserve the complementary strengths of the different entities, namely a non-governmental organisation (NGO) working in association with a world force for change such as the WHO (Kaufman 2001).

One of the first priorities of the TUFH project was to identify case studies from around the world. Studies were selected to illustrate endeavours to create 'Unity in Health'. As a result, there have now been important contributions to the global knowledge base provided by these case studies from many parts of the world.

THE LATIN AMERICAN EXPERIENCE

An outstanding example of this type of collaborative approach lies in the collective work that has been undertaken in Latin America. 'Una Nova Iniciativa na Educacao dos Profissionais de Saude: Uniao a Communidade' (A New Initiative for the Education of Health Professionals: Union with the Community) known as the UNI Programme and supported by the Kellogg Foundation. This very major project was built on the lessons learned from various initiatives in the 1960s, 1970s and 1980s. The UNI programme includes 23 projects in Latin American Countries, who are experimenting with models of health care reform.

The core of the UNI, 'ideario', consists of constructing viable models for the education of health care professionals and for health systems, using partnerships between the university, local health services and the community (Tancredi 1999). The identified projects are geographically distributed across 11 countries crossing Latin America from north to south, from Monterey in Mexico to Temuco in Chile and from east to west, from Natal in Brazil to Colima in Mexico. To achieve collaboration between Argentina, Bolivia, Brazil, Chile, Columbia, Ecuador, Mexico, Nicaragua, Peru, Uruguay and Venezuela was a daunting task. A total of 23 projects were approved and encompassed 15 different health specialties in the health professions or related areas. The projects embraced 103 undergraduate university courses (Chaves and Kisil 1999).

For example in Montevideo, Uruguay the representatives of the Family Health Care Student Practitioner Team worked with advanced students of medicine, nursing, physiotherapy, medical records, dentistry, psychology, social work and nutrition in order to develop an overall strategy for the provision of multiprofessional care for families in the local community. As a result, local polyclinics are beginning to emerge. The evaluation has been positive and has highlighted the necessity for interprofessional inputs in this type of setting. It has also enabled students to develop greater interaction between the professions. However, this programme was not without conflict, most particularly in relation to curriculum boundaries, competing schedules and opposition from traditional teaching teams. Nevertheless, the programme has demonstrated that it is possible to transform the format of multiprofessional teaching and learning in the field.

There is no doubt that the UNI programme was able to promote highly significant changes in the way in which services were provided and used (in project areas). These findings were highly positive and indicate that the idea of promoting a better understanding among academia, the services and the community are worth while. Sadly, a major weakness was highlighted in that it proved difficult to mobilise all the relevant professional groups to participate in the projects. This highly original and visionary initiative must now demonstrate that long-term change has taken place in relation to the training of health care professionals, the organisation and function of the health service and the role of the community in Latin America (Dussault 2001).

CONCLUSION

Developments on this scale are rare but the emerging body of expertise and the critical mass, which is coming together with the collaboration of countries and networks as described above, should point to a much greater capacity and ability to contribute to the development of a multiprofessional body of knowledge world-wide. This is particularly evident with the emergence of web sites and international databases.

This chapter has demonstrated a ladder of developments and a range of initiatives integrating the original multiprofessional aims of EMPE with the collaborative ideals of The Network. Furthermore, The Network intends to integrate its aims with those of the TUFH project in order to develop a powerful approach towards identifying individual health and community health needs world-wide.

The UNI programme has stressed the importance of the political environment. This is highly relevant to all new initiatives whether it be the developments in Paris, Linkoping, Exeter, EMPE, The Network, TUFH or Latin America. This crucial factor can inform and facilitate new advances or can become an insurmountable barrier.

It is hoped that the early developments, proposed amalgamations and integrated projects referred to in this chapter will benefit from the political will to enable them to succeed. These developments indicate how different organisations have come together in different ways to provide a driving force for change. At the same time, they have preserved their unique identities and specific fields of interest. The emergence of joint forces on a global scale, the creation of a critical mass of multiprofessional enthusiasts and the political will to provide sustenance could precipitate far-reaching changes in the provisions of multiprofessional systems of care world-wide. 'From little acorns mighty oaks grow'.

REFERENCES

Areskog, N. (1992) 'The new medical education at the Faculty of Health Sciences, Linkoping University: A challenge for both students and teachers', *Scandinavian Journal of Social Medicine* 20, 1–4.

Areskog, N. (1994) 'Multiprofessional education at the undergraduate level: the Linkoping Model', *Journal of Interprofessional Care* 8, 279–82.

Boelen, C. (2000) 'Education to create unity in health: an educational programme to support the TUFH Project', *Towards Unity for Health* 2.

Boelen, C. (2001) 'Refocus: towards unity for health', *Towards Unity for Health*, 3.

Bor, D. (2001) 'Report upon the Network and TUFH integration', Newsletter of The Network: *Community Partnerships for Health through Innovative Education, Service and Research*, 36.

Chaves, M. and Kisil, L. (1999) *The Network: Community Partnerships for Health through Innovative Education, Service and Research*, Maastricht: The Network.

Dussault, G. (2001) 'Preliminary education of the UNI programmes strategic dimensions', in A. Almeida, A. Feuerwerker and M. Llanosn (eds), *Education of Health Professions in Latin America*, Maastricht: Network Publications.

Goble, R. (1990) *The Barriers to Multiprofessional Education in Health Care*, Paper delivered to the 4th Meeting of European Network for Development of Multiprofessional Education in Health Sciences, Exeter.

Goble, R. (1991) 'Keeping alive intellectually', *Nursing* 4 (33) 19–22.

Goble, R. (1994) 'Multi-professional education in Europe: an overview', in A. Leathard (ed.), *Going Inter-Professional: Working Together for Health and Welfare*, London: Routledge.

Goble, R. (2000) *Observe: Theorise: Collaborate*, Paper delivered to the 11th Annual Conference of The Network: Community Partnerships for Health through Innovative Education, Service and Research, Bahrain.

Goble, R. (2001) *Interprofessional and Multi-professional Education*, Position Paper for the Network: Community Partnerships for Health Care through Innovative Education Service and Research, Maastricht: The Network.

Jones, R. (1986) *Working Together Learning Together*, *Occasional Paper 33*, London: Royal College of General Practitioners.

Kaufman, A. (2001) 'Facilitating information exchange among international foundations and local initiatives through a common clearing house', *Towards Unity for Health*, 2.

Pereira Gray, D. and Goble, R. (1998) *The Case for Multi-professional Practice*, Unpublished Paper, Exeter: University of Exeter.

Richards, R. and Saylad, J. (2001) 'Faculty of Health Sciences, Linkoping University, Linkoping, Sweden', in R. Richards (ed.), *Addressing the Needs of People: Best Practices in Community Orientated Health Professions Education*, Maastricht: The Network.

Schmidt, H., Neufeld, V., Zohair, M., Noonan, M. and Oganbode, T. (1991) 'Network of community orientated educational institutions for health sciences', *Journal of the American Medical Association* 5, 259–63.

Snadden, D. (1997) *The Multiprofessional MSc Degree in Primary Care*, Dundee: University of Dundee.

Tancredi, I. (1999) 'Preface', in A. Almeida, A. Feuerwerker and M. Llanos (eds), *Education of Health Professions in Latin America*, Maastricht: Network Publications.

Wallstrom, O., Sanden, I. and Hammar, W. (1997) 'Multiprofessional education in medical curriculum', *Medical Education* 31, 425–29.

World Health Organization (1991) *Targets for Health for All: The Health Policy for Europe*, Copenhagen: WHO.

Chapter 24

Conclusion

Audrey Leathard

SUMMARY

Some key outcomes for working together from policy to practice in health and social care are reviewed from both a national and international viewpoint, which leads to questions on evidence-based care and evaluation. The issues consider present-day terminology, professional perspectives and user views. The place of accountability, costs and boundaries are then brought into focus. The final section looks at ways forward for interprofessional collaboration through management perspectives, innovative ways of working and new initiatives, concluding with the place of service users in the twenty-first century.

SOME KEY OUTCOMES FOR WORKING TOGETHER IN HEALTH AND SOCIAL CARE BOTH NATIONALLY AND INTERNATIONALLY

Words and purpose

The introduction reviewed a wide range of words to denote working together. The key terms used most readily could now be listed as: collaboration; teamwork; integrated care; interagency, interprofessional but interdisciplinary, more particularly, in the USA. The front runner shifts from time to time, but partnership working is presently in the forefront.

As the defined term has been reduced to a few key words, the context might then be assumed to be set within a more manageable, simplified frame of reference. However, by the start of the twenty-first century, the reverse has been the outcome. The complexities of changing trends and structures as well as new programmes have opened up evermore questions and issues.

As one example, Chapter 4 from Australia illustrates contradictory developments where a tension exists between a move towards greater interprofessional integration, on the one hand, while the direction of change has also been reversed towards the re-emergence of professional boundaries, on the other.

The purpose of interprofessional collaboration also needs to be clarified. One positive view could be to enable better, more cost-effective services for patients and users; although both elements together could even contain contradictory factors. However, within a constantly changing structure for the provision of health and social care in the UK, service users might find it difficult to distinguish or pinpoint the effects or otherwise of working together for better care.

Outcomes

Such an overall purpose for interprofessional collaboration then raises more fundamental points about how outcomes are judged and evaluated: by whom; for whom; or whether based on process or outcomes or both. Evaluations have been largely limited to the field of public health (Health Action Zones and health improvement programmes) primary health care and services for older people (Chapter 13 by Glendinning and Rummery provides one valuable example). However, evidence-based interprofessional practice has yet to be applied to any overall evaluation format. Nevertheless, again from Australia (Chapter 4), the point has been made that the enthusiasm for evidence-based practice stems as much from the needs of particular professions and their contribution as from a 'detached pursuit of scientific inquiry'.

Furthermore, as Powell et al (2001) have set out, there are potentially several types of partnership. Within the management system, vertical performance management covers working together at local level, while horizontal partnership 'drills down' centrally determined performance levels and requirements. Once on this trail, Powell et al (2001: 55–6) perceive no end of dualities for partnership working: enforced versus voluntary; diffuse versus dedicated; based on objective or subjective measures; or led by sanctions versus incentives. However, in assessing outcomes, the 'evidence' is often lacking, more specifically with special initiatives as in the diffuse field of health inequalities; added to which both costs and ownership can also be ambiguous (Powell et al 2001: 44).

Rather differently, from Canada, Chapter 20 shows that quantifying teamwork learning is not easy, where ideally interprofessional education should accompany interprofessional collaboration. However, the greater part of the publications on interprofessional work have been largely concerned with primary health care, public health, nursing and social work. Neverthless, certainly in the UK for example, joint working between housing and social work departments also has an important part to play. Meanwhile, an increasing number of specific studies have been undertaken, as even this publication shows, in the field of interprofessional education (Chapter 19), teamwork

(Chapter 8), primary health care (Chapter 9), developing services for older people (Chapter 13) and for homeless people (Chapter 16).

Overall, to address outcomes effectively presents a complex task, made more intricate by the growing involvement of the private sector, despite the increasingly high level of commitment both to interprofessional education and practice by public service providers. When Gregson et al (1992) undertook one of the earliest pieces of research in the UK on collaborative working between general practitioners, health visitors and district nurses, the starting point was to observe that everyone thought working together 'was a good thing'. By 1997, New Labour considered partnership working a very good thing indeed, to be promoted by all manner of means (DoH 1998) right across the pathways of health and social care. One problem for assessment has always been to pin down 'a good thing': for whom, by whom, when and where (country-wide or specific courses/projects) and with what resources, in a complex field when relating policy to practice.

Some professional issues within an interprofessional context

The professions involved in joint working across health and social care services stand to gain much, in principle, from an interprofessional approach. The positive factors include: the sharing of knowledge and resources, enabling a more satisfying and supportive work environment; the widening of professional perspectives; encouraging overall service planning; achieving objectives more fully and economically; as well as maximising specialist skills. These factors have been known for a decade and have been shown to work effectively, especially in the field of primary care (Pritchard and Pritchard 1992).

Some 10 years later, certain issues still present some difficulties for professional groups, while new challenges have arisen. Hong Kong provides an interesting example (Chapter 22) of how professional concerns are to be overcome. Professional differences on service philosophy, principles and approaches to work have resulted in differing views about criteria. Past divisions and rivalry between health and social care professionals have also been based on claims to specific knowledge, skills and values, while the policy and organisational differences have reinforced the sense of separateness and tension. A consultancy study has now recommended an integrated long-term care system for older people in the provision of community care services in Hong Kong.

In the UK, differences in agency norms, language and communications, career structures, cultures, even dress codes have contributed to professional wariness in working together. Balloch and Taylor (2001: 23) have identified a key difficulty in that performance indicators are usually specific to the service involved rather than seeking to address the factors needed to enhance interagency and interprofessional working.

The generic worker

More recent challenges include, first, the place of the generic worker which, as Hugman points out (in Chapter 4), can be defined variously from practitioners who share skills, knowledge even identity, to practising across overlapping services (as illustrated in Chapter 7 on models). However, the outcome, as described in Chapter 4 from Australia, shows that genericism has become more of a force to deprofessionalise rather than to enable interprofessional working.

Blurring boundaries

Second, in the UK, the development of health care assistants holds certain parallels, which can lead to the 'blurring of boundaries'. From 1990, health care assistants formed a new grade of staff, known as support workers, who now average some 8 per cent of the nursing workforce. After six months of training, health care assistants can undertake, among other functions: counselling; drug administration; venepuncture; and sometimes being in charge of a shift (Leathard 2000). The health care assistant illustration thus highlights the potential blurring of professional boundaries. In this case the issue is between what health care assistants and nursing staff are expected to do (Thornley 1997), which has led the Royal College of Nursing to raise concerns about regulation that had been left to individual employers (Snell 1998).

Meanwhile, in the legal profession, significant changes have been made by the Bar Council to allow barristers to be hired directly by their customers (instead of through the intermediary of solicitors), which would remove the last important difference between the two legal professions. The question for the future was whether fusion would be far behind (Berlins 2002). Similarly, will rationalisation and service integration also lead to blending, blurring, fusion and amalgamation across the health and welfare professions in the course of time?

Professional regulation

A third issue of importance has been the regulation of the professions to practise in the health and community care services. Significant changes are taking place to reorder and rename the professional regulatory bodies. Table 24.1 gives a brief overview of the proposals and intended outcomes for the professions more particularly involved with interprofessional work in England. Arising from the changes set out in Table 24.1 (some of which were introduced by April 2002), one key factor will be the requirement for the National Care Standards Commission to pursue a strategy of working together with the provider to meet required standards in care homes. In the face of a net loss of 12,600 residential and nursing home places in 2000–2001,

Table 24.1 Changes in the regulatory bodies for health and social care in England for the twenty-first century

Former body	Newly named body
Health services	
United Kingdom (UK) Central Council for Nursing, Midwifery and Health Visiting to register the above professions for professional practice and to ensure standards	Nursing and Midwifery Council
Council for Professions Supplementary to Medicine to register 12 professions that include physiotherapists; occupational therapists; radiographers, for professional practice and to ensure standards	The Health Professions Council with 12 independent boards
General Medical Council to license doctors to practise medicine in the UK; to protect patients and to guide doctors	General Medical Council to stay but under notice
	National Clinical Assessment Authority to address poorly performing doctors where concerns are raised by patients or employers
Social services	
	The National Care Standards Commission to regulate service providers
Central Council for Education and Training in Social Work	The General Social Care Council to regulate the profession, register workers, publish codes of practice, regulate training and continuing professional development
	The Social Care Institute for Excellence: a not-for-profit company to disseminate information about best practice
The Social Services Inspectorate	The Social Services Inspectorate to continue to review the performance and quality of local authority social services departments

Proposed changes for inspection and audit: probable starting date 2004

Health services

Commission for Healthcare Audit and Inspection (CHAI)

Independent of the Department of Health: to investigate the performance of NHS organisations, as well as the registration and inspection of private and voluntary hospitals; to encompass all of the current and proposed work of the Commission for Health Improvement (CHI) and the Mental Health Act Commission (MHAC) with the national NHS value for money work of the Audit Commission and the independent healthcare work of the National Care Standards Commission (NCSC).

Continued

Table 24.1 continued

Social services

Commission for Social Care Inspection (CSCI)

To combine all of the work of the Social Services Inspectorate (SSI – a part of the Department of Health) with the Joint Review team of the SSI/Audit Commission and the relevant functions of the National Care Standards Commission in relation to social care.

Note:
The audit and inspection proposals for the future would seem to perpetuate the divisions between the health and social services in England.

the challenge will be to help to raise care standards in a fragile market (Brindle 2002).

A further challenge for setting standards, as the chief inspector of social services, Denise Platt has warned, is that the changes are set against a backdrop of massive structural and regulatory changes to meet the quality and performance targets of *The NHS Plan* (Secretary of State for Health 2000). Turbulent times could lie ahead for the eventual integration of health and social services as social work faces mounting vacancy rates (Gould 2001).

Above all, Table 24.1 contains no reference to any pursuit of the regulation of either interprofessional education or practice. However, the first step towards the need, albeit justification, for some form of interprofessional regulatory council would suggest the development of specifically educated interprofessional workers from the start of training. A subsequent danger might then be, however, that 'interprofessionalism' could become a specialism in itself. Nevertheless, for the moment, with regard to professional regulation and standard setting in England, the field has remained entirely uniprofessional. However, the possibility of a major shake-up of the disparate bodies inspecting the NHS might be required to integrate over time, according to the Secretary of State for Health (*Health Service Journal* 2002). More immediately, under the National Health Service Reform and Health Care Professions Bill (2002: 29), plans have been included for a Council for the Regulation of Health Care Professionals to promote best practice, the interests of patients and cooperation between regulatory bodies.

Meanwhile, in Hong Kong, as Chapter 22 has shown, proposals are afoot for an Interprofessional Practice Council responsible for professional practice standards for the different professionals involved in long-term care provision, although with objections from the Hong Kong Medical Council.

User views and perspectives

As Chapter 2 has shown, the views of users in the social care services in England have been significantly recognised and brought into the provision process. Then again, in the health and social support services for disabled people, Chapter 14 describes a field where user-controlled initiatives have made a major impact on policy at both national and local level to enable disabled people to lead independent lives.

In contrast, the place of the user perspective within the health service has become evermore complex as various bodies and councils are being introduced to enable users to express their views through such bodies as: patients councils; patient forums; a Commission for Patient and Public Involvement in Health; as well as independent patient advice and liaison services (PALs). Steps have also been taken to provide an additional independent advocacy service to support complaints (DoH 2001a) following the decision to abolish Community Health Councils (CHCs). New patient forums were to operate as independent statutory bodies to allow patient representatives the right to monitor local primary care services as well as a seat on primary care trust (PCT) boards. Together with local authority scrutiny, independent local advisory forums and specialist advocacy services, the successor bodies to CHCs were set to cost five times as much to run (Shifrin 2001a, 2001b).

With such an array of intended user involvement, the impact of any outcome from user views would be difficult to determine or assess overall. Further, little suggestion has been made as to how user views on partnership working could be expressed or taken forward. However, as Balloch and Taylor (2001) have argued, when partner agencies are not working effectively together, it is the user that suffers. As integrated health and social services become a reality, user representation and the involvement of user views will have to be fundamentally reconsidered to enable a meaningful outcome for collaborative working.

Accountability and costs

As health and social care services form into care trusts, to achieve integration or pursue partnership working more extensively, the question of accountability becomes a key issue. Who should be accountable to whom and for what? As matters stand, the professions and practitioners, as shown in Table 24.1, have their own regulatory bodies for accountability, but not on an interprofessional basis. However, as Balloch and Taylor (2001: 7) have pointed out, the place of accountability in partnership working is extensive, which has to cover the different expectations of managers, politicians, front-line staff, the needs of the community and service users. In such a wide field, not surprisingly, joint working involves major tensions. A balance has to be achieved between the flexibility needed when seeking to develop new initiatives, through interprofessional and interagency collaboration, but which developments have also to be held to the requirements for accountability where public expenditure is involved.

However, interprofessional working, as such, has rarely been costed (specific projects apart). Joint working might be seen, in principle, as a cost-cutting exercise, but little evaluation of the outcome has been undertaken, as the costs of health and social care overall are based within a complex arena of increasing needs, demands and changing structures. From 1997/8 (when the earliest forms of teamworking were already in existence) to 2000/2001, when partnership working played a far more significant part in service provision, the expenditure on the National Health Service in the UK rose from £26 billion to £59 billion (Matheson and Babb 2002: 137). Within the mounting costs, accountability and outcomes for interprofessional work have tended to remain obscure.

Then again, an important part of interagency working also involves the voluntary sector but which brings in a different equation altogether for accountability. A further complexity is introduced by the widening use of the private sector. Although, as Chapter 2 has shown, audits have been undertaken with regard to the private sector input into public health care, the place of intersectoral costs as a partnership issue has yet to be addressed.

Meanwhile, taking an overall view of partnership working, Powell et al (2001: 45) have warned that conflicts over resources and accountability are likely to lead to cost-shunting and power struggles. Further, drawing on the Audit Commission's (1998) findings with regard to effective partnership working, pooled budgets, joint finance and joint appointments were found to be easier to quantify than attendance at staff meetings and data-sharing. The final point to be raised, in the context of accountability, is the question of ownership and outcome. With regard to ownership, even though an equal partnership might be preferable, a more likely outcome is for a stronger and weaker partner to be involved even within a joint enterprise. An interesting form of public ownership is shown in Chapter 22 from Hong Kong, where the work of government-owned and financed social services are undertaken largely by voluntary agencies. In contrast, Chapter 21 shows the continued strong commitment to public funding and a welfare state approach to health and social care in Norway within the context of a welfare policy and education policy.

Boundaries

The disruptive effect of continual change and evolution is a first important factor in looking at service boundaries. As Chapter 13 on the services for older people in England has described, while local authorities are reorganising their structures and elected council membership, so organisational 'turbulence' threatens improved collaboration more particularly between local authority and primary care organisations.

Second, Chapter 4 from Australia, points out that the continuation of strong professional boundaries may have a justification but there is conflicting evidence as to the benefits for service users.

Third, Ambrose (2001) raises the question of the costs of boundaries between differing agencies. For example, within the field of urban regeneration, time and money are spent in contacting several agencies at the service interface. The costs are both financial and stressful in terms of the frustration and loss of time involved in settling issues. The way forward suggested is to establish close interagency working as well as to enable a more holistic approach in service delivery. The purpose would be to search for a cost-effective service delivery together with a more sensitive approach to user needs.

Fourth, as services in England look towards 'seamless care', the question then arises as to who should stitch the seams: the professionals and practitioners, the managers or the users? Or would a patchwork quilt be preferable where all stitch together? As Chapter 4 from Australia points out, the context is not necessarily simple where services differ between state and non-government services, as well as the differences in service provision between federal, state and local levels. Forces therefore pull in various ways across boundaries.

Finally, as Lonica Vanclay discusses with respect to supporting families in Chapter 11, collaboration is of central importance across boundaries, wherein leadership, trust, mutual respect, communication and shared, clear goals and objectives are among the fundamental policy drivers. Powell et al (2001: 56–7) would take the issues even further by suggesting that only a fully integrated health and social care service, set up on a cost-effective basis under the Department of Health, can achieve effective partnership working. Any such future development also needs to be matched by a more joined-up government approach at the centre to enable policy and resource streams to flow together to meet the needs appropriately at local level.

MANAGEMENT SYSTEMS FOR INTERPROFESSIONAL WORKING

The background

Across the 1990s, various organisational approaches have been used to manage interprofessional practice (Leathard 1994).

1   *The structural approach* has provided one way for health and welfare professionals to work together through the service structure provided, wherein specialist teams can be facilitated, as well as pathways created, to

enable collaborative mechanisms across the health and social services. In this context as one early example, Heptinstall (1990) concluded that Newcastle's services for physically handicapped and frail elderly people had stood the test of research and the judgement of the consumer. Care trusts have subsequently provided a twenty-first century approach to integration through the structure provided.

2 *The professional leadership model* has been dominant over the years, wherein the general practitioner (GP) leads a team of health professionals (in particular practice nurses and health visitors) and, to some extent, social workers. Differentials in pay, status, training backgrounds, language and value systems between the professional groups have caused tensions. However, as Geoffrey Meads has shown in Chapter 9, the professional leadership model has been undergoing a significant change as GPs have been turning to multidisciplinary teamwork. Further, this management model has also become modified by the place of primary care groups/trusts (PCG/Ts) boards (or governing bodies), which include representation from community nursing, social services (former health authorities), users as well as GPs drawn from the area. As PCTs have assumed a wider and more complex role in both commissioning and provision, so the professional leadership arena has had to absorb evermore demands and wider requirements.

3 *The egalitarian team approach* has become increasingly relevant to interprofessional work, as the need for health and social service personnel to work together across professional and sectoral boundaries is now a dominant feature in meeting user needs. One example of many would be reflected in the work of mental health teams (as discussed in Chapters 2 and 15). The essential approach to interprofessional teamwork has continued to emphasise the need to collaborate and coordinate activities, to allocate priorities, share information and organise the work schedule together. However, a more recent feature of significance has been the requirement to incorporate the views and place of users and carers. Within an egalitarian team, leadership tensions become less relevant, but wherein the team approach works well when functions and roles are clearly defined. However, when collaboration breaks down, then disastrous results can occur such as in the Victoria Climbie child abuse case in 2001 (Carvel 2001).

The managerial approach became a dominant feature in the first half of the 1990s to address the purchaser–provider split within the internal market. From 1997 onwards, the commissioning role for health care has remained in place both in the work of health authorities (until their demise in 2002), PCTs, and for local authorities commissioning for social care. The manager as coordinator has also sought to enable interprofessional teams to work together across boundaries. However, management has to reconcile contrasting pressures between the issues of competitive pricing, costs, quality, access and delivery in contrast to the interprofessional context of joint planning and working, which is underpinned by shared beliefs, common goals and collaboration.

Management systems for the twenty-first century

Various initiatives have now emerged with potential for new approaches to collaborative working in the future.

A whole systems approach

Looking at the change programmes and management approaches that encourage the 'right kind of' collaborative partnership across agencies and professions, Su Maddock and Glenn Morgan (1999), from the Manchester Business School, have advocated a whole systems approach.

The right conditions include:

- Management and practitioners sharing the same agenda on quality and funding issues
- Support for communication between users and front-line staff
- A senior management team with a unity of vision
- Involvement of actively committed medical staff
- Appropriate performance measures supporting change and staff development

For the whole systems approach to work, partnerships needed more than simply a commitment at the top but also to be given time to establish strong relationships, devolved power to make decisions, but with the necessary support to survive.

In the field of mental health, the importance of a whole systems approach has been highlighted by the Department of Health (2001b) with relevance to the Care Programme Approach (CPA). For the CPA, a coordinated programme is considered essential across the agencies involved to enable efficient and effective delivery of care in order to facilitate access for individual service users to the full range of community supports needed for recovery and integration.

In practice, a study based on the delivery of services to older people across the health and social care services in Brighton and Hove, Sussex, has shown the benefits of the whole systems approach (Callanan 2001). The positive features included:

- An improvement in both the services provided and in the multidisciplinary assessment and review
- Initiatives to identify gaps in services

- Enabling small changes which would result in significant improvements in service provision
- As well as improved flexibility to meet users' and patients' needs

Among the findings, one key theme has been the need to involve patients, users and carers in the decisions being made in the endeavour to achieve the coordination of services through a complex system. Above all, the whole systems approach has provided a focus for the development of thinking through effective partnership working (Callanan 2001).

Integrated care pathways

Integrated care pathways (ICPs) are structured multidisciplinary care plans that define the essential steps and expected course of events in the care of patients with a specific clinical problem over a set time scale (Barden 2002). ICPs focus on whole systems and managing components in an integrated package. The importance of care pathways for the future lies in their relevance to a range of current initiatives aimed at improving the quality of health care that include clinical governance, the new performance frameworks, evidence-based practice and the development of partnership working (Middleton and Roberts 2000). For patients, the benefits of pathways have been identified as covering, improved patient outcomes, better teamwork and improved consistency in care (Cottrell and Parker 2002). Furthermore, innovation has extended to better NHS and social service care links; concordats with the private sector, and partnership working with patients (Cottrell and Parker 2002). Network teams and structures have been set up, as in Nottingham, to provide seamless care, quality improvement, address unmet need and raise standards (Winter 2002).

Certain issues surround the recent development of ICPs such as visibility, the place of representation and local politics (Crump 2002), nor is there much evidence, as yet, of any ICP evaluation. However, NHS links apart, while the programme has not so far covered social care, integrated care pathways point an innovative way forward for joint working, whereby a clear interprofessional and interagency approach to care for a patient group is based on the available evidence and consensus of best practice. The potential could be extended to other aspects of specialist forms of care across the health and welfare services.

Care trusts

The Health and Social Care Act 2001 ratified the creation of care trusts (outlined in Chapter 2), which can hold budgets for both health and social care to enable an integrated service. The purpose of care trusts was to be an important vehicle to modernise both social and health care, to ensure integration and to be focused on the needs of patients and users (DoH 2001c). Widely hailed by politicians of all parties as a means of integrating health and social services, there was one major snag: that health care remained free at the point of delivery, while personal care provided by local authorities in England continued to be means-tested and based on charges (Pollock and Campbell 2001). However in Scotland, from July 2002, both nursing care and personal care were intended to be provided free at the point of use (Scottish Executive 2002).

Meanwhile, some 15 care trust pilots across 12 localities were to start work in England betwen April 2002 and April 2003. However, the Department of Health has never encouraged any notion of NHS functions to become integrated under local authority arrangements. Care trusts were to be essentially NHS bodies, which has caused suspicion among local authority social services in England who have viewed protecting social care funding levels in a care trust with some concern, although agencies were to remain accountable for their own services. While care trusts initially appeared to be a preferred model for joint working between health and social services, as primary care trusts concentrated on the delivery of improved services, so care trusts seemed to slide onto a back burner. Care trusts then began to be regarded as only one of a number of mechanisms to enable health and social care integration (Smith 2001, Stephenson 2001, Hudson 2002).

Seamless care

Creating seamless provision has been one favoured option. Two examples in practice have already taken place. In Sandwell in the west Midlands, the director of social services has been seconded to the local health authority as chief executive in order to develop a joint health and local authority trust through plans to merge various trusts and services in the area to secure integrated provision. One unresolved debate has been whether the move of the social services directors into health signifies the demise of conventional social services departments, but the developments in Sandwell are described as based on the needs of local circumstances (George 2002).

Similarly, the director of social services, in the east London borough of Dagenham, is one of a small but growing number of social services chiefs who either straddle or have moved across to run health service organisations. The outcome seeks to create an integrated infrastructure for social services and a local primary care trust (PCT) to cover human resources, finance and performance management, together with some of the commissioning roles from the discontinued health authority (from April 2002), while the local PCT embraces all health care provision except acute hospital and mental health care. However, the whole partnership agenda is intended to create a seamless web of health and social care (George 2002), but just how far vested or special interests were to play a part, in undermining the seams, remained to be seen.

Overall, in many parts of the country, community NHS trusts are expected to be absorbed into primary care trusts or new care trusts, which leaves for the moment only acute, general or some specialist hospitals to remain somewhat outside the trend towards integration. Meanwhile, the government's commitment to integrated working has been underpinned by the creation in the UK of 28 new strategic health authorities (see Table 2.3 in Chapter 2) whose full statutory powers were in place by the autumn of 2002. The strategic health authorities are to provide a national integrating force through, among other roles, the overall responsibility for managing the NHS, developing strategy and performance, in order to ensure service delivery and consistency of approach.

INNOVATIVE WAYS FORWARD FOR INTERPROFESSIONAL COLLABORATION IN THE TWENTY-FIRST CENTURY

This final section sets out new initiatives, some in action, others with potential, to point towards a future vision for interprofessional work at the start of a new century.

NHS Beacons

As part as part of the Modernisation Agency in England, the NHS Beacons Programme seeks to support the development of a modern, responsive health service. By identifying services that have been particularly innovative in meeting specific health care needs, the Beacons programme offers ways of sharing information and experience about good practice so that original ideas can be adapted to suit local circumstances elsewhere. (NHS staff from Scotland, Wales and Northern Ireland can visit the NHS Beacons Programme; Wales is even considering a similar development for the future.) Meanwhile, in England, the programme is based on a wide range of learning opportunities to match team and individual needs, through workshops, conferences, mentoring, visits and secondments. In keeping with modernisation, dissemination is via e-bulletins and a Beacons web site: www.nhs.uk/beacon; although communication devices from a previous era, such as fax, a postal address and a telephone number, are also available.

Of interprofessional significance, a number of projects discussed in the NHS Beacons Learning Handbook (NHS Modernisation Agency 2001) are particularly involved with health and social care agencies working together. For example, in the Royal Borough of Kingston upon Thames, 'Young Livin' has been developed with young people, the Children and Family Services and Kingston's Family Support Forum (a multi-agency partnership, made up of representatives of the Borough's voluntary and statutory agencies), to make local services more accessible to young people. Among the features, the programme has opened up and maintained with young people the creation of a young people's monitoring group. As a continually developing project, the intention is to include direct links with school nurse services and the child and adolescent mental health team. Along with other initiatives elsewhere, this particular Beacons programme was chosen for a Health and Social Care Award for innovation.

Another interesting example of working together locally can be seen in a Beacons site at Dorset HealthCare NHS Trust in partnership with patients, carers, general practitioners, social services and the independent and voluntary sectors. The Beacons programme provides comprehensive community-based mental health services for older people with dementia and functional mental illness to include assessment, rehabilitation, respite care, continuing care and support to carers. Among the achievements of successful partnership working has been the outcome of an integrated Community Mental Health Team. The dissemination activities include: customised arrangements (such as speakers on partnership working with social services and carers); secondments; workshops; and a web site to be available shortly. (Modernisation certainly requires a web site.)

In spreading good practice, the NHS Beacons Programme covers a range of arenas such as: cancer care; health improvement; human resources; palliative care; primary care; intermediate care, among others, together with Department of Health funding for a Health Action Zone Innovation Scheme. Applications for new Beacons on specific themes are invited in line with national priorities and objectives. Collaborative working is woven into the various programmes according to the type of work in hand. Overall, innovation and initiative are the core factors that both promote and underpin the sharing of good practice as well as partnership working for the future.

NATIONAL SERVICE FRAMEWORKS (NSF)

From 2001, the new century heralded a major commitment, on the part of the Department of Health, to modernise the NHS and social services, which required these agencies to work together to provide integrated services to improve the quality of life for all. By July 2001, some seven areas had been selected to form part of the NSF programme that included cancer, coronary heart disease, diabetes, long-term conditions, mental health and care for older people.

As one example, the Department of Health (2001d) set out a programme of action and reform to address the failure to meet the needs of older people and to deliver higher quality services. The National Service Framework set out to provide, significantly, the first ever comprehensive strategy to ensure fair, high quality, integrated health and social care services for older people. In a 10-year programme of action, the intention was to link services to support independence and promote good health, specialised services and culture change so that older people and their carers were treated with respect, dignity and fairness (DoH 2001b).

Then again, as Tony Leiba has pointed out in Chapter 15, the National Service Framework for Mental Health required the Care Planning Approach to be fully integrated into the mental health services to enable health and social services to work together to secure appropriate provision for users, carers and their families. As the Department of Health (2001b: 1) stated for the Mental Health NSF, a coordinated approach from the relevant agencies was essential to ensure efficient and effective care delivery. No one service or agency was the key focus, as service users themselves provided the focal point for care planning and delivery.

Overall, the significance of the National Service Frameworks for interprofessional collaboration is the central place given to developing more effective links between health and social services. The Health Act 1999 had already introduced new partnership flexibilities to enable health authorities and local councils to improve services at the interface of health and social care. From April 2001, local strategic partnerships were to be established across the country to improve the quality and governance in a particular locality through bringing together the public, private, voluntary and community sectors and service users to provide a single overarching local framework, through which more specific local partnerships could operate, such as through the arrangements for implementing the NSF for older people (DoH 2001d: 8). The way forward for the future of the NSF programme was to be through a full commitment to partnership working.

NEW WAYS FORWARD FOR INTERPROFESSIONAL WORKING IN AN ELECTRONIC AND TECHNOLOGICAL AGE

As Scott Reeves and Della Freeth (Chapter 6) have shown, the use of electronic technology offers a number of wider opportunities to enable new forms of collaboration. The significance of the technological context is that interprofessional issues can be addressed without the need for professionals to be on site together. The release of time and space then opens up many possibilities.

Homeworking

For example, homeworking is one device on the increase in twenty-first century in the UK. Datamonitor market research has shown that one in four Britons are choosing to work from home instead of commuting to a place of work and the number is increasing. The study reveals that homeworkers tend to be better paid, more highly qualified and efficient professionals whose status above their office-bound contemporaries enables them to undertake homeworking. However, this new and increasing development in the UK has been made possible by new technology such as the Internet, emails and a rapid rise in the number of new phone and computer connections (Winnett 2002). The relevance for interprofessional work is that homeworking is likely to become a significant feature of networking within the specific context of health and social care.

Networking models for professional practice

The wider place of networking opens up a new vision of working together in the twenty-first century. The Community Practitioners and Health Visitors Association (CPHVA) has been active in setting up professional networking models for developing practice, through the work of their Professional Officer, Research and Practice Development, Cheryll Adams, who has most kindly discussed the initiatives with me for this publication. Under the headings now set out, for *purpose*, *networking* and *intended outcomes*, the possibilities have drawn on work from the CPHVA practice field of post-natal depression and maternal mental health, which have been extended by myself to apply to the potential for interprofessional practice through the gain from the use of new technologies.

Interprofessional networking for developing practice

Purpose

- To provide a national network of information
- To further sharing and joint working
- To improve practice both for professionals and users
- To address different challenges in practice, drawing on professionals with a common interest

Networking

- Facilitating through a members' association based on CPHVA
- Seeking an expression of interest through CPHVA publicity

- Forming a database
- Gathering information from members' telephone calls, mail and emails
- Ascertaining areas of interest to support professional practice
- Targeting areas of need for professionals and users
- Drawing on the National Electronic Library for Health (NeLH) where a future possibility could be to link up with the Library to promote practice development

Intended outcomes

1 To reduce duplication of effort
2 To speed the transition of research into practice
3 To improve efficiency and effectiveness in practice delivery
4 To promote equity in service delivery
5 To lead teamworking bringing in a wider group for networking: mid-wives; psychiatrists; GPs; community psychiatrists; nurses; social workers; and voluntary organisations
6 To share information gained interprofessionally
7 To extend knowledge and professional application for users
8 To improve on collaborative practice for post-natal depression and maternal mental health for CPHVA but could be extended far more widely
9 To draw on a common understanding of issues for the benefit of patients/ users
10 To develop e-learning
11 To act as a model for networks in other practice areas
12 To engage special facilitators to coordinate and to enable effective practice

Figure 24.1 now sets out a future vision of a networking approach for the development of interprofessional practice, which could be linked to a wide use of the new technologies, as well as based on partnership working and inter-professional collaboration.

Future implications

- The potential for the future could involve a management section, suggested in Figure 24.1, but which is not in position as yet even for CPHVA networking
- Networking models have a powerful resonance for the twenty-first century that reflect ways of working with and supporting health and social care professionals by using the new technologies to further patient care and users needs
- Even more significant for the future is the possibility that e-networking

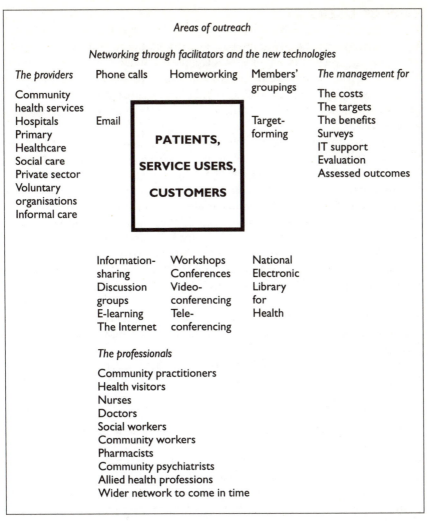

Figure 24.1 A future vision of a networking approach for practice development to support interprofessional practice in action.

could lead to a rethinking of the complex and costly structures for the delivery of health and welfare services to enable simplification and support through new forms of technology to cut through bureaucracy towards more effective service delivery in practice.

However, as Cheryll Adams has pointed out to me, the emphasis is now on the 'what' not the 'who' which has major implications for the next decade as professional boundaries are expected to be broken down in response to new needs within an electronic age.

SERVICE USERS

By the twenty-first century, patients and users had been placed at the centre of service delivery. Taking user involvement and empowerment seriously requires, as Turner and Balloch (2001: 167) have pointed out, that agencies work in partnership with those for whom services are provided which, for professionals and front-line staff, can be a threatening and confusing experience.

Looking across the health services in England, with the demise of the Community Health Councils scheduled for 2002/3, a new patient protection strategy is intended to include a range of measures to involve service users discussed earlier in this chapter under user views and perspectives. Further, the intention of the NSF Programme is also to involve service users and their carers in the planning and delivery of care. Then again, the National Health Service Reform and Health Care Professions Bill (2002) has set out proposals, under Section 19, for a Commission for Patient and Public Involvement in Health. The Department of Health's (DoH 2001e) health improvement and modernisation plans also envisage the creation of a patient-centred NHS that brings in the voices of patients, their carers and the public at every level of the NHS to act as a powerful lever for change and improvements as well as to build on the local authorities' own mechanisms for engagement with local communities.

Meanwhile, Turner and Balloch (2001: 177) have considered the extent to which users of social services have been sufficiently empowered to work in partnership with professionals. The conclusions suggest that the outcome is limited. The developments to encourage the growth of users' networks, the extension of direct payments and user involvement in defining outcomes have encountered a reluctance by local authorities and professions to share in decision-making, while user empowerment has not achieved power-sharing. As Colin Barnes has shown in Chapter 14, however, the increasing influence of user involvement in the field of disability has become more positive. The 'intensifying' growth of user-controlled initiatives in the last 20 years has made a significant impact on policy-makers at a national level with a direct outcome on both statutory and voluntary provision at a local level.

Overall, Turner and Balloch (2001: 177) conclude that despite the limitations where user involvement is concerned in the social services, the place of patient involvement in the health services is even further behind. In striking contrast the user, in the private health sector, becomes a consumer who pays the bill or who is insured to cover the expenses whereby a greater level of choice is thus made possible. In social care, a similar situation arises for private residential and nursing care, but little influence can be exercised by the consumer on the nature of the service, other than by the withdrawal of the customer from the paid commitment and receipt of service as, with an increasing shortage of residential and nursing care places, the consumer may have little choice or influence on provision.

One final point then remains for the twenty-first century. Rather than a range of different programmes to attempt to involve the service user in the separate developments between the health and social care services – whether towards empowerment, power-sharing, or simply through making the views of users known on service provision: one further option is still left open. As partnership working has taken centre stage in policy developments for health and social care: the possibility then opens up for an interprofessional collaborative endeavour, linked to evaluated outcomes, towards enabling patients and service users to become part of an integrated user forum to discuss views as well as to engage in an involvement with a whole systems approach. Through a shared pathway of commissioners, providers and users across health and social care, the potential is then created for all parties to work together to improve services, in response to the views of customers, to meet the needs of the twenty-first century.

FINALE

Drawing together the three main parts of this publication, the policy section has shown that interprofessional collaboration has become a crucial factor in the development of health and social care provision, underpinned by management involvement, driven by the new technologies, but evermore involved with ethical issues. In linking policy to practice across professions, sectors and communities working together, the service user has become the central focus of action and endeavour. Finally, with regard to learning together, one key outcome has been the increasingly international and global nature of interprofessional education, which sets the context for the new millennium.

REFERENCES

Ambrose, P. (2001) 'Holism and urban regeneration', in S. Balloch and M. Taylor (eds), *Partnership Working: Policy and Practice*, Bristol: The Policy Press.

Audit Commission (1998) *A Fruitful Partnership, Effective Partnership Working*, London: Audit Commission.

Balloch, S. and Taylor, M. (2001) *Partnership Working: Policy and Practice*, Bristol: The Policy Press.

Barden, P. (2002) 'Integrated care pathways – a tool for modernisation and redesign', *Integrated Care Pathways*, Harrogate: Harrogate Management Centre.

Berlins, M. (2002) 'Why barristers may soon kiss monopoly money goodbye', *The Guardian*, 6 February, 15.

Brindle, D. (2002) 'Handle with care', *The Guardian: Society*, 6 February, 4.

Callanan, A. (2001) 'The whole systems' approach', in D. Taylor (ed.), *Breaking Down Barriers: Reviewing Partnership Practice*, Brighton: University of Brighton.

Carvel, J. (2001) 'Climbie inquiry to prosecute witness', *The Guardian*, 4 December, 13.

Cottrell, K. and Parker, G. (2002) 'Developing pathways collaboratively', *Integrated Care Pathways*, Harrogate: Harrogate Management Centre.

Crump, N. (2002) 'Creating integrated care pathways in practice', *Integrated Care Pathways*, Harrogate: Harrogate Management Centre.

DoH (Department of Health) (1998) *Partnership in Action: New Opportunities for Joint Working between Health and Social Services*, London: Department of Health.

DoH (2001a) *Assuring the Quality of Medical Practice*, London: Department of Health (www.doh.gov.uk/assuringquality).

DoH (2001b) *National Service Framework for Mental Health*, London: Department of Health (www.doh.gov.uk/nsf).

DoH (2001c) *Care Trusts*, Health and Social Care Joint Unit, London: Department of Health.

DoH (2001d) *National Service Framework for Older People*, London: Department of Health, March.

DoH (2001e) *Involving Patients and the Public in Health Care: Response to the Listening Exercise*, London: Department of Health.

George, M. (2002) 'Shared aim', *The Guardian: Society*, 6 February, 10–11.

Gould, M. (2001) 'A poisoned chalice', *Health Service Journal* 111 (5770) 9–10.

Gregson, B., Cartlidge, A. and Bond, J. (1992) *Interprofessional Collaboration in Primary Health Care Organisations*, Occasional Paper 52, London: Royal College of General Practitioners.

Health Service Journal (2002) 'Inspection bodies face integration', 112 (5788) 4.

Heptinstall, D. (1990) 'A progressive partnership', *Social Work Today* 8 March, 8–9.

Hudson, B. (2002) 'Silence is golden', *Health Service Journal* 112 (5792) 18.

Leathard, A. (1994) *Going Inter-Professional: Working Together for Health and Welfare*, London: Routledge.

Leathard, A. (2000) *Health Care Provision: Past, Present and into the 21st Century*, Cheltenham: Nelson Thornes.

Maddock, S. and Morgan, G. (1999) *Conditions for Partnership*, Manchester: Manchester Business School.

Matheson, J. and Babb, P. (2002) *Social Trends*, No 32, London: The Stationery Office.

Middleton, S. and Roberts, A. (2000) *Integrated Care Pathways*, London: Butterworth-Heinemann.

National Health Service Reform and Health Care Professions Bill (2002), London: The Stationery Office.

NHS Modernisation Agency (2001) *NHS Beacons Learning Handbook*, Vol. 4, Petersfield: NHS Modernisation Agency (www.nhs.uk/beacons).

Pollock, A. and Campbell, F. 'Bye-bye Bevan' (2001) *The Guardian*, 26 January, 20.

Powell, M., Exworthy, M. and Berney, L. (2001) 'Playing the game of partnership', in R. Sykes, C. Bochel and N. Ellison (eds), *Social Policy Review 13: Developments and debates: 2000–2001*, Bristol: The Policy Press/Social Policy Association.

Pritchard, P. and Pritchard, J. (1992) *Developing Teamwork in Primary Health Care: A Practical Workbook*, Oxford: Oxford University Press.

Scottish Executive (2002) 'Free personal care timetable extended', News Online, Edinburgh: Health Department, Directorate of Health Policy.

Secretary of State for Health (2000) *The NHS Plan: A Plan for Investment, A Plan for Reform*, Norwich: The Stationery Office.

Shifrin, T. (2001a) 'CHCs' successor bodies "set to cost five times as much to run"', *Health Service Journal* 111 (5739) 4.

Shifrin, T. (2001b) '"Patient advocate" plans taking sting from CHCs', *Health Service Journal* 111 (5737) 6.

Smith, P. (2001) 'Care trusts on back burner as interest drops', *Health Service Journal* 111 (5764) 8.

Snell, J. (1998) 'A force to reckon with', *Health Service Journal* 108 (5597) 24–6.

Stephenson, P. (2001) 'Route planner', *Health Service Journal* 111 (5766) 14–15.

Thornley, C. (1997) *The Invisible Workers*, London: Unison.

Turner, M. and Balloch, S. (2001) 'Partnership between service users and statutory social services', in S. Balloch and M. Taylor (eds), *Partnership Working: Policy and Practice*, Bristol: The Policy Press.

Winnett, R. (2002) 'More Britons opt to work from home', *The Sunday Times*, 26 January, 28.

Winter, N. (2002) 'Creating integrated care pathways in practice', *Integrated Care Pathways*, Harrogate: Harrogate Management Centre.

Index

Employment Action Zones 162
empowering: 45, 85; practice/s 112; services
    112
empowerment 8, 112–14, 354, 355
Engel, C. 4, 44, 48, 49, 99–100, 293
English National Board for Nursing,
    Midwifery and Health Visiting (ENB) 274
Epp, J. 287
Epsom Health Care and St Hellier trusts 106
ethical: 69–78; and legal framework 268;
    basis 77; consequences 69; considerations
    82, 84–5; dilemmas 47; framework 268;
    issues 4, 69–78, 89, 266, 355; obligations
    69; position 77; practice 71, 73, 76;
    priorities 244; requirements 84; sauce 70;
    standards 70; theory 151
ethics 69–78, 257, 300
ethnic minority: agency 252; Chinese 310;
    communities 256; families 160; groups
    207, 215, 252, 256, 260, 267; needs 256,
    221; (voluntary) organisations 206, 256
Etzioni, A. 8
Europe 325, 328, 329
European: centres 324; members 329
European Network for the Development of
    Multiprofessional Education in Health
    Sciences (EMPE) 324, 325, 328–32
European Network on Independent Living
    (ENIL) 206
European Union 35
evaluate/d/ing/evaluative 34, 38, 96, 100, 123,
    183, 189, 192, 219, 220, 226, 266, 277, 282,
    284, 292, 293, 312, 322, 327, 328, 336, 355
evaluation/s: 8, 20, 34, 35, 38, 51, 81, 82, 88,
    89, 93, 102, 109, 110–11, 115, 146, 147, 148,
    149, 150, 159, 167, 175, 178, 179, 187, 188,
    215, 220, 226, 265, 268, 275, 276, 282, 283,
    285, 286, 293, 316, 328, 332, 335, 336, 342,
    346
Evans, T. 35
Evers, H. 313, 317
evidence-based: 28, 29, 336; care 335;
    practice 38, 46, 58, 273, 336, 346
Ewles, L. 27, 153, 154
Exeter (UK) 324, 328, 332
Exworthy, M. 144

family/lies 57, 103, 111–13, 158–69, 173–4,
    204, 209, 212, 214, 215, 217, 220, 229,
    240–1, 243, 245–7, 268, 313, 315, 322, 332,
    343, 350; carers 240, 241, 320; centre/s 159,
    164, 165, 175, 257; health/care 140; 331
Family Health Service Authorities (FHSAs)
    18, 105, 107
family life 159, 244
Family Matters, Counting Families In (2001)
    241
family: medicine 318, 320; members 159,
    167, 314; policy 163; services 161, 164,
    313; studies 288

Family Policy Unit 163
Family Rights Group 250
Family Support Forum (Kingston, Surrey)
    347
Family Support Grant Programme 163
family support (services) 4, 158–65, 167–9,
    173
Family Welfare Assocation (FWA) 158,
    164–9
Farmer, E. 174, 175
Farrell, M. 5
Faulkener, A. 255
Finkelstein, V. 209
Finland 88
Finnegan, E. 13
Firth, B. 182
Firth-Cozens, J. 218, 219,
Fish, D. 78
Fisher, A. 71
Flynn, M. 255
Flynn, R. 19
Fowler, P. 61, 64
France 36, 325
Freeman, M. 4, 121
Freeth, D. 4, 79, 84, 220, 265, 272, 274, 277,
    281, 282, 350
Fruin, D. 209
funding/fundholding practices 17, 19 *see
    also* GP fundholders/fundholding

Gardner, R. 255
Garside, P. 122
General Medical Council 74, 339
general (medical) practice/s 12, 14, 15, 21, 96,
    122, 134, 135, 140, 161, 166, 187, 188, 190,
    192, 194–7
general (medical) practitioner/s (GPs) 3, 13,
    14, 15, 18, 22, 31, 33, 37, 39, 59, 62, 65, 70,
    74, 75, 94–5, 104, 105, 112, 134–7, 140,
    143, 165, 186–94, 214, 319, 337, 344, 349,
    352
GP (general practitioner) fundholders/
    fundholding 17–18, 19, 20, 22, 33, 105,
    186, 188
General Social Care Council 29, 339
General Nursing Councils (GNC) 275
generic: 62 134, 289; practitioners 62;
    services 228; worker 60, 61, 62, 338
genericism 60–2, 338
George, M. 34, 347
geriatrics 320
geriatric assessment teams (Hong Kong)14,
    312, 314
gerontological education 318
gerontological care 318, 320, 321
gerontology 319, 320, 321
Gerrish, K. 322
Gibbons, J. 158
Gilbert, J. 4, 270, 280, 282, 291
Gillam, S. 27, 29, 110–11

Routledge, P. 151
Royal Association for Disability and
   Rehabilitation 206
Royal College of Nursing 338
*Royal Commission on Health Services (*1964)
   287
*Royal Commission on Long Term Care of
   Older People* (1999) 245
Rummery, K. 4, 115, 186, 187, 188, 189, 336
Russell, H. 147
Russell, J. 252
Russell, L. 252

Sackett, D. 46
Safer Cities 147
St Giles Trust 225, 226, 225, 228, 235
St Mungo's Community Housing
   Association 227, 235
Salford University 271
Salmon, G. 86
Sapey, B. 201, 207
Saunders, P. 150
Saving Lives (1999) 22
Saylad, J. 327
Schmidt, H. 330
Schmitt, M. 274, 295
Schluter, N. 137
school nurse/s 19; services 349
SCOPME (Standing Committee on
   Postgraduate Medical Education) 270
Scotland 10, 37, 134, 202, 205, 206, 347, 348
Scott, D. 252, 256
Scott, R. 253
Scottish Executive 201, 240, 347
Scriven, A. 147, 169
Seaton, B. 287
Secretary of State for Health 16, 21, 22, 23,
   25, 28, 29, 30, 31, 32, 32, 33, 34, 35, 37, 69,
   70, 95, 105, 108, 136, 212, 213, 215, 218,
   230, 340
Seebohm, F. 160
Seebohm Report (1968) 12
semi-professionals 6, 8, 143
Senge, P. 135, 150
shared learning 5, 122, 321, 265, 266, 304,
Shapiro, J. 203, 235
Shaw, I. 6, 267
Sheaff, R 189
Sheffield University 179
Shelter 225
Shepherd, D. 215
Shields, P. 216
Shifrin, T. 30, 32, 34, 341
*Shifting the Balance of Power within the
   NHS: Securing Delivery* (2001) 38
Shore, B. 58, 59
Sigmoid Curve 93, 113–15
Simpson, A. 127, 130
Sims, D. 275
Smith, D. 36

Smith, J. 38
Smith, P. 347
Smith, T. 153
Snadden, D. 325
Snell, J. 338
social and health: care 346; personnel 299
social care (services): 3, 4, 18, 21, 25, 28, 33,
   37, 39, 108, 109, 110, 112, 160–1, 186–98,
   204, 216–20, 239, 241, 275, 341, 344,
   346–7, 354; agencies 256; collaboratives
   136; needs 12, 14, 239; professionals *see
   also* professionals; provision 313;
   qualification 275; sector 313; trusts 109;
   workers 29, 61, 218 *see also* social services
Social Care Act (1964) (Norway) 297
Social Care Institute for Excellence 339
social centre 314
social educators 301
social exclusion 27, 37, 147, 160–2
Social Exclusion Unit 21, 162, 163
social inclusion 151, 268
social input 127
social model 30, 205, 206, 208, 209, 275
social needs 216, 314, 317
social networks 159, 313
social policy 151, 257, 297
social regeneration 147
social sciences 318
social security/system 102, 112, 297, 313
social service/s: 3, 12, 13, 16, 18, 21–2, 25–7,
   30, 31, 33–5, 39, 65, 96, 101–2, 104,
   108–10, 112–13, 128, 137, 140, 147, 160,
   175, 182, 186–98, 212–15, 217–18, 221,
   224, 255, 257, 312–14, 318, 339–40, 342,
   344, 346–7, 349, 350, 354; assessments 187,
   214; director/s/chiefs 347; professional *see*
   professional/s representatives 179, 190,
   191, 193, 194, 196, 197; Westminster 228
social services departments (SSDs) 15, 20,
   24, 34, 96, 105, 175–6, 181, 187–9, 191–2,
   206–8, 221, 225, 347
Social Services Inspectorate (SSI) 24, 28,
   33,183, 209, 220, 339–40
social support/services 159, 298
social welfare (services) 60, 298, 310, 315,
   318
Social Welfare Department (Hong Kong)
   311, 313, 314
social work: 14, 47, 59, 61, 65, 72, 88, 101,
   104, 148, 161, 164, 176, 192–3, 227–8, 232,
   234, 266, 272, 274, 281, 288, 399, 300, 302,
   304, 318, 319, 320, 320, 332, 336, 340;
   education 299, 318; posts 275;
   practitioners 140; service/s 142, 188; staff
   15; teams 194
social worker/s 3, 8, 13, 14, 15, 22, 31, 33, 39,
   72, 122, 127–30, 143, 161, 164–5, 174–5,
   182, 187–9, 192–4, 209, 212, 214–15, 220,
   234, 251–2, 266–8, 301, 304, 312, 318, 319,
   344, 352